Advance praise for *P*

"A riveting account of the scenarios facing the post-coronavirus society. I'm amazed at the way Trond Undheim combines a deep dive into our dystopian reality with optimism if action is taken."

— Gary Epler, M.D., Harvard Medical School

"Trond Undheim is that rare genius who builds the future even as he is predicting it. This is the book the world in lockdown has been waiting for."

— Sir John Hargrave, bestselling author of *Mind Hacking* and *Blockchain for Everyone*

Praise for *Disruption Games*

"An intriguing learn-from-failure investment manual with a hard-edged practical side."

— Kirkus Reviews

"Excited to hear MIT legend, star speaker and moderator Trond Undheim's new book, Disruption Games is available for pre-order. I cannot think of a better guide to the disruptive world that founders and executives inhabit."

— James Mawson, CEO and Founder, Global Corporate Venturing

"[...] a comprehensive walk-through for anyone interested in business innovation [...] this book could be helpful for business owners looking to change or adapt but are unsure of the best way forward [and] is especially useful at the moment when the world is changing more drastically than we would have ever imagined in such a short space of time."

— LoveReading.co.uk

"[...] a fantastic book that is full of helpful information and insight for industry professionals and budding entrepreneurs [...] one of my favorite business books [...] it should probably be read a few times to absorb everything it has to say."

— Arthur Thares, Reviewer, *Pacific Book Review*

"Disruption Games excels in specific examples, approaches, and game-changing plans for addressing both success and failure. It is recommended reading for any forward-thinking businessperson interested in not just learning from business failures, but embracing and growing from them."

— D. Donovan, Senior Reviewer,
Midwest Book Review

"Even though I was an experienced founder, I have to say the partnerships Trond facilitated when he ran the startup program at MIT ILP were instrumental to our launch and success."

— Natan Linder, Cofounder, Formlabs (3D printing) and
Tulip Interfaces (advanced manufacturing app)

"Trond is extremely knowledgeable about the use of technology to reach any customer base."

— David Molchany, Executive Partner,
Gartner Executive Programs

"Trond is thorough, analytically strong and has the ability to push boundaries for himself and others."

— Constantijn Van Oranje-Nassau,
Special Envoy, Startup Delta

"Through MIT, Trond has worked with some of the best startups in the world. Read this book for insights on what it took for them to succeed. Part business, part personal development, Disruption Games provides a blueprint of practical ways to jumpstart successful innovation through examining failure."

– Brent Hoberman, Cofounder, Founders Forum, Lastminute.com, Made.com

"Trond is absolutely trustworthy, full of good ideas and has got the energy and the optimism to walk on trying to get things done."

– Jochen Friedrich, Technical Relations Executive at IBM

Praise for *Leadership from Below*

"It is a book containing real strategies for real people, based on a philosophy of leadership and a way of thinking that at first seems so obvious, yet at the same time remains so elusive to most of us."

– Espen Moe, PhD, Author of *Governance, Growth and Global Leadership* (2007); Professor of Political Science at the Department of Sociology and Political Science at NTNU

"Leadership from Below presents an important set of skills and concepts that anyone can use to maximize his or her potential influence and impact in an organization."

– Barbara Larson, MBA, Executive Professor, Management and Organizational Development at the D'Amore-McKim School of Business, Northeastern University

"A must-read for any young manager looking to apply the lessons of eBay, Google and Facebook to the real world."

– Julian Herbstein, Founder and CEO, Magic Fitness

PANDEMIC AFTERMATH

HOW CORONAVIRUS CHANGES GLOBAL SOCIETY

TROND UNDHEIM

atmosphere press

Published by Atmosphere Press

Cover design by Nick Courtright

Pandemic Aftermath
2020, Trond Undheim

atmospherepress.com

For my children, Naya, Jax, and Zadie. I wanted to leave you a better world than this. Failing that, I wrote this book so that we together may save what's left.

For the immunocompromised, the elderly, those with preexisting medical conditions, and to those who live in places that predispose you to coronavirus vulnerability because of poor air quality, poor health security, or poor leadership, I also dedicate this book to you.

CONTENTS

INTRODUCTION

THE PANDEMICS OF YESTERDAY AND TOMORROW

"Surviving Ebola was not only a matter of avoiding contagion or receiving treatment, but a broader social matter of living through the crisis in a dignified and meaningful way."

— Dr. Jonah Lipton, London School of Economics

We are currently witnessing the most drastic rewriting of the rules of society since the industrial revolution. Other observers had previously thought that it was the technological revolution of the past few decades that deserved this same stature, but recent months' events surrounding the severity of the 2019 coronavirus pandemic and the increasing spread of the virus and the COVID-19 disease that comes with it would seem to beat it hands down.

Interestingly, the world is being brought to a halt by a much more virulent member of the family of virus that includes those that cause the *common cold*. In fact, all coronaviruses have spiky projections on their outer surfaces that resemble the points of a crown (*corona* in Latin), a word that now has become a loaded term. The more familiar human coronaviruses, including types 229E, NL63, OC43, and HKU1, are in and of themselves poorly understood because they don't kill. As different and potent as novel coronavirus (COVID-19) is, had we bothered to figure out more about the common variants, we might not be in this situation. Coronavirus is a common pathology in animals, so animal health professionals were more familiar with it.

However, as will become apparent throughout the book, it is the confounding of coronavirus with another common disease, the flu, that has created the most damaging blind spots. Either way, we have, from the outset, grossly underestimated this virus, its mode of transmission, virality and effects on the body and, ultimately, the damaging effect on our society.

Half of all deaths happen by way of infectious diseases (Tisoncik, 2012). One would think we should be more worried about it than we are. Devastatingly, some of the confusion has been transmitted by public health authorities who have introduced but not explained (or at times fully understood the implications of) paradigms such as “herd immunity”, “epidemiological modeling”, and “social distancing”. The analysis of these terms as they affect large populations have more to do with wide spectrum social science than with narrow medical reasoning.

Some leaders, notably female heads of state, have so far shown outstanding leadership (Greer, 2020). It’s too early to tell if their great initial results will hold up in the long term, but it is likely. One may also wonder if there are characteristics countries with female leadership have in common that enable this success, but that’s a longer discussion that requires more data than currently available. I’ll be the first to look at that data and bow down to female crisis leadership. Intuitively, it makes sense, thinking of the importance of trust, empathy, and interpersonal skills, long thought to be more prevalent in women. At least one scientific study by Caprioli & Boyer (2001) showed that “the severity of violence in crisis decreases as domestic gender equality increases.”

Unfortunately, there have also been leading politicians across the world who have brought a short-term focus on “economic growth”, their own special interest agendas or simply the instinct to try to appease voters at all costs. When politicians embody behavior that is *antithetical* to understanding long term societal evolution it leads to confusion and further aggravates a crisis. At times, such politicians have piggybacked on the epidemiologists and modelers, acting confidently on poor data, making a bad situation worse, other times they have completely ignored the experts, which typically also leads to bad outcomes. In fact, in general, leaders don't appear incented to act on major, long term challenges.

Let's look closely at why this is so and what we can do about it. A key part of my remedy is to put COVID-19 into the context of the aftermath of two other massive diseases that scorched the earth, the Black Death and the 1918 influenza pandemic, to compare, contrast and imagine.

Over the course of the first half of 2020, it has become more challenging to disagree with the notion that we are all, at least at the moment, living in a "risk society" where the state of emergency threatens to become the norm. Sociologists Ulrich Bech (1992) and Anthony Giddens (1991) brought up this challenge already in the 1990s and attributed this fact to a host of conditions intertwined with globalization, which I'll explore throughout the book.

Around COVID-19, those risks lead to a host of questions that, most commonly, would need to be answered by domain experts: How dangerous is the virus? Why are there such differences in death toll within and between countries—and will this difference persist? How long will we need to socially distance? When will there be a vaccine? What will be the new normal? Except that, in this situation, there are few experts that have the whole picture. Everyone—from Nobel Prize winners down through presidents and prime ministers to state epidemiologists—is still figuring it out. To some extent, the answer is still in the lab, with the caveat that, unfortunately, the lab isn't small; it is the world as we know it.

In the book I'm going to use "coronavirus" and "COVID-19" interchangeably, given the lack of great options due to the confusion caused by a poorly chosen official name for the virus.

Just to be sure this is clear, the WHO International

Committee on Taxonomy of Viruses (ICTV) announced "severe acute respiratory syndrome-related coronavirus 2 (SARS-CoV-2)" as the name of the new virus on February 11, 2020, which connects it to SARS, which was unhelpful in a myriad of ways. That disease was different in terms of infectious period, transmissibility, clinical severity, and extent of community spread, and radically different in terms of social outcome and historical significance. The WHO was afraid the connection to SARS would create "unnecessary fear" in Asia, but the opposite may be the case, since I would say an appropriate amount of fear would have been helpful. Arguably, the name has contributed to obscuring the fact that this disease was novel in a plethora of society-shattering ways and should have been narrated more closely to previous deeply scary diseases such as HIV/AIDS and Ebola virus (EBOV) in order to better reflect its genetic and societal punch.

I also note that the WHO announced "COVID-19" as the name of this new disease, which connects it to the year it began (2019) but obscures the fact that the full impact was felt in 2020. Finally, experts are aware of 5000+ existing strains of coronavirus in animal populations (Qiu, 2020), so clearly that term isn't perfect either since it is, unfortunately, bound to be the generic name for a plethora of future infectious diseases.

I make this distinction to foreshadow that the naming of a disease is an early and important step in shaping the narrative. The direction of a disease narrative has a deeply meaningful impact not only on how decision makers see the challenge but also on how people in general see it, how we react, and what we end up doing about it.

As social scientists like Bruno Latour (1983) have shown, beyond the biological impact of a virus (its genetic makeup), which, for instance, makes it deadly if certain conditions are met, a virus doesn't in and of itself have the power to change the world.

In nature, microbes hide, and the result is largely invisible and messy, and sometimes catastrophic. In contrast, in laboratories microbes get exposed, isolated, nurtured, and can be (for the most part) contained and mobilized in useful ways. The resulting sociotechnical networks consist of microbes, scientists, and experimental results, mediated by sponsors who invest in the potential treatments, and are (if we are lucky) subsequently followed by antiviral drug compounds and vaccines, which, in turn, need health workers to administer them and patients to accept the treatment.

In that process, the (now) assembled, *technical* entities have agency in the same sense as social actors, in that they can be credited with being the source of actions (disease outcomes and cures, even, as well as disease trajectories, e.g., "we have the disease contained"), but only because they are enacted and now have a clear role to play in the mixed blessing that is the contemporary public health landscape.

Before the work of Louis Pasteur, these powers of the microbes were only latent, according to Latour (1983). Since they became activated in the real world outside the lab, as long as you followed "a set of laboratory practices—disinfection, cleanliness, conservation, inoculation gesture, timing and recording," it got extended to every French farm, and in the years to follow, across the world.

If we make the analogy to the world's current struggle with coronavirus: before we get efficient cures or vaccines, the world needs to "get behind" the properties of coronavirus, so we can properly support the work going on in laboratories, not just financially but in agreeing to enlist in human trials already now, and in being willing to codevelop the response through joining a common narrative. Even before vaccine candidates emerge, the negotiation with the antivaxxers begins, because without "herd immunity" through vaccinating a high percentage of the world's population, there is no end in sight. And in all this, we need to be prepared for disappointments along the way, given the long timelines and uncertain success of vaccines.

The nuances of that process of discovery, its subtle narration, and its corresponding societal impact are still poorly understood today and remain the source of many of the problems that surround how infectious diseases become pandemics as well as whether they are contained or not. The problem isn't to *get* to the facts, but to successfully *negotiate* what the agreed facts are going to be.

Coronavirus is now subject to a global fight for the narrative that will ultimately hold. In the first phase, the unique narrative framing power was held by Chinese doctors in Wuhan who initially characterized it as a "strange influenza" (that characterization stayed with the virus for quite long and characterized the early response) although one of them, Wuhan doctor Li Wenliang, shared a WeChat about the new "SARS-like virus." This was followed by the local government who continued calling it "pneumonia of unclear cause" or "viral pneumonia," followed by the Chinese national government, who eventually brought in the WHO calling it an "unknown illness" and subsequently map the virus genome and starts calling it a "coronavirus."

From that point onward, public health officials held significant sway, emphasizing that the disease broadly was about "poor public hygiene," but only until national politicians attempted to get on top of the debate, at which point the question of "economic impact" became inextricably linked to the core of the narrative. Some attempted to frame it as a "Chinese" problem or a "problem with China," and initially call it the "Wuhan virus" (from its origin, despite the fact that there are numerous viruses with that name already) or "Chinese virus" (which would be highly imprecise).

Others have brought up the disease as a "consequence of globalization" or simply "urbanization" and particularly the "growth of megacities." There's also the case to be made that it is "caused by superspreaders," whether they be individuals or cultural practices such as mass gatherings to watch sports, listen to concerts, or engage in religious worship or business practices such as congregating in offices and having meetings.

As the nature of needed measures trickled down to regional, local, and city level, those authorities became even more important in shaping the way people understood and acted around the disease.

In the middle of all of this, health workers, from doctors to nurses to emergency medical technicians (EMTs), have been called in as "expert witnesses" and have so far largely focused on "equipment shortages." Media has also inserted itself with the considerable framing power it represents, although largely without a point of view beyond "this is about us, the media, getting the deserved attention." Months into the disease, economic experts are starting to dominate the debate. A likely next phase would involve a broader set of experts.

Already, the inclusion of nonprofits and celebrity spokespersons in the public narrative has brought in the notion that it is also about "race" and "disadvantaged groups" or even simply about "poverty." The security angle is that the disease is important because of how it "enables terrorism" or "foments organized crime." Extreme social media memes such as #BoomerRemover start to appear (presumably referring to the fact that the disease often attacks the older among us as a group). The meme is even factually wrong since it is the Silent Generation (born 1925–1945) that suffer the most, then Baby Boomers (born 1946–1964).

After that, subject to what happens to social movements ability to congregate in any meaningful way (but even through online means), the public response is likely to take center stage and the others (including government representatives of any sort) are likely to have to respond more than generate the thrust of the narrative (and response). The two—narrative and response—are deeply connected and likely cannot be viewed in isolation. To uncover what's at stake, I will use techniques that make things visible, tangible, and knowable. Coronavirus is, of course, about all of these things and more. But a clearer picture can only be obtained from looking at infectious diseases in a historical perspective.

The consequences of the Black Death

The Black Death (1347–1353) killed 75 million to 200 million globally over 4 years, peaking in Europe from 1347 to 1351, cyclically wiping out huge chunks of the population in the centuries to follow and remained quite active until 1750. There are still a few cases every year on each continent even today.

Quarantine is a word based on the word *quarantena*, Venetian dialect meaning 40 days, and first imposed during the peak of the Black Death (1347–1351). Quarantine replaced the earlier notion of *trentino*, a 30-day period, which was found to be ineffective.

The Black Death is commonly believed to have been the result of plague, an infectious fever caused by the bacterium *Yersinia pestis* which would have been transmitted from rodents to humans by the bite of infected flea. However, over the past few decades some holes in that theory have been found (Mackenzie, 2001). Notably, the rapid speed of spread as well as the quarantine practices (quarantining humans not rodents or fleas) at the time would indicate the presence of a more virulent agent than what we find in the plague that reoccurs from time to time in our own society (Scott & Duncan, 2001). Other culprits, such as anthrax, hemorrhagic viral fever, and louse-borne typhus, have been proposed. For our purposes, the type of microbe is only relevant insofar as it points to how little we know about such a defining moment in human history. We must hope the current calamity can be better understood.

The initial social and economic effects of the Black Death were largely negative, including people abandoning their friends and family, fleeing cities, and shutting themselves off from the world. Funeral rites, one of the few public gatherings of those times, became perfunctory or stopped altogether, both because of the risks involved in gathering and because of the futility of making a big point out of the ordinary. There was, understandably, an atmosphere of fear, grief, and hopelessness in the years that followed.

After the immediate effects, discrimination ensued, as people sought to blame particular social groups, notably the Jews. Arguably, they were slightly less affected because they lived in ghettos and practiced cleanliness beyond the average of their times. That fact plus their general industriousness, which also made them cope better, became a reason for envy.

The Middle Ages was also a very violent time in human history. Military inventions that were developed during that period include the lance, the longbow, the crossbow, the flail, and armor, including chainmail.

Work changed in innumerable ways. The immediate impact was that work ceased due to lack of motivation, lack of funds to mount projects, as well as labor shortages. However, after the initial shock one discovered that the remaining workers had more tools and land to work, and became more productive, producing more goods and services. As a result, wages increased. This is familiar to economists who study the effects of labor demand, even today.

Eventually, people moved on and life continued, but it was permanently slightly different. The plague created a change in medicine, farming, and housekeeping. Peasants were able to change the way that they were perceived and treated.

Numerable innovations, both incremental and radical, could be attributed to its aftermath. Metal cookware among serfs became commonplace, courtesy of more gracious landlords. Innovation of labor-saving technologies, including the one-stilt plough and switching out oxen for horses, started to change agriculture. Arguably, many of the technical inventions that resulted in miniaturization and even the printing press in 1454 were indirect impacts of the plague, as there was an increasing demand to be kept informed. The lesson here might be that elite information control is the first thing that goes south in the aftermath of a huge crisis, as everyone realizes the premium on timely, accurate information to organize themselves, be productive and take care of their loved ones. The emergence of literacy among the ruling classes including merchants, and eventually trickling down to larger swaths of the population followed.

The harnessing of time was another development. Public clocks started becoming common in places like Italy, which allowed time to be divided up more efficiently than simply following the patterns of the sun and moon.

Ironically, the Black Death is thought to have originated in Asia, perhaps among the Golden Horde and to have arrived in Europe through Italy, which is a grim yet interesting, perhaps instructive, parallel to today's events. One could without doubt say that the Black Death was the first truly negative consequence of the flow of people and goods across great distances. On the other hand, it also contained the seeds of the industrial revolution that has spurred so many positive changes and altered the very platforms that fuel progress in our society.

However, the Black Death was in no way the only factor spurring these technological and societal changes, and many of the technologies and innovations we may simplistically wish to claim were direct results of the opportunities provided by the aftermath of the plague were actually either in place earlier (like advanced wool or silk manufacturing and windmills) or indeed took centuries to gain ground (like the creation of townships with elaborate governance). Even agriculture was already becoming more efficient before the plague and evolved gradually throughout the whole period.

Furthermore, it is important to point out that not only did the Black Death not determine all changes that took place but also *not everything changed* either. The Black Death, for all its impact, did not change the status of women in the labor force very much and arguably did not create substantially more, different, or better jobs for women (Humphries, 2014). The separation of the home and work spheres was also kept very distinct for centuries to come, with a strictly gendered division of labor, where work in the fields was performed by men and household labor was performed by women. In the UK, labor law put in place further restrictions that hampered women's entry into the labor force. The *Ordinance of Labourers* (1349) and the *Statute of Labourers* (1351) included a ban on wage increases and restrictions on movement in search for work, forcing women into permanent labor contracts, according to Oxford historian Jane Humphries (2014).

These qualifications are important to note as we ponder the impact of disease on society. Neither progress nor decline are linear, nor are they shaped by one factor alone. Disruptive change also doesn't linearly lead to progress. Claiming otherwise will bring us into a lot of trouble.

Since the Black Death, there have been at least nine known pandemics, in 1729, 1732, 1781, 1830, 1833, 1889, 1918, 1957 and 1968, according to CIDRAP (2020), but they are without any discernible pattern. Additionally, the key planning challenge is that pandemics defy common postwar political timelines. For example, according to FullFact (2019), the average term of a UK government since the Second World War is 3.7 years. Parliamentarians typically sit for 3-6 years, depending which country we are talking about. Members of the U.S. House of Representatives serve two-year terms and are considered for reelection every even year, U.S. Senators however, serve six-year terms and the U.S. Supreme Court is a lifetime appointment. Monarchies typically don't have term limits (Queen Elizabeth II has ruled since 1952) but are mostly ceremonial roles these days. Prime Ministers don't typically have term limits but must wield support from Parliaments with three to six-year terms as well as political parties which each have their own election cycles. Would a system with meaningful power that lasts for decades better deal with a pandemic? Perhaps worth to ponder.

The impact of the 1918 influenza

The nation-state was first invented in Europe with the principle of territorial sovereignty agreed at the Treaty of Westphalia in 1648, which spurred wider expansion. Over the centuries, as borders were drawn in various ways, gradual internationalization, and eventually the waves of globalization during the 20th century, made the world increasingly connected. This connectedness has had tremendous network effects, mostly positive.

However, toward the end of World War I and in the immediate aftermath, another tragedy hit. The Influenza of 1918, the slur being "Spanish flu," although that was only where Patient 0 was first detected, took little more than 1 year to kill 50 million to 100 million people worldwide.

Why did it kill so many people? Barry (2004), Roos (2020) and others point to many factors. I'll just quickly look at scientific, political, logistical, psychological and geographical reasons, since they are the most relevant for the analysis to come.

The *scientific* reason might be that it was a new, deadly strain of influenza which triggered a "cytokine storm", a fancy medical term for the fact that some infections causes the immune system to turn against itself. The *political* reason is that it happened in the middle of a world war and public officials and media were afraid to sound the alarm or put in place strong quarantines for fear of crippling the war effort. The *logistical* reason might be that there was a severe nursing shortage since they were mostly sent out to help with the war effort—and nurses are more useful than doctors when all you have available is palliative care. The *psychological* reason might be that people (and city leaders) stubbornly refused to account for a possible second wave of infection and let down their guard, stopped social distancing, and got hit with something far worse. The *geographical* reason might be related to industrialization and urban population density. In Chandra et al.'s (2013) study of the 15 million who died in India during the outbreak, researchers found clear density thresholds, which put Calcutta as well as large parts of the coastline plus the Gangetic plain under much higher death loads than other parts of India.

When hundreds of thousands die of flu every year even today, they die from a strain of that flu. It's unclear where that flu originated from, although France, China, and Britain have been suggested and the state of Kansas in the US is notorious for having the first known case. What we do seem to observe is that today's strain typically originates from Southeast Asia.

The Black Death, The Great Influenza and COVID-19

The ultimate tale of what will happen with COVID-19 is too soon to tell, but that it perhaps will enter into world history as an event comparable in scale and impact to the Black Death and the Influenza of 2018 is now becoming apparent to some of us, if not all of us. The reason is not just its immediate impact in 2020 but stems from considering the fact that a novel and deadly pathogen is, again, in community spread, and will likely not leave us very quickly, perhaps not for decades or even generations, even if a cure or vaccine is developed relatively soon. Either way, three distinct pandemics will mark the last 750 years of human history. This fact must give us pause. It matters. It is worth a moment of silence to gather your thoughts. What's next?

Even if this particular virus doesn't in the end stand up to the Black Death in its significance (there's always the chance), I'm quite certain that some emergent pandemic in the near future will. When reading onward, please keep this larger picture in mind just in case it becomes hard for you to imagine that what is happening in 2020 as such could have the magnanimous consequences I chart in the following pages.

Black Swans and beyond

How similar is the COVID-19 outbreak to either of these pandemics? What's different about the COVID-19 situation isn't so much the pathogen (although the way particular microbes become fixed in people's mind as the "only" threat they can see is a story in itself) but the fact that it happens to a global society that considers itself highly advanced. It is one thing that a deadly flu virus can kill millions immediately after a world war that has left the international community with open wounds and poor capacity to respond to any new crisis. It is a whole other thing to fathom that an only slightly more pathogenic and slightly more contagious virus can wreak the kind of havoc that COVID-19 already has done to the world's top economies as well as its top healthcare systems, including the US and the UK. This is even before we have taken in the (necessarily) huge toll the disease will have upon the developing and emerging markets around the world, particularly upon its megacities.

Lebanese American author (and former Wall Street trader) Nassim Nicholas Taleb's 2007 book *The Black Swan* coined a term that has come to encapsulate the random appearance of highly improbable events that have high impact on an aspect of our society. Understandably, people were quick to announce that coronavirus was a Black Swan event, as if that made it more acceptable. Subsequently, others were even quicker to point out that it was *not*.

Taleb describes how humans rationalize the Black Swan phenomenon to make it appear less random. Fittingly, his basic observation originated in an earlier book of his, *Fooled by Randomness* (2001). Examples Taleb gives of Black Swan events include the rise of the Internet, the personal computer, World War I, the dissolution of the Soviet Union, Black Monday, the Dotcom Bubble, and the September 11, 2001 (aka 9/11) terrorist attacks. Later events that would conceivably fit the definition would be the 2008 Financial Crisis (e.g., 15 September 2008 when Lehman Brothers filed for bankruptcy and DOW began its 54% plunge) or Brexit, which was announced in 2016 and completed in 2020.

Now, the coronavirus may or may not be a great fit for the term Black Swan. Arguably, it was not unpredictable, but has rather been foretold by journalists, documentary authors on infectious diseases, public health officials, and activists. The problem was perhaps not that we did not know it could happen but that it actually did. The way it happened was by stealth mode, at first in a place full of secrets but with a centralized polity that was well positioned to quell it, China, although it escaped. The experts were not worried because it was neither pandemic influenza nor hemorrhagic fever. People were not too worried either because 1918 is a long time ago. In fact, it was the year my maternal grandmother was born.

As with previous times of great upheaval, it is clearly difficult to see the full ramifications of change when we are in the middle of it. However, there is considerable urgency in making the attempt. I want to note that taking a deep interest in this phenomenon does not, like Taleb, make me a "catastrophist." Unlike Taleb, who has made millions advising private equity on Black Swan risks, I have no special interest in seeing such a thing happen or indeed a credible plan for profiting on it.

Rather, my main argument is that, in a much more

substantial way than with previous pandemics, or indeed any other single events, the entire society will now potentially be re-jiggered to respond better to the next one. Or indeed, the world might just adjust itself without the need for a coordinated central command, due to the existence of a critical mass of an informed, mobile, and knowledgeable public. This contrasts to the Middle Ages' illiterate population and 1918's relative dearth of a worldwide consumer market capable of surge response and independent market shifts based on social dynamics alone.

A pandemic is also not a single event, but an avalanche of connected events. And, even if it is not, and gets quelled quite soon, which is of course also a possibility, we would have to live with the awareness that we are taking an increasingly calculated, knowable risk by continuing as if nothing had happened.

Bouncing back, better and different

The question is, of course, what does that mean in order to return to normality? But before that, why do I think that this pandemic will lead to such drastic change in the very fabric of society? Isn't it the case that we will "bounce back," as US President Trump has said on many an occasion?

I'm looking at the severity of the crisis; the emerging data on the impact on key societal areas of work, life, and play; and the fact that the crisis is unfolding on a global scale contemporaneously.

Moreover, the world's "confidence" that it has made major progress in economic development, quality of life, technology, and myriad other areas has never been greater. The fall from grace, or the readjustment, is poised to be of similar magnitude. While some will forget what happened, many will not, and the institutional fabric around us will make quite serious readjustments. Just in terms of magnitude, let's say 9/11 was at a level 5 in terms of a global crisis—and caused a rethinking of air travel, building security, international relations, terrorism, and interstate cooperation and information sharing, and much more. If so, COVID-19 is at a level 8, and is likely to cause far greater changes, a host of intermediate changes as well as a plethora of long-term changes that might be hard to imagine right now.

The only more severe event I can think of at this time (short of an alien attack, which I, even with my futurist hat on, consider quite unlikely) would be a true extinction event related to the uncontrolled spread of a much more lethal pandemic (say an Ebola-like pathogen), nuclear war, or a global environmental disaster and ensuing ecological cataclysm with severe, lasting implications for air quality. We may, of course, have to be prepared to handle those as well, but this might be the second chapter of the story and hopefully some time into the future. But can we gamble on it?

Learning to respond

Pandemic Aftermath introduces anybody who cares about the future of our society to key strategies to understand the impact of the coronavirus pandemic on the world, learning from our collective failure to anticipate and respond effectively with the express idea of disrupting existing modes of response.

While the coronavirus pandemic is widely seen as unexpected, for example, the ultimate Black Swan event, in contrast, I would argue that the key failures were only partially foreseeable—a fourfold lack of response coming from the domains of foresight, government, media, and innovation. However, my perspective is optimistic and future oriented.

The book offers five ways to look at what happens next (i.e., scenarios) based on my study of the forces of disruption that brought on the pandemic, and also potentially could remedy its consequences or even enable segments of society to thrive on it.

Charting the forces of disruption

The first portion of the book is nonfiction. The second portion is a scenario-based novel: the book charts new territory by interweaving the grim reality of 2020 with a first-person exploration of the next decade as if we were already in it.

Given that there is so little certainty right now, a nonfiction book seemed premature, but given the real stakes, a fully fictionalized approach of the near future seemed incomplete.

Understand the forces of industry disruption. A crucial skill in this new situation is to learn to track changes in emerging tech, policy, business, and social dynamics as a strategic framework that presents clear priorities to chase, interrelationships to be aware of, and gaps to fill.

How did COVID-19 become a pandemic? The book traces the virus from its inception in Wuhan, China, through Europe and the US and throughout the world, emphasizing superspreader incidents, bottlenecks, and other key inflection points.

How did key stakeholders handle it? Next, I move to considering how coronavirus was handled across the world, diving into who the main actors turned out to be, what they did, and what the immediate consequences appear to be.

What are the impacts of the virus and the measures? Finally, I consider what the appearance of the virus means for work, education, politics, and our planet as the world moves on from the shock and starts to consider its aftermath.

Scenarios for the next decade

Why already ponder what's next? The world is, arguably, still in the middle of fighting the virus and its impact. What could possibly be said about the future? Well, the truth appears to be that if we don't already start planning for the next virus—or even just for how to live with the current virus long term—we will face even more earth-shattering negative consequences.

Responding to this need, I have drawn up a few *immediate scenarios*—new ways to think about the future. Scenario thinking is *usually* a way to prepare for an imagined future. Instead, I would argue, these sweeping societal changes will happen much faster. I have drawn up five. In this case, each of the scenarios are quite near term; in fact, we are living in versions of each of them right now. Crafting solid scenarios can help us, as citizens, policy makers, or business leaders, decide which path we want to chart for what lies ahead. Or, as it were, distilling key facets of the reality we are already living, we might learn to live with it a bit better. Leaving aside the details, let me also state that different parts of the world seem to respond differently to this crisis. Therefore, the potential is that we will shatter into regional or national worlds. We will get into that in the last section of the book.

Broadly, I see five scenarios for our post-coronavirus future. The five scenarios considered are: borderless world, nation-state renewal, two worlds apart, Hobbesian chaos, and status quo.

Scenario I: Borderless world.

In this scenario, we consider what it would look like if world leaders were able to fully implement globalization as well as solidarity and implementation strategies to fix the weakest links (e.g., health systems in Africa).

Scenario II: Nation-state renewal.

This scenario considers a situation where borders close down and people stop traveling huge distances, perhaps because of a principle of proximity where long-distance travel and contact with more than 50 people a week is discouraged, perhaps outlawed.

Scenario III: Two worlds apart.
This scenario considers a radical acceleration of the separation of the top 0.01% of population from the 99.99%. It foresees entire new cities purposefully constructed to avoid contagion, filled with the world's most expensive real estate, governed by their own laws.

Scenario IV: Hobbesian chaos.
This scenario considers a possible next decade where survival of the fittest becomes an extreme reality. Rule of law ceases to exist, and clans and ideological movements sweep through the earth with constant struggle and fight for scarce resources as a result.

Scenario V: Status quo.
This scenario considers the possibility that nothing much at all will be different as a result of COVID-19. That is, after a period of readjustment, society and the world economy, on most dimensions, will not be significantly altered by this pandemic experience. Science will largely continue as before, as a slow evolution most akin to the table game Chutes and Ladders, up and down, through triumphs and failures. Technology will make progress at the same pace as before (nonlinearly and in surprising ways). Businesses will operate in the same way. Governments will operate as before, nation-states will not change, international organizations will still battle for relevance. Social dynamics will not change. Consumption patterns will go back to what they were before.

Broadly, this book will:

- provide a conceptual framework for the sociopolitical reality of coronavirus;
- help you imagine the next decade's technology,

society, and physical proximity; and
- provide a blueprint for leadership, far beyond public health.

In sum, the choices before us as a global society, which of course largely means the choices nation-states and their voting citizens make, are important and far outshine public health considerations as such. The question before us is how to live through the crisis—and live beyond it—in a dignified and meaningful way. I'm writing this book with at least that question in mind. I fear not everyone will have that perspective, given that the survival instinct and self-protection, as well as the opportunities envisioned by taking a more egotistical approach, would also become quite evident in the time to come.

We should not only be planning for the pandemics of tomorrow (which we should also do) but also for the society of tomorrow. Doing so simultaneously will require a different dialogue and ambition level than the world has had over the past 50 years, at the very least. There is no time to lose.

Disclaimer

The author shall in no event be liable for any decision taken by the reader or any organization based on this book. Under no circumstances shall the author be liable for any damages whatsoever arising out of the use or inability to use the book for forecasting or other purposes. The entire risk arising out of the use of the book remains with the reader.

Learning from historical pandemics

There are two precedents to COVID-19: The Black Death and the Influenza of 1918.

What were the three most important long-term consequences of the Black Death?

1.______________________________

2.______________________________

3.______________________________

What were some important societal changes after the Influenza of 1918?

____

Scenarios for the next decade

What are your first thoughts about each of the five scenarios?

Do they scare you? Fascinate you? Surprise you? Bore you? Mobilize you? What's your core feeling around each of them? (Please don't look at each chapter yet.)

1. Borderless World______________________________

2. Nation-State Renewal______________________________

3. Two Worlds Apart______________________________

4. Hobbesian Chaos______________________________

5. Status Quo______________________________

Forces of pandemic disruption

The coronavirus pandemic is so much more than a public health crisis. It will arguably change global society. Right now, we are not sure exactly how. But we can look at which areas will be impacted.

Can you name some (ideally 4) forces of disruption described in this chapter?
Use your own words.

1. ______________________________

2. ______________________________

3. ______________________________

4. ______________________________

CHAPTER 1

THE ORIGIN OF THE CORONAVIRUS CRISIS AND THE EARLY DAYS

Coronavirus originates in Wuhan, China, in December 2019, or so it seems. On December 10, Wei Guixian, one of the earliest known coronavirus patients, starts feeling ill. On December 16, a patient is admitted to Wuhan Central Hospital with infection in both lungs but resistant to antiviral flu drugs. Staff later learned he worked at a wildlife market connected to the outbreak. Early on, experts seem to both be blaming bats and pangolins (also called *scaly anteaters*). If so-called *zoonotic spillover* from wildlife to people turns out to be indicative of the transmission to Patient 0, it would not be the first time. Just think of flu (Swine flu, Avian or Bird flu), filoviruses (Marburg, Ebola), and previous coronaviruses (MERS, SARS).

Only as late as December 31, China tells the World Health Organization's China office about the cases of an unknown illness, and on January 11, China reports its first death. On January 13, the first coronavirus case is reported in Thailand, the first known case outside China. Cases in Japan and South Korea follow.

On Jan. 15, the patient who becomes the first confirmed US case, a man in his 30s, leaves Wuhan and arrives in the US, carrying the coronavirus. On Jan. 21, the US Centers for Disease Control and Prevention confirms the first coronavirus case in the United States. On Jan. 24, China extends the lockdown to cover 36 million people and starts to rapidly build a new hospital in Wuhan. From this point onward, strict measures continue to be implemented around the country for the rest of the epidemic.

On Jan. 28, the US government's lead medical expert on

infectious diseases, Dr. Anthony Fauci says, "The driver of respiratory outbreaks is symptomatic people, not asymptomatic carriers." At the same press conference, Alex Azar, secretary of the Department of Health and Human Services (HHS), says, "Americans should not worry for their own safety."

On Jan. 30, the WHO declares a global health emergency and the following day President Trump restricts travel from China.

A surge of cases in Italy and beyond

In February, a cruise ship in Japan, the *Diamond Princess*, quarantines thousands and hundreds test positive for the virus. On February 7, a Chinese doctor who tried to raise the alarm died, making it clear (to some), that healthcare workers would be a significant casualty in the time to come. On Feb. 11, the WHO officially names the disease that the virus coronavirus causes: COVID-19. On Feb. 14, France announces the first coronavirus death in Europe. On Feb. 19, the Champions League soccer match between Atalanta and Valencia gathers 44,000 people at the Giuseppe Meazza stadium in the San Siro district of Milan (we will look at superspreading events in Chapter 3). On Feb. 21, the virus appears in Iran from an unknown source, although beyond some questionable infection numbers, the outside world still knows very little about the progression of the crisis in Iran. On April 1, Iran accuses the US of "medical terrorism" because of the sanctions they claim block financial transactions and discourage nations and organizations from dealing with Tehran.

On Feb. 23, Italy sees a major surge in coronavirus cases and officials lock down towns near the source of the outbreak, the town of Codogno, southeast of Milan, in the region of

Lombardy. The Italian outbreak seems to be exacerbated, possibly caused, by a single "superspreader." On Feb. 24, the potential economic toll of the crisis becomes apparent, as the Trump administration asks Congress for $1.25 billion for coronavirus response. Simultaneously, the CDC warns of an impending outbreak. By the end of February, Iran emerges as another epicenter of the crisis and the cases spike and spread across Europe. Other continents, notably South America and Africa, have only sporadic cases at this point. On Feb. 29, the US records its first coronavirus death and announces travel restrictions.

The Austrian village of Ischgl, an Alpine ski destination and party hotspot in Tyrol, remained open even as other nations issued travel warnings of potential coronavirus exposure. Thousands of revelers returning from vacations in Ischgl spread infections across much of Scandinavia. On March 8, Norway said 40% of its infections were traced to Ischgl. Out of 1,198 infected, 491 had the virus from Austria, mainly from Tyrol, as reported by Euractiv. That same day, I'm still weighing traveling to London and Oslo on my book tour for my innovation book *Disruption Games* on March 24–April 5. Separately, I start worrying for my mother, who lives in Norway, is particularly susceptible to infection, and is of the age that puts her within the demographic group of elderly people public health authorities in Norway and the US by now say we should be worried about.

Travel bans, social distancing, and school closings

Generally, undocumented, asymptomatic, or presymptomatic infections are believed to be roughly half as contagious as individuals with severe symptoms, according to new research by scientists at Columbia University Mailman School of Public Health.

On March 11, Trump's prime-time speech to the nation announces an EU travel ban, shocking European officials, and on March 13 he declares a national emergency, making another $50 billion in federal funds available. At this point, I cancel my trip to Norway (and the UK), out of concern I'd be put in quarantine (in some country) or might be unable to get back to my kids because of travel bans. On March 13, the UK, led by its Scientific Advisor, Sir Patrick Vallance, and its Chief Medical Officer, Chris Witty, announces they will take a herd-immunity approach to the virus, which means they will not actively stop the population from getting the virus but rather scale it up or down with the goal of reaching 60% immunity as fast as the health system can handle. Sweden signals a similar approach.

Sweden, as the only Nordic country to do so, tries a "modern" approach to pandemic epidemiology and has so far (mid-April 2020) called for citizens to hold themselves accountable for social distancing, work from home when possible, keep gatherings to less than 50 people, and avoid crowded places like bars and restaurants. However, the country has stopped short of imposing formal restrictions, urging its citizens to "behave like adults" instead of ordering lockdowns. This "extreme trust" in its citizens is possible because Sweden is a thoroughly transparent society with 10.2 million citizens who *mostly* trust their politicians, public health officials, as well as the media.

However, Sweden also has a large immigrant population that definitely don't always have the same level of trust. This is one of the X factors in Sweden's chosen approach with "an astonishing high rate" of deaths noted by local researchers among Stockholm's Somali population, according to the *Huffington Post*.

Swedish state epidemiologist Anders Tegnell has outlined a strategy based on the disease being "a marathon, not a sprint." He gambles on the notion that coronavirus will be "impossible to stop" so it's better to let it "run its course," establish herd immunity in the population (he assumes around 50% contagion is enough), and protect the immunocompromised and elderly as well as they can. That way, he keeps his cards close, always has more stringent measures to pull out, and he avoids the grim economic consequences of a shutdown for as long as possible.

Part of his plan has backfired, since Sweden has not been able to keep coronavirus out of old people's homes, and indeed elderly homes have suffered high death tolls. Critics question Sweden's approach as the death toll in mid-April passes 1,300 and Sweden has a 17-times-higher death burden than other, comparable Nordic countries such as Denmark (321 deaths), Norway (150 deaths), and Finland (75 deaths). A full 2,300 Swedish academics signed an open letter to the government in April 2020 calling for it to reconsider its approach, citing the "lack of consent" among the population to this extreme laissez-faire approach.

By most accounts Norway has had a relatively mild experience with coronavirus. Among locals, a plethora of explanations have been offered: the quality of the health system, the overall good health of the population, the relative lack of antibiotics resistance (touted as a miracle cure for all medical ills—and relevant for the bacterial pneumonia that is the add-on to COVID-19), the lack of air pollution (apart from in the three largest cities), the low smoking rate, the (relatively) low obesity rate, and an interesting one, the fact that the population has had the bacillus Calmette-Guérin (B.C.G) vaccine which was compulsory until 1995 and part of youth vaccinations until 2009.

Scientists are now testing a possible, and highly surprising possibility that previous (live) vaccines could have a "nonspecific" vaccine effect beyond the disease it was meant for by inducing "trained immunity" (Curtis, 2020). Note that BCG vaccination of the newborn was started in Sweden in the

1940s and was stopped on April 1, 1975 and is subsequently given only as selective vaccination of groups at higher risk.

However, as Norway gradually opened up again, with kindergartens opening by mid-April 2020, the first test of its strategy may be around the corner. If cases simply spike when reopening, what good was the lockdown? If cases don't spike, can Norway conclude it was smart or simply lucky? What we do know, is that Singapore had a significant second wave of infections almost immediately after its successful shutdown of the first wave.

The context, of course, is that we are comparing two of the world's top public health systems. Norway does not have a lot of spare ICU capacity in principle but does have lots of options to create extra ICU beds, given its advanced infrastructure. Sweden has elderly (nursing) homes with less requirements for trained nursing staff (nursing care is provided by nurse assistants not nurses), low control by the state due to an expanded role of for-profit providers, Norway has elderly homes with a higher degree of trained nursing staff (nurses) and stronger municipal government involvement (van Buul et al., 2020; Segaard & Saglie, 2017).

Who will be right in the long run? Sweden's Tegnell is writing the minority report, but, on the other hand, most models assume that, without a vaccine, the virus will eventually run its course across the population. To be blunt: if this works, it's exciting and also promising for open democracy, for common sense (in Swedish: *folkvett*), and for a different, "contemporary" take on epidemiology. But if it fails, it's catastrophic.

Because, in the end, this is also a question of ethics. Is it okay to let a vulnerable population be exposed this way if you can at least slow it down, hoping for a cure, a vaccine, or even just not to overburden the health system?

On March 15, the CDC recommends no gatherings of 50 or more people in the US. At this point, most universities across the US have closed down and schools have started to close, including the New York public school system. During this week, the virus shows exponential growth in Norway, which is somewhat surprising in one of the richest countries pro capita with a stellar-reputation public health system and advanced sanitary and hygienic practices.

On March 17, France imposes a nationwide lockdown, prohibiting gatherings of any size and closing its public parks. The same day, the EU bans travelers from surrounding countries, and Imperial College (2020) issues a new report stating their previous simulations were wrong and a quarter of million people could die if the government trusted their earlier estimates and continued the herd-immunity strategy.

On March 18, New Zealand, a country of five million people, closes its borders to foreigners. They go on to become one of the more successful countries in handling the first wave of COVID-19 in spring 2020, choosing an "elimination" strategy, aiming to completely get rid of the disease as opposed to merely contain it (but can it last and can their economy take it?). On April 27, the country already reduces the alert level from 4 (lockdown) to 3 (restrict), signaling a gradual return to normalcy. Being a remote island, with a population living in low-density cities, this is obviously a unique advantage. But the economic costs are significant and evolving, and elimination requires an enormous testing effort and subsequent contact tracing and isolation of found cases. The ultimate success of an elimination strategy cannot be proven in the short term.

On March 19, California Governor Gavin Newsom issues a statewide stay-at-home order, projects 56% of Californians could get coronavirus within 8 weeks. By late April, backlash follows the closing of Californian beaches with even local officials claiming closures is "retribution", according to the LA Times (2020).

"Social distancing" is on everyone's lips. The misnomer,

which more aptly refers to physical distancing, is the preferred public health strategy in free and open societies and sounds a whole lot better than mandated quarantine. The public, however, have little experience with it. To most people it means trying to keep a few feet of distance to the next person, which is great in theory but hard when you live in a city and need to deal with narrow crosswalks or find yourself exercising in a highly trafficked park or hiking on a trail. Physical distancing is bound to be among the most interesting sociological phenomena to come out of the crisis. What will its long-term impact be? Is there even a way that such a thing can last more than a few months? Which social groups and personality types will abide by the rules the longest? Who will revolt? Time will show. Even in the original *Big Brother*, the Dutch reality competition television franchise created in 1999, house isolation only lasted for a season and only one person remained for that long. COVID-19 isolation practices in some ways represents the biggest reality show ever attempted.

A *New York Times* op-ed article points out that the most realistic expectation, in fact the best-case scenario, would be that the US needs two to four rounds of social distancing: "The best analogy is pumping a car's brakes on an icy road. Either doing nothing or slamming on the brakes leads to an accident. Pump the brakes—pushing on the brakes, then easing up, and then applying them again—and after three or four times we slow down enough to stop." (Emanuel et al., 2020). As the US makes an 18-month plan to handle coronavirus, this pumping effort looks increasingly more likely to be implemented, given that a total shutdown of the US economy would be detrimental to the economy (and to Trump's reelection effort), and that every week and month that passes, more of the US manufacturing muscle can be mobilized to handle the shortages and health workers can be redeployed or called out of school or retirement.

Throughout March, President Trump has pushed for a

vaccine, stating that it is near, being tested, and will resolve everything. Nobody has told the public that, according to a recent review by Pronker et al. (2013), the average vaccine has a market entry probability of 6% and takes over 10 years to develop from the preclinical phase to availability. Even with 20 vaccines being tested and some already being tested on people, since individual probabilities cannot simply be added up, the percentage of each of them is still 6% and the total probability is not higher that the vaccine path will succeed. Also, vaccines that fail or are seen as ineffective will only spur the antivaxx movement and will backfire for future vaccination programs. Having said that, the attention and stakes this time is higher than ever, so the money and urgency might spur a quicker, more successful outcome than the average—if we are lucky.

On March 28, Illinois reports the first known death of an infant with the coronavirus in the US, perhaps starting to shatter the impression public health officials initially gave people that the disease was not a threat at all to infants, kids, young people, even healthy adults.

On April 20, Trump announces that all immigration to the US will cease both to "protect the US from the invisible disease" and to "protect jobs for our American citizens."

China on the offensive

On March 19, after rigorously implementing mandatory quarantines since January in the affected regions and deploying social distancing everywhere else, China reports no new local infections, seeing a potential end in sight in that massive country alone. China's ruling Communist Party goes from being on the defensive to a public relations offensive involving calling out poor national response in other countries as well as sending medical equipment to Italy and elsewhere.

This approach comes as the large country takes on (and envisions) a larger international role, given the vacuum left by the US having enough with its own problems and being led by an openly protectionist and nationalist leader. The Chinese propaganda part is, so far, clearly more successful at home than abroad, although Serbian President Aleksandar Vucic blasts the EU and, according to ABC News, says, "European solidarity was just a fairy tale." On April 15, EU Commission President Ursula von der Leyen offers a "heartfelt apology" to Italy for "not being there on time," as MEPs debate coronavirus response.

On April 17, China revises the coronavirus death toll in Wuhan, the city at the heart of the pandemic, upward by 50%, according to Chinese state media. The reason given is that it now accounts for "patients unable to reach hospitals" as well as "difficulty linking information" between the various hospital types, regular, private, and temporary.

UK briefly courts herd immunity, then reverses its path

On March 21, Italy records its highest death toll in a day at 627 deaths, now surpassing China as the nation with the most COVID-19 deaths in total, Italy at this point having had 4,032 coronavirus-related deaths. At this point, a limited deployment of the military is accepted by regional authorities in the Lombardy region in order to enforce a lockdown. Simultaneously, there are bright spots and strategic containment moves that seem to work. In the small northern Italian town of Vo, one of the communities where the outbreak first emerged, the entire population of 3,300 people was tested—3% of residents tested positive, and of these, the majority had no symptoms, researchers said.

On March 11, British Premier League soccer team

Liverpool plays a Champions League match against Atletico Madrid on the legendary Anfield Road with 52,000 spectators, 3,000 of whom are coming in from Spain, which is at the early peak of its epidemic. Liverpool's manager calls the fact that the match went ahead a "criminal action." Spain locks down 3 days later.

Meanwhile in the UK, on March 20, Britons wake up to a surprisingly grim reality after, in a stark reversal of earlier assurances, all pubs in the United Kingdom were ordered closed by Prime Minister Boris Johnson. This is widely seen as ending the British PM's maverick stance in the crisis, aiming for herd immunity. While nobody is officially talking about Britain's departure from the European Union these days at 10 Downing Street, having Brexit coincide with a pandemic has drastically reshaped Britain's expectations to escape unscathed from 2020. On the other hand, Brexit enabled a more potent (and quicker) monetary rescue, as the Bank of England cut interest rates to a record-low 0.1% and added 200 billion pounds ($230 billion) to its asset-purchase program (often called QE or quantitative easing) in its latest emergency action. Even so, the pound is at this point at its lowest level since 1985 against the dollar.

On April 19, a senior Whitehall source admits to The Guardian that "all the government's pandemic planning was based on a flu scenario. And then it turned out to be something different and far, far worse and the response was completely inadequate." Coronavirus is not the flu. Having the wrong scenario in mind can be deadly.

On March 22, Germany prohibits gatherings of more than two people and German Chancellor Angela Merkel is in self-quarantine following a visit to an infected doctor as the number of confirmed cases in that country rises to more than 23,900 with more than 90 deaths. My German friends seem concerned with the European Union's seemingly relative lack of effective tools to handle the crisis, and the fact that national borders now are closing across Europe. The whole idea of Schengen was open borders. We have a brief Facebook interchange on the mixed merits of a borderless regional entity during such a crisis. Clearly, this question will not go away.

Strict regimes in Singapore and Hong Kong

On March 22, Singapore bans tourists but also ensures that treatment related to COVID-19 would be free. On March 23, Hong Kong follows suit and also bans all alcohol sales in bars, in the 8,600 restaurants, bars, and clubs holding liquor licenses, initially for a 2-week period. Eleven confirmed COVID-19 patients were known to have visited or worked in bars and restaurants in the city's nightlife district, according to Lan Kwai Fong, from the Centre for Health Protection. This is the second blow to Hong Kong's tourism industry, as its 2019 protests also took a toll. Hong Kong already places wristbands on those infected, prosecutes mandatory quarantine orders swiftly, with offenders facing a maximum HK$25,000 (US$3,205) fine and 6 months in jail if convicted. Also announced, a hotline to allow the public to report those suspected of violating home quarantine.

Despite early success, while keeping its schools and malls open and enjoying a semblance of normal life, Singapore, a country of 5.7 million people, experiences a second wave already by early April, and infected cases spike from 100 to 2,000 as people stop respecting social distancing plus an outbreak among the country's significant share of migrant workers. The Punggol S11 dormitory houses more than 300,000 migrant workers from Bangladesh and India, who live in cramped rooms with bunks for up to 20 men, sometimes "packed likes sardines" (Business Insider, 2020). Cannot even Singapore contain coronavirus from community transmission? The world is watching, as one of the countries in Asia ranking as the world's safest city in the 2017 Global Smart City Performance Index. On April 3, Singapore closes schools and offices, starts recommending all citizens to wear face masks, and hands out masks to all households.

However, while the World Justice Project's (WJP) Rule of Law Index 2017–2018 ranked Singapore first for order and security, the 2020 Index sees Singapore in 12th position, as it struggles in the "open government" category (https://worldjusticeproject.org/). Could transparency be among the key factors that determine the fate of each country in this crisis? If so, the WJP would indicate we should look to Norway, Denmark, Sweden, Finland, and The Netherlands, with Germany not far behind, in the overall ranking.

Showdown between Trump, public health officials, and state governors

By mid-March, a myriad of national and global media reports that the tone of Trump's coronavirus press conferences starts to look a bit more like presidential election campaign rallies. On March 23, Trump tweets "WE CANNOT LET THE CURE BE WORSE THAN THE PROBLEM ITSELF" (capital letters in original). In the middle of the accelerating pandemic, Trump actively pushes for a change and a return to economic normalcy. It is becoming increasingly clear to many observers in the media and otherwise, that he is, quite blatantly, talking about how the problem affects himself, his businesses, and his reelection concerns. Trump's other obsession is blaming China, arguing that if we called it the Spanish flu (the politically correct term now is "the 1918 Influenza"), why can't we call it the "China virus"?

What is the precedent? Well, there's Marburg virus, a hemorrhagic fever named after a German university town. The 1957 outbreak (the so-called "Asian flu") and the "Hong Kong flu" in 1968. Hendra virus carries the name of the

Brisbane suburb where it was first discovered. Zika is a forest in Uganda. Fujian flu is named after a Chinese province. Ebola carries the name of a river in the Democratic Republic of the Congo. However, while one could legitimately wonder whether Wuhan virus would be an apt name following this tradition, China virus is not a candidate.

As the United States, the most prosperous country in the world, grapples with what it means to have ineffective federal leadership at a time of global crisis, state leaders act somewhat more decisively. A showdown between two fronts is brewing: that between federal and international public health authorities and the White House and that between the White House and the hardest-affected states. On March 24, Massachusetts, where I live, goes under stay-at-home orders for 2 weeks, following states such as New York, Connecticut, Louisiana, Delaware, Ohio, and California. A showdown is brewing between Trump and Maryland Governor Larry Hogan, a Republican who is also the chair of the bipartisan, and powerful, National Governors Association. Representative Liz Cheney, the No. 3 House Republican, also voices that there can be no functioning economy if the hospitals are overwhelmed.

On April 8, ABC News claims there is a November 2019 intelligence report containing analysis of wire and computer intercepts, coupled with satellite images by the US military's National Center for Medical Intelligence (NCMI), which is part of the Pentagon, warning of a "cataclysmic event," something the Pentagon denies the day after.

On April 11, for the first time in US history, all 50 states plus the US Virgin Islands, the Northern Mariana Islands, the District of Columbia, Guam, and Puerto Rico, is under a federal disaster declaration.

On April 14, Trump announces he will freeze funds for the WHO, citing what he thinks is a China bias. The US has contributed $893 million to the WHO's operations during its current 2-year funding cycle. The day after, Finland responds to Trump's announcement with increased funding to WHO. The same week, every other Western leader at a virtual G7 summit expresses strong support. The Gates Foundation also announces an extra $150-million donation. On April 19, the One World: Together at Home global broadcast and digital special to support frontline healthcare workers and the WHO raises a total of $127.9 million, providing $55.1 million to the COVID-19 Solidarity Response Fund and $72.8 million to local and regional responders. On April 23, China pledges an additional $30 million to WHO and on April 24, Chinese video-sharing social networking TikTok, used to create short dance, lip-sync, comedy and talent videos (my teenage daughter is an addict and dances even during dinner), pledges $10 million, too (Zhu, 2020).

On April 15, Trump announces that the US is investigating whether the virus came from a Wuhan lab, the Wuhan Institute of Virology, and was released as an accident, not as a bioweapon. He appears to echo Fox News (2020) reporting that same day that the virus could be part of China's effort to demonstrate that its efforts to identify and combat viruses are equal to or greater than the capabilities of the United States. This is a theory that a plethora of scientists have denied.

What's clear, though, is that the *Washington Post* has reported on State Department cables from 2018 demonstrating concerns about the safety and the management of the Wuhan Institute of Virology biolab.

There are different sets of biocontainment precautions required to isolate dangerous biological agents in an enclosed laboratory facility, depending on the pathogen you are handling. The WHO operates with Bio Safety Levels (BSLs) from BSL-1 (least safe) to BSL-4 (safest). Wikipedia lists over 50 BSL-4 lab facilities around the world, including Wuhan Institute of Virology.

Generally, the early epicenters of the US outbreak were the

Life Care Center in Kirkland, Washington, near Seattle, as well as in Boston after a fateful Biogen meeting that included travelers from China. At the end of March, a lot of the attention shifts toward California and especially toward New York City, which at some point has almost half of the infections reported in the US. Throughout April, the focus moves from Louisiana to South Dakota as coronavirus continues its spread across the continent.

On April 13, Smithfield Foods plant needs to close as 238 of its employees test positive for the virus, representing half of South Dakota's outbreak at the time, sending shocks through the US food supply chain, as the plant accounts for 5% of the nation's pork production. At the Tyson Foods poultry plant in Camilla, south-west Georgia, despite several COVID-19 deaths, the US president invokes the Defense Production Act (DPA) to mandate meat processing plants stay open during the pandemic. As of 2 May, at least 20 meat packing workers have died from the virus nationwide and 5,000 have become infected, according to unions quoted in The Guardian (2020).

There are reports of farmers having to pour out milk or plow down their harvest due to reduced demand. The sense that this is becoming a looming food security disaster spreads across the US.

For us as a family, this is more of the same, as we, short of federal or state guidelines, had already imposed a strict self-isolation the past 10 days based on a strict implementation of local town guidelines and our own personal sense of duty and analysis of the situation. I admit to and take personal responsibility for having hoarded food for the past 2 weeks to protect my family. I estimate we could survive for 1 week before I need to restock on basic groceries, or 3 weeks if we only eat dry food and water from the fridge's coal filter. However, my hoarding is more related to staying away from grocery stores to avoid contagion than thinking they truly will run out of food.

My wife and I are determined to reduce infection exposure to zero for the next few weeks. The three trips I have made to the grocery store have all been wearing *one* of the three N95 masks left over from last time I repainted my house (I later discover there are only two masks left) as well as protective eyewear from various other home improvement projects of mine. Every time, as I come home, I take off my clothes, put them in the laundry and immediately shower. It seems the virus can also spread through human hair, although, at the moment, little seems to be known for certain.

As time goes by, we realize that at least one of us might have had coronavirus during what we thought was a flu during March. Several of the kids also have flu symptoms. Despite this, we continue our self-quarantine, and the official advice gets stricter, too.

On April 15, my wife has to go in to complete a complex root canal filling, which was already initiated before the outbreak. As a result of the risk of new exposure, when she got back from the dentist, despite having been in 6-weeks' strict self-quarantine, we decide to put her into isolation in her own bedroom and bathroom for as many days as we can bear.

Moreover, even after 2 months of COVID-19, our family is reevaluating our options for work, education, play, and life in the next few years. Will my job opportunities still come through and will ongoing negotiations continue? How long can existing employers hang on to us? Will our children manage this online school environment long term? Can we sustain a life in 100% isolation from other people, and if so, for how long? Will there be major interruptions in the food supply or other consumer goods, beyond the relative shortages of dairy products, cleaning supplies, and toilet paper? How long can my mother in Norway handle a self-imposed 100% isolation? What kind of a life would that be? These thoughts bring strong emotions. What a change a few months can make!

If these kinds of disruptions are happening in a comfortable upper-middle-class life in Boston Metrowest, USA, in a wealthy suburb in the world's most powerful country, I cannot imagine what kind of planning it would take to be a service worker, a healthcare worker, or live with one family member who actually has contracted the disease under more trying circumstances. It also highlights to what extent the efficiency and implementation of these changes and constraints depend on a *voluntary social contract* between the people you are closest to. In the end, how we discuss, negotiate, and trust ourselves, the news we read, and the governance around us, all plays a part in creating the outcome.

Cultural resistance to social distancing

Beyond the US, by end of March, other national governments are more united in their messaging, although most governmental bodies have slightly differing messages. Common for all jurisdictions, whether global, national, regional, or local, is that they struggle to enforce these tight new restrictions. In the US, spring breakers from Florida to Virginia ignore social distancing even as many will soon return to shelter-in-place policies in their own home state where their parents and grandparents live. Beach goers enjoy the great weather in California despite the shelter-in-place order there. Miami bans recreational boating after boat parties take place over the weekend, and Washington, DC, closes roads after visitors ignore social distancing as crowds flocked to view cherry blossoms.

Leaner government, a trend in the Western world for decades, means less experts, less excess capacity in public service and in hospitals, and has, arguably, led to more efficiently run public services. At least this is how the new public management thesis has sold the development.

However, throughout March, the story across Europe and

in the US has been of various public health bottlenecks: hospital capacity; the population's patience with extreme measures; economy backlash; cultural resistance; shortages of basic medical equipment, such as gloves, masks, disinfectant, and eye protection, as well as advanced medical devices, particularly ventilators. In the US, the entire national emergency stockpile of ventilators is 12,000–13,000, which is an amount the Mayor of New York already at this point says he will need at the present time.

According to WHO, it took 3 months to reach 100,000 coronavirus cases worldwide, the second 100,000 took 12 days. Around mid-April, worldwide cases pass the 2 million mark and death toll stands at 125,000 with the disease found in 213 countries, areas, or territories.

Cultural resistance to government mandates is nothing new. It regularly happens around gun control; there's even a famous lobby group dedicated to it in the US. It happens around vaccines, and this is bound to arise with the current outbreak as well.

Social movements are always born out of a perceived crisis. Toward mid-April 2020, there begins to circulate reports about "social distancing deniers" holding long protest marches and drives in several US cities, including in the state of Michigan. Whether this will turn into a veritable protest movement similar in scope to the Tea Party or Occupy Wall Street remains to be seen, but it will be a key factor that plays out in any scenario. By the way, it could also work the other way, with support movements (perhaps online) that unite the front in support of government policy, and, ultimately, in support of better governance. Again, time will show.

As Republican Governor Brian Kemp of Georgia announces the state will reopen for business on April 24, before that state has reached its epidemic peak, experts warn that Americans must be made aware of the likelihood the country will have a resurgence. As of May 2, Georgia has a total of 28,302 infected, 5,387 hospitalized and have recorded 1,173 deaths, mostly concentrated in four adjacent counties in the metro Atlanta area (Georgia Department of Public Health, 2020).

On April 19, an iconic picture taken by a Reuters (2020) photographer shows a healthcare worker standing in the street as a counter-protest to those demanding the stay-at-home order be lifted in Denver, Colorado.

On April 21, CDC chief Robert Redfield warns second wave this winter will likely be worse because of flu season. He is forced to backtrack a bit on his statement, but the cat is now out of the bag—the troubles won't end by summer.

Medical equipment shortages spark public actions

Elon Musk tweets he thinks ventilators can be easily made, and New York governor Andrew Cuomo responds he takes him up on the offer. Further tweets on March 21 reveal Musk is now in touch with US medical technology manufacturer Medtronic to discuss how to make ventilators. By end of March, it is announced that Tesla's New York factory, having initially been shut down, is reopening to start manufacturing ventilators.

Around the world, private sector as well as individual initiatives arise that offer to produce medical equipment on the kitchen table or by repurposing existing manufacturing facilities. Distillers start producing disinfectant. Famed New York designer Christian Siriano offers to sew masks. Soldiers are building hospitals, perfumers are making hand sanitizer, and doctors and nurses are being called back from retirement. Stories out of Italy speak of equipment shortages, having to prioritize who to save based on age and other criteria on the fly (without any national guidance), and increasing despair among medical professionals. It seems clear that the pandemic is out of hand in Italy. Countries like the UK and even the US start talking about "flattening the curve" to avoid continuing on Italy's trajectory. The early exponential growth of the COVID-19 pandemic in Norway, despite having a top public health system, came as a shock. Norwegian officials disagree on how to interpret this situation. However, Norwegian authorities are open about what they know and don't know about the disease. Erna Solberg, Norway's Prime Minister, tries to reassure the people that few young people and children need to worry about the disease. At this point, data on this aspect is scarce and comes from a Chinese and Italian disease context not fully understood, but does seem to be a reasonable interpretation. Cases of children on ventilators start to appear in the media, although usually with the "reassuring" message that they had a preexisting condition. However, as of April 6, according to Reuters, the Norwegian Health Minister declares coronavirus epidemic "under control", claiming to have brought the famous "R naught" down from 2.7 to 0.7, meaning each infected person infects less than one person on average. The question is, will the situation last as social distancing measures are gradually relaxed?

Beyond a public health crisis

By mid-March it is becoming clear that the coronavirus pandemic is more than a public health crisis. It will have lasting economic effects on the Western world, for sure, and who knows about the developing world yet. Sanguine observers point out that if the disease develops clusters in Asia, or in vulnerable spots like refugee camps (wherever they are—even in Greece), near instant devastation is to follow.

The cultural consequences of the crisis now start to become apparent. *Techonomy*, the newsletter, publishes an article asking: "Are We Ready for a Do-Not-Touch World?" Short answer, we are *so* not ready. Cultural responses include a stunning DIY face-mask craze (do you prefer origami style using cleverly folded paper, or bra style, using cutouts from cheap brassieres?) and the Spanish ceremonious 8 p.m. clapping for medical workers from their balconies.

The human toll during a quarantine is significant; even a simple task of going grocery shopping becomes a stressful event. In Italy, throughout March, people who were out shopping were forced to wait in line at the entrance to make sure the store was filled with only a handful of shoppers at a time. My friend Dani in Naples, Italy, where I studied and learned how to relax but also how to think, and how to speak Italian and some semblance of sign language to accompany the cultural meanings, tells me a visit to the supermarket takes 2 hours. I start to prepare for the same.

What about individual responses? We still know little about what is happening to individuals. There are no studies, little reporting and little access to trustable data. Among the privileged upper-middle class, the crisis has so far been a mix of very serious issues (elderly relatives sick or worried) to work disruptions and childcare issues (as well as dealing with worried children).

However, to take my own example, it has so far largely been an opportunity for growth: I've learned to edit music and sound in Apple's Garageband app; I've begun writing on two books and have spent time re-jiggering the marketing efforts of another book; I've started a levain culture to make better bread and pizza (turns out it only takes 5 days plus daily nurturing of 3 minutes/day); and I've started painting my house (when would be a better time than during a stay-at-home order). I've also been spending lots of time with my kids, playing games, preparing food, and watching movies together. Finally, and perhaps not unique to me, who knows, I've been working actively to repair poorer aspects of my marriage, given that we are locked into the same house. I'm also quite irritable and I am quick to get mad at the kids. Also, I talk about coronavirus all the time and my wife as well as my 13-year-old daughter scold me for it. I can't help it. I cannot stop thinking about it. Moreover, I keep writing, almost as a therapeutic practice to stay sane in all this madness. I know there's psychological precedent, not that I care, or have a choice.

In contrast, essential service workers continue to keep the world's grocery stores, public transit, hospitals, and logistics network operational, generally not sporting personal protective equipment. These workers don't have the ability to work from home. They are starting to run out of money given that their income and hours are typically shrinking, and expenses are constant. The unemployment rate is unevenly distributed, and disadvantaged groups suffer more. A debate about the role of race in the COVID-19 epidemic starts to rage in the US, forcing state and federal government to come out with numbers to demonstrate case and death rates by ethnicity. Huge discrepancies are apparent and the way that America's racial disparities translate into health outcomes goes from being a grim fact to a visible trail in the morgue.

The super-rich attempt to isolate themselves as best they can and make plans to ride out the crisis in purpose-built bunkers and with private planes including medical personnel at bay. Madonna, an otherwise apt reader of the zeitgeist, issues an Instagram video with rose-petal-covered breasts from her bathtub stating "COVID-19 is the great equalizer" and receives predictable backlash on this stance. The brief video, however, remains as iconic as anything she ever did, just perhaps not the way she intended.

What the emerging sociology of the coronavirus epidemic is going to be is still only speculation, but the data that is emerging speaks of a diverging set of data from further individualization, isolation, and conflict to community and a new sense of togetherness at various levels of society (which brings us to the importance of considering the scenarios).

Reopening the economy?

China is the first country to contemplate reopening their society for business, having successfully fought the pandemic for 3 full months. Policy makers have promised loans, aids, and subsidies. Wuhan, the city of what's thought of as the first outbreak, gradually opens after a 76-day lockdown. The world takes note that the historical 40-day quarantine is doable.

Adjustments will be made to keep some measure of social distancing in effect even during a return to normalcy. Measures include that residents with a government-assigned green Quick Response (QR) code on their mobile phones—meaning they're healthy and safe to travel—have been allowed to go back to work as long as they have a letter from their employer. New health clearance codes are put in place for travelers. It's a bit unclear what this will look like in practice, but the gist is that you can only travel if you have a clean bill of health (no fever, etc.). In Wuhan, the government has given each person a QR code, which will have an individual's health status linked to it. This barcode is a machine-readable optical label that contains information about the item to which it is attached. Presumably, this is in digital form or on a piece of paper and not branded to the individual. As the government restrictions slowly are eased, businesses implement their own safeguards as well. Some are set to operate at 50% or lower capacity. Hygiene is increased. Vigilance is observed. Government is watching.

The challenge is that imported infections are a "new" threat to China and might entail a completely different set of measures than the ones previously undertaken to curb the domestic outbreak. China will soon experience how different travelers are. For one, they don't have a home to stay quarantined in. Secondly, they travel for a reason—to see people—so their motivation will be the opposite of social distancing. Thirdly, they will have traveled through airports and have been in close proximity to a lot of people on airplanes and public transport, so any superspreaders would have an equally devastating effect as it did in other economies when Chinese superspreaders were the problem.

Paradoxically, for some who only see negatives, China was by March/April 2020 beginning to look like a safe haven. The only large economy to have successfully battled coronavirus once, the sense is that even if it resurges, the government has the experience to curb another outbreak if it occurs. However, the highly likely next waves of infection loom in China as well.

As governments around the world have implemented initial rescue packages and ponder new ones, there is considerable anxiety about when, whether, and how the world economy will return to some sort of normalcy. Many predictions about for how gradual or quick the recovery will be and who the winners and losers are likely to be abound. Some businesses have already gone bankrupt and may never be in business again. Others have just temporarily taken a hit but would be able to return once the markets reopen. Entire new segments of opportunity might open as well.

Dr. Anthony Fauci, the leading US expert on infectious diseases, on March 26 makes one of his more memorable statements: “We don’t set the timeline, the virus sets the timeline” which instantly becomes a meme. However, the statement doesn’t seem to (overtly) influence the US President’s thinking, although one can never be sure.

The proponents of the earlier mentioned “pumping the brakes” approach to social distancing initially only considered the public health consequences. Around the world, economists are now trying to predict what will happen as a staggered pattern of gradual reopening and closing of various geographies and sectors will happen throughout the second quarter of 2020 and beyond.

Consequences for the global economy and various specific

sectors are catastrophic, certainly short term. Given the uncertainty, I'll explore specific impacts in the scenarios (giving some wiggle room), but here's a factoid from education: on April 14, Harvard, arguably the world's most reputable and endowed educational institution, announces salary and hiring freezes, discretionary spending reductions, potential deferral of capital projects, and leadership salary cuts, according to *The Harvard Crimson.*

Will the pandemic also become a humanitarian crisis?

Around the world, aid workers are holding their breath. The reason is clear. Acceleration factors for a pandemic generally include things like population density, unemployment, lack of sanitation, poor personal hygiene, having a poorly developed health system, and illiteracy. Ring a bell? These things are especially acute in failed states, but, more generally, there are at least 100 countries around the world that score poorly on well-accepted public health metrics such as the Global Health Security Index. One might particularly want to watch Venezuela (which arguably has become a failed state over the past decade under the regime of President Nicolas Maduro).

On April 16, Brazilian President Jair Bolsonaro fires Luiz Henrique Mandetta as minister of health after a public dispute over how to handle coronavirus, following weeks of unrest across Brazil, setting that country on a downhill trajectory.

In Africa, we'll be paying close attention the situation in people rich Nigeria, with its vulnerable population of 190 million. Already, cases of chloroquine poisoning are recorded there. On April 18, Abba Kyari, the Chief of Staff to the President of Nigeria, dies of COVID-19. Ten African countries have no ventilators at all, the *New York Times* reports.

Secondly, at the bottom of the Global Health Security Index in the 197th position, Somalia, with a population of 17.4

million, is a country to watch. They had their first reported case on March 16, although their international contagion is more limited. Reports say the virus goes from "fairy tale to nightmare." The Al-Qaeda-linked extremist group Al-Shabaab is also an actor to watch now.

Other surrounding East African countries would be similarly challenged. All in all, the most populous African nations—Nigeria, Ethiopia, Egypt, the Democratic Republic of the Congo, South Africa, and Tanzania, each with over 50 million inhabitants—stand to lose the highest percentage of people to the pandemic, should they each get a full-fledged outbreak.

In Asia, North Korea would be the worry, although they are quite isolated, apart from trade with China, which now may turn out to be a protective factor. India is definitely a question mark with its enormous population and densely populated cities with areas with poor sanitation, as is Pakistan. Iran is already a worry, but Iraq, with its war-torn soil, could also become a pandemic hotspot. On April 18, during the lockdown, a Bangladesh funeral for a religious leader, an Islamic preacher, attracts 100,000 people. Madrasa leaders had assured authorities strict social distancing rules would be followed. The incident happens 2.5 hours by car from the megacity of Dhaka. Bangladesh has 160 million inhabitants. The start of the month of fasting of Ramadan is set to begin 5 days later, on April 23, putting even greater strain on lockdown efforts.

On March 24, India, with 1.4 billion inhabitants, steps up its fight against coronavirus as Prime Minister Narendra Modi announces a complete lockdown of the country from midnight, arguing if they don't take this step, the country will go back by 21 years (a bit unclear what he meant by that). At this point, India has 550 cases of coronavirus and 10 deaths. Vast slum areas in the outskirts of India's megacities Dehli and Mumbai are perfect breeding conditions for superspread of the disease. Urban air quality is at the bottom of the world rankings. The country's urban economy is powered by seasonal migrants who typically travel back and forth through long distances. Already, before the disease has hit to any extent, the government has issued a decree calling in volunteer, retired doctors and army medical workers. India deploys a "cluster containment strategy," attempting to contain outbreaks to smaller geographical areas.

At the end of the day, the response to a pandemic is not something only the leadership controls. Cultures are more or less ready for the measures that get attempted. In South Korea, for instance, remarkably, they first lost control and subsequently regained it with no lockdown and simply strong application of social distancing, enhanced by using novel digital technologies for contact tracing, according to a study published in the *Lancet*. The South Koreans successfully implemented advanced contagion protection through technology monitoring those who are found to be infected retrospectively for the past 14 days through surveillance cameras and mobile phone and credit card usage. Imagine the kind of detailed data they then had to commence their contact tracing. Culturally, and resource-wise, not a lot of countries would be able to do the same. Singapore's "corona detectives" are also known to conduct excellent contact tracing efforts.

On April, 21, an initial 148 refugees in Greece test positive for COVID-19, all asymptomatic (Fallon, 2020). On April 22, the UN's World Food Programme (WFP) warns the coronavirus pandemic will cause global famines of 'biblical proportions' pushing an additional 130 million people to the brink of starvation and 1 billion into 'dire situations' since 821 million people are already chronically hungry, with 55 countries at risk (Picheta, 2020). On the horn of Africa, the worst locust infestation in 25 years already threatens crop yields. On April 29, 2020. the International Rescue Committee (IRC) estimates up to 1 billion infections, leading to up to 3.2

million deaths, in 34 conflict-affected and fragile countries. The same day, the International Labour Organization (ILO) reports nearly half of global workforce at risk of losing livelihoods, with particularly devastating impact on the 1.6 billion workers in the informal economy. With no access to savings and no safety net in the community or in government, these workers have few options to take care of their families and themselves, they will have "no food, no security and no future".

The future of pandemics

Many scenarios for the future development following this pandemic could exist at this point. Many predict growing isolationism on trade, increased xenophobia, and higher domestic production of goods to protect national supply chain vulnerabilities. But what about the cultural consequences? We shall examine those in Chapters 2, 3, and 9.

There are also many strong ideas out there about how the world could be better prepared in the future. One, put forth by actor and activist Sean Penn, is to reconceive the military as a health force. Another is to curb the growth of regional trade blocs (e.g., EU, Mercosur) that hamper the development of truly global institutions (UN). Most public health specialists forecast that intermittent suppression is the only way forward for both the current and future global pandemics, since eradicating them might just be too hard. The time to come might also entail a rethink on which institutions need to be considered critical infrastructure (including Internet providers, grocery chains, disinfection manufacturers, 3D printing companies, who else?).

At this early stage in the pandemic, here's what seems clear to many people: there is a long list of unacceptable truths:

- No country had adequate pandemic readiness plans (i.e., policies, training, contact tracing software, stockpiles, spare ICU capacity, ventilators, lab capacity, medical workers, masks, virus test kits).
- The WHO is inefficient, under sourced, lacks authority, and fails at sufficient global coordination (although many choose to see the glass half full and cling to them as the only comfort in a sea of failing single government initiatives). It's also clear that "something like the WHO," but better, is drastically needed for the next time.
- Governments will remain key in pandemic response but will increasingly have to find a much quicker way to establish public private partnerships upon demand.
- Vaccines taking 15–24 months to develop is too little, too late, with devastating consequences on public health and the economy.

We shall summarize the key global failures uncovered so far in the crisis and attempt to indicate what we potentially could learn from those mistakes in Chapter 3.

The origin of the coronavirus was initially set in people's mind as Wuhan, China. Recent developments have brought some doubt to the question—could it also have been circulating independently in Italy, or perhaps even have originated there? Or, could it have circulated in the human population for years—in many places?

Regardless, the initial 6 months of the coronavirus pandemic has been focused first and foremost on regional response (Wuhan, China and Lombardy, Italy) and subsequently morphed into a national focus (China, Italy, UK, Spain, the US), as governments mobilized to a varying degree. In the next 6 months, the focus is likely to shift to what happens in emerging economies and particularly in the world's top 10 megacities (to which we will turn in Chapter 3, as it directly relates to the hyper incubation condition for super spreaders and associated events).

After that, as we will explore in our scenarios (see Chapters 4–8), the focus will likely, again, shift. This time the emphasis is bound to be on a myriad of multilevel governance issues (pulsating quarantines, supply chain disruptions, mass unemployment, violence, and deaths induced by social isolation) that stem from a forever changed risk environment. One does not have to be a fatalist, or a futurist, to predict that survival of the fittest will be a key ingredient in the initial aftermath. The real question, however, is what happens in the intermediate term and also long term.

In the first 6 months of the COVID-19 crisis, the myopic focus on medical equipment shortages, which are real enough for healthcare workers and definitely impact regional death tolls, has nevertheless monopolized the public discussion so that we seem near incapable of seeing the larger issues unfolding.

However, the exact way it plays itself out, and whether survival instincts will be more or less pronounced, or will be tempered by reasonable, moderate governance principles, depends on how governments (intergovernmental, regional, national, city, local) choose to discuss, decide, and handle the implementation of key guiding principles. What will the "winning" public health strategy to coronavirus be? What will be the overarching political response? What will happen to the world economy as it contracts throughout the year? Is this a global recession, a depression, a great depression, or god forbid, even worse? We will look at some of the factors but, given the scant evidence, mostly explore the scenarios that enable us to prepare without exact predictions.

Also, it will depend on social dynamics, such as what key segments of the population (the working classes, the upper-middle class, the elite) overwhelmingly do as their crisis response. For instance, do they stop shopping for luxury goods? How much do they cut spending overall? Will they even stop spending on some types of groceries and turn to ready-made food (or the exact opposite)? The evidence is not yet there, but short term, the food industry desperately needs to know how to best adapt their supply to the new forms of demand.

I shall leave many of the short-term issues behind, only to revisit them in the scenarios. The reason is that the larger issues go far beyond immediate death tolls, or even unemployment. I will now turn to a framework that puts this into context.

The origin of the coronavirus crisis

Toward the end of 2019, a "strange influenza" appeared in the city of Wuhan, China. It will change the world. Was there any way this could have been prevented?

____

If you were a public health official in each of these countries, what would you have done, once you heard the news from Wuhan?

1. China ____________________
2. Italy ____________________
3. The UK ____________________
4. Spain ____________________
5. The US ____________________
6. Hong Kong ____________________
7. India ____________________

In the first few months, a few surprising medical shortages became apparent. Which ones?

____

The coronavirus pandemic affects nearly everyone on planet Earth. What are your feelings around it? How have you been affected so far?

CHAPTER 2

THE SUPERSPREADERS OF CORONAVIRUS ACROSS THE GLOBE

The phenomenon of superspreaders takes on considerable importance during any pandemic. We know from previous pandemics that individuals or contexts have had an outsized impact on the spread of a disease. Superspreading events have occurred during many infectious disease outbreaks, such as measles, tuberculosis, HIV, Ebola, and SARS.

For instance, commercial sex workers were quite significant in spreading HIV. A good amount of the spread of SARS in Hong Kong happened at the Prince of Wales hospital, as well as the Amoy Gardens residential complex alone. In Sierra Leone, a single traditional funeral was associated with 28 laboratory-confirmed cases of Ebola. Doctor shopping (e.g., visiting several doctors to get a diagnosis or test) has been associated with spread of disease in situations where medical care is stretched or the condition in question is relatively unknown among healthcare providers.

In the annual flu outbreaks, kids are generally recognized to be potential superspreaders due to being in close proximity to each other even if they have runny noses and not washing their hands. In a situation with asymptomatic spread and where kids seem to be less susceptible to get the disease in a very serious way themselves, this could be an important factor not to overlook. Public health officials used this argument in closing schools surrounding COVID-19.

In fact, the 20/80 rule has been invoked to point out that a smaller percentage of individuals are responsible for most of the spread, although the evidence for the exact percentage is scant. When we talk about *superspreader*, we are also usually reserving the term for even more extreme spread, perhaps down to 0.1% of the population or even just case by case.

Defining a superspreader

How do you define a superspreader? Lexico.com says a *superspreader* is "a person infected with a bacterium, virus, or other microorganism who transmits it to an unusually large number of other people." In a BBC UK town pandemic study, they defined it as spreading a disease to three people. During the 2003 SARS outbreak, a superspreader was classified as someone who directly infected at least 10 people, the CDC says. Five people were identified as such.

A crucial metric called R0, pronounced R-naught, represents how many people an average person with a virus infects. The R0 of the SARS-CoV2 so far seems to hover around 2 to 2.5, according to the World Health Organization, although that estimate is only as good as the data it is based on. However, in the case of SARS-CoV2, that's not much more than the average, which in the first 6 months of the outbreak has fluctuated between two and 10, depending on the country, and the measures they took, so a superspreader would have to be somewhat more prolific than that, perhaps infecting 20 or more?

Given the rapid moving and extreme circumstances, we don't always have full knowledge about all such incidents or phenomena. Even today, years later, many stories of superspreaders remain anecdotal single source reporting in one news outlet (and many copycat mentions) with little follow-up research.

Had we had such knowledge before or during the superspreading event itself, we could obviously have tried to stop them. In the case of COVID-19, asymptomatic transmission seems to play an outsized role compared to other outbreaks where initial symptoms may be more notable. The exact prevalence is unclear. Early on, this was not even considered a factor by public health authorities.

In many cases, history shows that there always were voices trying to stem such events, but those voices were quelled by other, stronger voices, who may have simply pointed out that such horrible events are "unlikely" or that it would be "too costly to cancel" or would "unnecessarily worry the public."

It is notable that the 2020 Tokyo Olympics were postponed until 2021 because of coronavirus. However, given that it is the largest mass gathering in the world, the decision could potentially save many lives. The irony is that we will, likely, never know for sure. Any simulation is likely to be inaccurate.

Risk factors for superspreading

I think it makes a lot of sense to focus on superspreader *potential* in addition to focusing on identification and contact tracing once superspread has occurred. Analysis of superspreading events during previous pandemics have generated a huge list of risk factors including co-infection with another pathogen, immune suppression, changes in airflow dynamics, delayed hospital admission, misdiagnosis, and interhospital transfers. Behavioral patterns also play a huge role; the risk behavior even by a single infected individual who exhibits high viral shedding can have devastating consequences.

Starting with hospital transmission, it is clear that infection control is the deciding factor in whether hospitals become sources of superspread (Frieden, 2020). It starts with appropriate protective equipment (masks, gowns), since spreading disease among healthcare personnel is an obvious recipe for getting a situation out of control. Implementing clever triage procedures (which may depend on each situation and capacity) is the next step, since without knowing which overall risk category your patients are in, any spike would render a triage process ineffective. Rapid and accurate diagnosis is also crucial, since a quick triage on the phone or in the reception can only do so much, and always will have a larger margin of error. Isolation protocol and appropriate facilities to carry it out are also critical, such as isolation rooms and (worst case) partitions to protect against respiratory droplets, as well as proper ventilation systems. This is obviously especially important in case of airborne diseases.

Currently there is some debate on the extent to which COVID-19 is airborne. The early WHO guidance of 6 feet of social distancing is somewhat of a hybrid position and does not fully take into account potential aerosol spread, particularly indoors. We will leave this matter for now and come back to it in the scenarios in Chapters 4–8.

Subsequently, flow patterns and procedures for patients, visitors, and staff need to be well thought out and need to scale or adapt to spikes in demand, at which point proper security becomes crucial. On-site testing with lab feedback within 1–2 days is also important, otherwise you might be isolating patients where there is no need to do so.

The evidence from superspreading events outside hospitals indicate that crowding can be a factor all in itself and cases have been recorded in soccer stadiums, hospitals, fitness centers, cafeterias, shopping malls, on public transport, in ski resorts, weddings, and many, many more crowded events or spaces. In theory, being near any crammed public place where people are less than a few feet away from each other or are sharing utensils or touching the same surfaces, especially indoors, has the potential to escalate the situation.

Environmental factors, such as population density and the availability and use of infection prevention and control measures in healthcare facilities, also play a significant role in superspreading events. Factors such as cough hygiene and whether people wash their hands thoroughly (or at all) have both cultural and individual origin.

If public authorities face choices on whom to vaccinate, it has been commonly thought that health workers should be first in line. However, if we could identify systemic factors that enabled us to create a psychographic profile of the superspreader, we should then go ahead and vaccinate, quarantine, or at least ask potential superspreaders to change their behavior and practice social distancing. I will now move to consider the individual profile of a superspreader and then move to systemic conditions.

The profile of a superspreader

What might the profile of a superspreader be? Let's see, so far, we have studied a marathon runner, a wedding guest, a birthday guest, and a skier—what do those people have in common beyond exposing themselves to large groups of people? Do they share any psychological or demographic traits? Are they in a specific socioeconomic group? Do they have any biological identifiers?

The term *virus shedding* was not commonplace outside the medical and public health communities before March 2020 and refers to a phenomenon that measures the different degree of contagion that occurs in any viral disease depending on the individual, stage of the disease, and myriad other factors that are still relatively poorly understood.

The scientific establishment has little data on what causes some people to be "supershedders," individuals who release unusually large amounts of virus from their bodies, so anybody coming into contact with them is more likely to become infected. We are not even sure that some do so more than others; perhaps it is just stages in the disease. However, if it were found to be the case, and we could identify causes and indicators, it would be a major breakthrough. Experience from both the SARS and MERS outbreaks has definitely confirmed that some patients, associated with worse outcomes, had significantly higher viral loads than others.

Patient 3 in the UK was Steve Walsh, a businessman from southeast England in his 50s, who contracted coronavirus at a conference in Singapore. He subsequently traveled to France where he stayed with his family in a ski chalet in the Alpine resort of Les Contamines-Montjoie. Five people who were known to have been in the chalet have tested positive.

Religion: South Korea's religious sects and quick recovery through technology

Discovering that there may be several superspreaders in close proximity is the ultimate fear. On February 17, an unidentified 61-year-old woman presents at the hospital in Daegu City, then the epicenter of infections in South Korea. Becoming Patient 31 in the country, she tested positive. As it turns out, she had previously attended worship services with at least 1,000 members of her secretive religious sect known as Shincheonji. Within days, numbers skyrocketed to 1,600; half of the cases were linked to the Shincheonji sect, arguably "a doomsday church cult," a Christian new religious movement established on March 14, 1984, in South Korea by Lee Man-hee. Daegu, a southeastern city, is by the end of March where roughly 70% of confirmed cases are concentrated. Nobody knows how Patient 31 got infected. The Seoul Metropolitan Government has filed a formal complaint against the congregation, accusing it of murder and specifically of violating the Infectious Disease and Control Act.

In India, a Sikh religious leader coming back from a trip to Italy and Germany before he went preaching in more than a dozen villages in Punjab state, having ignored a mandatory quarantine, has now died from the virus, prompting lockdown of each village. He had also visited a large gathering to celebrate the Sikh festival of Hola Mohalla, a 6-day festival that attracts around 10,000 people every day, shortly before he died.

Nineteen people are confirmed having tested positive as a

result and another 200 have been tested. These villages were put under even tighter restrictions than the strict 21-day nationwide stay-at-home order imposed by the government. The health department in Punjab tracked 934 of his direct and indirect contacts by going door-to-door and is testing them. Forty thousand people in 20 villages have been asked to stay in self-quarantine, as reported by *India Today*.

Sports: Italy's curious and tragic experience with coronavirus

A "strange pneumonia" was seen in Lombardy in November of 2019, according to Italian doctor Giuseppe Remuzzi. This fits into Chinese propaganda to muddle the origin of the virus, since Lombardy is home to Italy's largest Chinese population. Could the virus have originated in Italy, not in China? Regardless, genetic analyses in Italy indicate that the epidemic there was started by two people, one of whom, a marathon runner, gave it to 43 other people, including his pregnant wife, two doctors, his GP, three bar-goers, and a 77-year-old woman who died. Thirty-eight-year-old "Mattia" (which may or may not be his real name) went to a hospital in Codogno, northern Italy, three times starting on February 14 with flu-like symptoms before he obtained antiviral drugs and was diagnosed, initially just with pneumonia, on February 20. On Feb. 19, the Champions League soccer match between Atalanta (the city of Bergamo's team) and the Spanish club Valencia gathers 44,000 people at the Giuseppe Meazza stadium in the San Siro district of Milan, very likely further escalating the disease.

Life science: The Biogen meeting in Boston

In late February, employees of Cambridge biotechnology company Biogen attended a company meeting, gathering 175 company executives. The ill-fated Biogen management meeting at the Marriott Long Wharf hotel in Boston on Feb.

26 and Feb. 27 has so far been linked to 97 COVID-19 cases in Massachusetts and multiple cases in other states, which obviously escalated from there. The state of Massachusetts Department of Public Health initially traced 80% of the state's cases to the single Biogen conference. Just a few days later, media reports just over half of Boston's cases up to March 16 seem to stem from the Biogen event as the disease spreads further, perhaps through second-order spread, perhaps through other sources. Contact tracing appears to confirm the cluster of cases tied to Biogen and includes people in North Carolina, Indiana, New Jersey, Tennessee, and Washington, DC, as well as in Europe. Biogen notified authorities of the potential coronavirus outbreak nearly a week later. Biogen has cut ties with a US employee who allegedly hid her coronavirus symptoms during a flight to Beijing. The company's foundation is now committing $10 million to relief efforts.

Sports fans: Thai boxing

On March 6, a Thai boxing fan entered the Lumpini boxing stadium, unaware that he was infected by a relative who had traveled to Italy. He infected 50 other boxing fans, from several provinces, who then spread it to their provinces, before they were all quarantined.

Commuters: New York City gets it by morning

On March 5, 50 guests gathered at a home in Westport, Connecticut, for a 40th birthday party. The party was in honor of a man about to return to South Africa who tested positive for COVID-19 when he arrived in Cape Town and alerted partygoers. Half of the guests have been confirmed to be infected. This outbreak is obviously also connected to what later becomes the New York epicenter, given the fact that Westport is a commuting distance to Manhattan. By end of March, that outbreak is past the point of contact tracing.

On March 6, a New York attorney from La Rochelle takes

his regular commuter train into Grand Central Station using the Metro-North Railroad and walks to his office nearby. At least 20 cases have initially been linked to the man, as the family's temple, Young Israel of New Rochelle, get ordered to close and his son's school, Yeshiva University, closes too.

La Rochelle rapidly becomes New York state's corona hotspot, as New York city gradually also becomes a massive epicenter. Later, it emerges that it perhaps is the Metropolitan Transportation Authority (MTA) subway, the nation's largest urban transit system, with over 4.3 million people riders every day, that has escalated the immensely negative trajectory of New York as compared to other cities in the United States. The economic consequences of a full subway shutdown are immense, but the fact that by April 18, 2,496 subway workers have tested positive, and 4,365 are currently quarantined due to illness or exposure is also a serious issue, as reported by the *New York Post*. Governor Cuomo refuses to consider a shutdown, pointing out that the subway is essential to moving medical professionals and first responders.

Skiing: Austria and France export an après-ski bug

The Austrian village of Ischgl, an Alpine ski destination and party hotspot in Tyrol, remained open even as other nations issued travel warnings of potential coronavirus exposure. Thousands of revelers returning from vacations in Ischgl spread infections across much of Europe. Norwegian Prime Minister Erna Solberg attributes the early exposure her country got through these ski tourists being infected to the successful national response, because it was concentrated and visible.

Social events: the fateful wedding in Uruguay

On March 7, Carmela Hontou, a 57-year-old fashion designer from Uruguay, flew back from Spain, had lunch with her 84-year-old mother, and that night went to a wedding with 500 people in the district of Carrrasco, in the outskirts of Montevideo. She infected 44 people.

The potential of superspreaders is the X factor in any pandemic. Containing them early is also the key for society to have any kind of expectation that pandemics will not break out on a regular basis, even in societies with a top-notch health system.

Should we demonize the superspreader? Probably not generally, although risk behavior should be questioned in a time of pandemic.

Predicting superspread

Recently, epidemiological software has been using machine-learning algorithms to try to predict the spread of disease (which we will look at closely in Chapter 3). Canadian startup BlueDot picked up unusual flu activity in Wuhan, China on December 30 already, and flagged it to the authorities. The Boston-based Healthmap initiative similarly tracks disease globally.

Common for these platforms is that they base themselves on a mix of media reporting, self-reporting, and machine-learning algorithms. The future importance of dashboards and web-based tools, improved data sharing, and real-time information to support critical decision-making is unquestionable.

However, while they are currently somewhat useful early in an outbreak, the current avalanche of cases and news have all but overwhelmed the systems, as can be seen from the dots all over the map and the fact that most of them cannot keep up with the media stories coming in. Should we wish to be prepared to use these systems for actual decision-making, we need to build more scalable systems that are ready for prime time.

For a futurist trained in social science, the notion that spread of disease cannot be predicted is, at face value, not acceptable. I simply refuse to believe it can be the case. If we can, with some success, predict or at least create scenarios for most other important phenomena, why not disease?

Forces and factors of disease prediction

Without assuming we have much reliable data, let's make a small attempt to model the emergence of the COVID-19 pandemic based on the forces of disruption framework's conceptual tools alone. We will try to predict high-probability locations, professional groups, and psychographic profiles for superspread, as well as health outcomes.

A caveat here is that this is no substitute for an epidemiological model with actual empirical data points beyond a conceptual overview. However, most decision makers will not have access to an advanced, ideal typical epidemiological model, and even if they do, they are not likely to have the time to put in all the parameters all the time, as the picture is constantly changing. Strategy research in the corporate sectors has often shown that the needs among decision makers is typically for more mundane decision tools with 80/20 range effectiveness.

There are indicators to be found within each of the forces of disruption affecting pandemic superspreading events. While the picture is still emerging, the overview that follows indicates some of these factors.

Forces affecting pandemic superspreading events

Science & Technology

# of Scientists per capita, # of Clinical trials, Availability of Medical technology (# of ventilators)

Policy & Regulation
Global Health Security Index (country), City rankings (capital status, population, urban density, innovativeness), Year founded, Government effectiveness, # of ICU beds

Business Models & Startups
Airport size, # of Industrial strength areas, Supply chain disruptions, # of Relevant startups identified

Social Dynamics & Consumers
Demographics (average age), Cultural preparedness, Consumption patterns, Disposable income, Resistance, Protest, Individualism, Collectivism, Illiteracy, Political affiliation, Generation, Historical response to previous hardship

Ecosystem & Health
Air quality, Gene pool, Health demographics, Individual health factors

Just briefly on social dynamics, Yale sociologist Nicholas Christakis showed in his book *Connected* (2011) that biological and social phenomena spread in social networks in an interrelated manner. Namely, biological contagion (whether you might get influenza) might relate to social contagion (whether you are likely to get the flu vaccination).

The power of people and places—modeling superspreader events

The model looks at the most salient factors that might impact the spread of disease and the health outcomes based on superspreading in disease epicenters. For each, I will simply assign a value as positive (+) or negative (-); for some factors, the extreme parts of the scale might shift from negative to positive and vice versa.

I will heavily weigh factors that impact the network effects that are likely to occur in locations with a lot of people and especially with people who are travel around extensively, or in locations with particularly high density of people (with little choice in the matter).

Next, I will introduce the granularity of the analysis: country, city, profession, psychographic profile. Let's assume that only the top population centers globally will matter for this 80/20 type analysis, which leaves us with only a few countries per continent, namely:

Global Top-Population Centers
North America: USA
South America: Brazil
Africa: Nigeria, Ethiopia, Egypt, the Democratic Republic of the Congo, South Africa, Tanzania
Asia: China, India, Pakistan, Iran, Iraq
Europe: France, Germany, UK, Italy, Spain

We will then proceed to add a few more countries at the bottom of the scale for other reasons, such as their poor ranking on one of the lists we use (Health security, notably). Hence, we will add Venezuela because it is currently a failed state, we will add Somalia because it is a proxy for all of poor health security in East Africa, and we will add Norway because Scandinavian countries have a strong welfare state and an excellent health system, yet early indicators tell a tale of a virulent COVID-19 in Norway, the reasons for which are poorly understood. China is particularly interesting because of its control over its citizens, which cannot easily (or desirably) be replicated by others. Two widely used mobile phone apps, AliPay and WeChat, which nearly have replaced cash in China, helped enforce the restrictions, as the government was able to keep track of people's movements. In some cases, they even were able to stop people with confirmed infections from traveling, using a traffic light system of color codes green, yellow, and red on people's cell phones. The downside of such desire for information control, for countries outside China, is a less-than-complete desire and willingness to clearly communicate key data and developments internationally, at a pace this disease seems to require.

Pandemic outcome in megacities

Megacities emerge as a particularly powerful incubator for superspreading events and catalyzing individual superspreaders, enabling veritable outbreaks from a single case alone (see the Appendix, Part D, for further analysis).

As air quality and other factors enter the picture as causal agents, the death toll in New York and other Western megacities becomes understandable. This is not just a disease affecting the developing world. It is to prove catastrophic for any dense metropolitan area that is unable to put in place effective quarantines or social distancing before a major outbreak happens.

What becomes clear is that different megacities have different risks but that all major population centers have the potential to become incubators of superspread. Beyond that, nobody is saying that rural areas are "safer" in any way, given the relative lack of medical facilities in sparsely populated areas around the world. Rural hospitals represent about half of US hospitals. CNN (2020) reports rural hospitals are facing "financial ruin" during the coronavirus pandemic, as they have empty beds because people are scared of getting infected by coming to the hospital or because non-essential procedures were canceled as a precaution (some states started to allow them again starting in April). This adds to an already dire revenue decline; at least 170 rural hospitals have shut down since 2005 due to reductions in federal aid. Rural America, notably in Oklahoma, Missouri, and Mississippi, have a huge amount of elderly with preexisting conditions, smack in the middle of the coronavirus sweet spots. Many are uninsured. In 2019, nearly 11 million people—about 3% of the US population—lived in counties that had no hospitals—so-called hospital deserts.

For those interested in exactly what this analysis reveals, and which cities come out on top, take a look at the Appendix, Part D.

Policies that stem superspreading

Does old-school geographical containment (quarantines, stay-at-home orders) on a town, city, region, state, or national level work? Or, does the evidence from superspreader events prove that it is not the locations themselves that are the problem, but rather surgical, statistically rarer microinteractions within them? If so, perhaps we need to attack the behaviors that cause superspread, and curb the exact mechanisms instead of isolating entire cities and countries? Perhaps a question for another day in many countries right now, but definitely a question for the immediate future, given that the world economy, and the politicians who want to be reelected within it, cannot sustain this avalanche for many more weeks and months.

In summary, barring the ability to predict superspread events or individuals, speed of response seems to be the single most effective protective measure against superspreaders. Having said that, we are likely to see varying degree of vigilance surrounding mass events in the time to come. The potential risk of spreading disease should always be a factor to consider when putting on an even of 50 people or more, even absent an active pandemic threat. When it comes to events of 500 people or more, or even more for megaevents of tens of thousands (e.g., town festivals, sports events, concerts) or millions of people (e.g., the Olympics, citywide street celebrations), extreme vigilance will need to be exercised.

For entire countries or regions with poorly performing health systems with low capacity, the problem is even larger, and superspreading events can become near-extinction events for vulnerable parts of the population such as the elderly, the incarcerated, or people with preexisting diseases and/or severely compromised immune systems.

The crystal clear conclusion from our very preliminary analysis of superspreading events is that the logical global, national, or even regional response to an outbreak would be to take the most drastic action in the largest cities, as well as among the most vulnerable populations, especially in those social institutions (e.g., elderly homes, hospitals, jails, schools) known to easily transmit any contagion, including the seasonal flu.

Curiously, in the current COVID-19 outbreak, most action has either been state or countrywide and sweeping, instead of surgical and focused. If outbreaks become more commonplace, which they may well do, given how many viruses now are in community transmission, this is not a sustainable strategy.

Individual superspreaders, the nature of superspreading events, as well as categorizing superspreader locales, are each poorly understood at present. The somewhat myopic view of epidemiology and public health should not be the only view of these events.

We need not only to map the systemic risks but also evaluate exactly how an intermittent and scaled approach to restarting society and bringing capacity and risk up and down, *depend* on the dual challenge of building public health system resilience and at the same time making political choices between saving lives and saving the economy.

For that to happen, we need a much more fine-grained

understanding of the causes and effects of each of these types of events and the interrelationships between them. These systems analyses are highly complex, but that must not deter us. Choices will be made on an operational basis about each of these things regardless what we do about it, so we might as well take a deep approach to the problem. My discussion will pick up after the scenarios, which will illustrate how super-spreading might pan out given various parameters of the aftermath.

Superspreaders of infectious diseases

Disease does not spread evenly during an outbreak. Can you name the characteristics of a superspreader (a person, in this case)?

____

Specific venues that are prevalent in contemporary society seem to accelerate the spread of disease. Can you name a few of them?

1. ______________________________________
2. ______________________________________
3. ______________________________________
4. ______________________________________

The growing issue of megacities

People love to live in cities. The economic and cultural opportunities in huge cities are enormous. However, the risks of a big pandemic outbreak in a megacity are significant.

Name a megacity you have visited and describe how you think it would deal with a pandemic, both short term (the first month) and long term (the next few years).

CHAPTER 3
FORESIGHT FAILURES BY FUTURISTS, GOVERNMENT, MEDIA, AND INNOVATION

People argue that COVID-19 was a foreseen disaster. That's *not* the case. But not for the reasons typically given. However, pondering exactly what went wrong in foresight attempts from across the board (futurists, government planning, media commentary, and/or private sector innovation) is now of uttermost importance. This is not to shift blame—that's not terribly productive at this point—but to reflect on what went wrong to avoid anything like this in the future. I'll explain why.

Mapping the unforeseen: simulating the next decade

Simulating the next decade has never been an accurate science. Many futurists have given up on true foresight and prefer scenario thinking. I am also in that category (mostly). What this means is that I recognize that seeing exactly what the future holds is the kind of wisdom humans don't yet possess (or at least I don't). But what are simulations? They are models containing specific parameters that we subsequently let loose in order to see what would happen.

Scenario thinking is usually a way to prepare for an imagined future. Scenarios are designed to provoke thinking, to help us relate to a diverse set of future events that may or may not happen. It is often said that no scenario should be thought of as complete. For more on scenario methods, see the Appendix, Part A.

In this case, each of the scenarios are quite near term; in fact, we are living in versions of each of them right now. Crafting solid scenarios can help us, as citizens, policy makers, or business leaders, decide which path we want to chart for what lies ahead.

Mapping the unforeseen is a balance act. I am aware that this book will be available even after this decade is over, so the answers to "what really happens" will perhaps be there by then. On the other hand, it seems certain that we are moving into a decade that is far more uncertain than anybody imagined just a year before the 2019/20 pandemic hit. "*Certain to be uncertain*"; in other words, that's not being very confident.

This is where scenario thinking comes to the rescue. But remember, the biggest mistake made when crafting a scenario is to make it too obvious. I've been part of numerous scenario exercises. I've reviewed many scenario drafts. Based on that experience, I've attempted to make each scenario complex enough that it doesn't only tilt in one direction. I need to allow some interpretability. Is this really a desirable future? What is wrong in this picture? Because life itself is never that easy. We cannot pretend it is, even in fictional account–therein lies the responsibility of any writer or, indeed, of any futurist.

Even if the scenarios you are about to read and experience turn out to be far-fetched, the aim is that they still have the power to stimulate thinking and feeling, which may become relevant in the coming decade. Also, we will never fully agree on what the next decade holds, even when we are in it, or looking back at it. Such is the destiny of human history writing.

However, just to give you a little snapshot of how our commonplace assumptions are changing by the minute, in one of my more drastic scenarios, I have a little segment about oil prices stabilizing at $15/barrel. That seemed quite extreme, yet on April 21, 2020, US crude oil plunged to –$37.63 a barrel, which means that sellers have to pay someone to take the oil off their hands.

Is it possible to simulate the next decade? Quite definitely, no. However, what we can and should do is try to imagine what we might face. Without some level of foresight, we are doomed to walk blindly into potentially worse circumstances than we find ourselves in right now. Conversely, with concerted effort, science and technology and collaboration is far enough advanced that we have the tools to round up a response to near everything that might come our way, at least in the vein of diseases. What will be crucial to that effort is to not only understand but cater to the desires and needs of a far greater width of the human population. Not only would they be affected by our emerging choices they might also object to them in forceful ways which makes our own response futile or less efficient.

Despite how advanced we think our current society is, few of the traditionally forward-thinking institutions, nation-states, think tanks, media, or innovators, neither corporations nor startups, seem to have been able to foresee this pandemic, despite what they say now.

That being said, arguably, the mere fact that a global pandemic could spread havoc even in Western societies was a "catastrophe foretold," for instance, by Bill Gates.

Media, experts, and other prophets

In a recent article, Shapiro (2020), echoing historian and author John M. Barry's *The Great Influenza*, claims the US media "covered up" the Influenza of 1918 pandemic for fear of undermining the US Great War effort. However, by minimizing its effects they ensured that their readers didn't trust them and also stoked deep fear among their loyal readers. How about the press coverage of pandemics over the past decade? Does it stoke fear or ignorance, and why?

WHO/European Commission joint pandemic workshop (2005)

Pandemic influenza preparedness planning workshops were common during the time of Avian influenza. A striking report on the second joint WHO/European Commission workshop, October 24–26, 2005, reveals that the following case scenario was played out:

> *In recent weeks, increased and sustained transmission of influenza A/H5 in several of your neighbouring countries has forced WHO to raise the pandemic alert level to phase 6. Your country has been without cases so far, but in the past few days increasing numbers of patients with symptoms suspected of being influenza A/H5N1 have been admitted to hospitals in your area. The population has reacted with thousands of telephone calls to local authorities and health services about risks and recommendations to protect their families and themselves. Immediate action is required to control the situation.*

In retrospect, this scenario is interesting but quite abbreviated, as was the scenario exercise, given that "participants were divided into four groups" and had a quick discussion of either coordination, surveillance, scaling up health systems, and nonpharmaceutical or pharmaceutical interventions.

Lots of shortcomings are noted and the recommendations are quite specific as to what needs to be done better, including good things that frontrunner countries seem to have implemented. For example, "the finance ministry should be included in pandemic planning," "a checklist needs to be developed specifying what is expected from each institution (church, school, restaurant, etc.) regarding social distancing measures," and "possible inequities in access to healthcare and supplies for minority groups during the pandemic need to be addressed." However, again, the two organizations focus on themselves, recommending that "the roles of WHO and ECDC in the event of an outbreak need to be clarified."

The APSED framework (2005)

In September 2005, for the first time, the Asia Pacific Strategy for Emerging Diseases, or APSED (2005), was developed to provide a common framework for the 48 countries and areas of the Asia Pacific region. It boiled down to working harder on health security, focusing on eight areas: (1) surveillance, risk assessment, and response; (2) laboratories; (3) zoonoses; (4) infection prevention and control; (5) risk communications; (6) public health emergency preparedness; (7) regional preparedness, alert, and response; and (8) monitoring and evaluation.

While each of these areas may be important, the specifics of how urgently and with how much resources they would have to be implemented are lacking.

The Atlantic, a US periodical publication that has been unusually active around the pandemic, points to the 2018 demarcation of the 100th anniversary of the flu pandemic of 1918, which killed 50 to 100 million people around the world and claims there was lots of press about the potential of a repeat. Let's see.

However, if we take the example of the *Lancet*, the famous medical journal, their entry is short. They simply write, "This year marks the 100th anniversary of the 1918–1919 global influenza pandemic, which infected 500 million people and claimed more than 50 million lives. Since 1918, there have been further pandemics and today influenza remains a global threat." While that statement makes clear that influenza still can kill, there is nothing in that statement that qualifies the pandemic threat as anything more than a severe, but regular seasonal influenza (which is what many mistook COVID-19 for).

The OSI scenarios (2006)—a UK effort

Back in 2006, the UK Office of Science and Innovation (OSI) wrote a government scenario report called *Infectious diseases: preparing for the future*, focusing on the UK and sub-Saharan Africa, and looking "10–25 years into the future." This turned out to be a pretty accurate time frame, given that 16 years later we are facing a major pandemic. Their work involved 300 stakeholders from 30 countries. However, the main risk they identify regarding zoonotic disease coming into the UK is foodborne infections, while in Africa they are concerned with livestock infecting immunosuppressed Africans with HIV/AIDS.

The causes they identify are the rate and scale of global change in agriculture, trade, demographics, species translocations and invasions, microbial adaptation, and other complex factors. Their mitigation strategies are astonishingly vague, for instance suggesting "better contact" between veterinary and medical communities. Really? That's your remedy?

The 2011–2013 ASEF-ASAP scenarios

In the years after the 2009 Swine flu, the *Accurate Scenarios, Active Preparedness* (ASEF-ASAP) project of 2011, funded by the Government of Japan, convened a panel of high-level stakeholders from across Asia and Europe to develop pandemic scenarios. From the consulting firm Prospex, who ran the scenario facilitation, we learn that "ASEF brought together a broad range of stakeholders and experts including experts from international organisations like the WHO, WFO, UNOCHA, transport and nutrition companies like Lufthansa and Nestle, physician and patient organisations and NGOs such as CARE and the Red Cross." According to Prospex, "Together, over the course of 2 years, they developed scenarios that capture the possible outbreaks and environments of the future."

The resulting set of three scenarios for the future of pandemic preparedness—Grey Paradise, MosaInc., and GloCal Blocs—have nonsensical names that are hard to relate to, which is the first problem with them. The second "mistake" (in my estimation) is that they cover 30 years, which makes them nonspecific and without actionable timelines within any one government's time horizon. Within a span of 30 years, some countries will not even exist anymore and will be overtaken by others.

Third, the driving forces and uncertainties defined by the project are manifold and unspecific. Deriving any kind of logical pattern to compare these three scenarios on therefore becomes difficult, if not impossible.

Fourth, looking more closely, the actual storyline of each scenario (spanning 30 years) is around 1,400 words, which is not long enough to describe a credible, compelling societal development over a generation.

Fifth, the scenarios don't cover what happens after some pathogen appears at the scene, but instead stop short at discussing the potential risk of a whole host of potential plagues. The result of that is that even if they happen to cover a pathogen that in the future turns lethal (and they do have a discussion on zoonotic pathogens), that discussion is so short and meaningless that it has few lessons for future outbreak response.

Sixth, there are no human storylines within each scenario. As a result, we have trouble identifying with them. Nobody identifies with "the WHO" unless they happen to work there or with "governments" (even if they work there).

Seventh, there is no intrigue or violence. The closest they come is to write that "violence looms" without any further specifics.

Eight, these pandemic scenarios took no account of tech development or physical infrastructure changes throughout the 30 years [*sic*] of the scenario duration. How can that be? It's simply not believable.

Lastly, each of these scenarios is so boring and non-provoking that it doesn't engage us. The UN never collapses, things never get all that bad, and scientific progress continues unabated. Boring. Not necessarily true. Either way, scenarios for public health futures need to be sufficiently provocative to engage a wide set of folks who would not otherwise have given such scenarios a second thought.

If I rapidly recharacterize them, they deal with authoritarian Asian government dominance versus Weak governments / Strong civil society versus Myriad national bloc actors. What's more unclear is how the scenarios were used. From reading the report it seems they were largely put on the shelf after a single workshop developing and discussing them. This is not how to efficiently use scenario methods.

Langenhove (2012) comments on the weaknesses inherent in that the integrated system of detection, monitoring, and response depends very heavily on a centralized communication system, which is true.

The ASEF-ASAP report (p.51) rightfully points out that "all countries...focus on influenza-type epidemics" but then they go into minutia such as "many Asian countries use terminology that is not coherent with the terminology used by WHO." Again, a very myopic, self-serving view.

However, the report does mention zoonotic diseases as a trend in pathogens.

None of the reports have focused to any degree on asymptomatic transmission, which seems to be a blind spot in both public health policy reports and the research. This is despite the role it has played in previous diseases such as typhoid, C. difficile, influenzas, and HIV/AIDS.

EU pandemic foresight scenario (2011)

Another more recent pandemic foresight study (Suk &

Semenza, 2011) proclaimed the European Union a hot spot for the emergence of infectious diseases for its exposure to the three broad groups of drivers they identified: globalization and environmental change, social and demographic change, and health system capacity. Europe, the US East Coast, Australia, and scattered places in Asia also report higher incidents than elsewhere according to Jones et al. (2008), and human population density was a common significant independent predictor of Emerging Infectious Disease (EID) events in all categories, even controlling for spatial reporting bias by country.

Rand Corporation on pandemics (2012)

Some think tanks have written intelligently about pandemics for years. Rand Corporation's (2012) report *Threats Without Threateners* put it quite bluntly: "Only pandemics hold the risk of destroying American society within a foreseeable future" and says the case for including pandemics within the scope of national security is "compelling." With hindsight, that statement was prophetic.

However, reading on, it's clear that the Rand folks haven't thought through a serious scenario, as they write, "While national responses may entail restricting liberties through quarantines, limits on travel, and the like, those would, in most cases, be a temporary means of containing the spread of disease." Little awareness here of the potential need to extend quarantines for months and with disease outbreaks that last for years, which is what we will be facing from 2020 onward. Rand also, mysteriously, still puts pandemics in the category of "chronic" and not "acute" conditions.

Bill Gates' pandemic warning (2015)

Bill Gates' genius lies in making great impact on global health through his foundation. He is also a celebrity, one of the few true geek celebrities we have left. In an infamous 2015 TED

Talk, "The next outbreak? We're not ready," Bill Gates warns that "although there is no need to panic" (well, there was), the world now needs to put ideas from scenario planning to vaccine research to health worker training into practice relatively soon. "If anything kills over 10 million people in the next few decades, it's likely to be a highly infectious virus rather than a war," Gates says during the talk, "Not missiles, but microbes." Today he looks like a prophet. However, stating publicly that pandemics could be bad doesn't constitute genius nor does it describe what COVID-19 has done to the world.

In truth Bill Gates said only what most other experts in public health would agree to. However, pandemic readiness is expensive and tends to get deprioritized by public officials, which is what happened, TED Talk or not. I think media and elites often overestimate the impact of a TED Talk. TED is an American media organization that, since 1991, posts talks online for free distribution under the slogan "ideas worth spreading." Some talks gain viral traction. Contrary to what one might think, doing one doesn't always change the world. As of now, post-coronavirus, the talk has near 32 million views, but I don't know how many views it had before the crisis. His new TED Talk, "How we must respond to the coronavirus pandemic," recorded on March 24, for instance, has only 5 million views. The YouTube consensus, at the moment, is that if a video gets more than 5 million views in a 3-to-7-day period, it can be considered "viral."

New York Times' coverage of the Centennial of the 1918 Great Influenza (2018)

Looking back at 2018's *New York Times*, I found that already on January 8, an op-ed states "We're Not Ready for a Flu Pandemic"—so great. On August 14, they publish an article by Zachary Siegel titled "Is the U.S. Knee-Deep in 'Epidemics,' or Is That Just Wishful Thinking?" which turns out to be about suicides and overdoses. Later in the year, on October 22, there is an op-ed on "A Centennial of Death: The Great Influenza Pandemic of 1918," which recommends us all to get the flu shot and quoting another doctor, saying, "In the modern era, we think it can't happen, but we should be aware of it, we should remember it, and think of it as something that is out there waiting to happen." On November 28, they publish a piece by Malia Wollan under the rubric "tip" with the headline "How to Survive a Flu Pandemic." One tip is from a former CDC official who advices "practice cough etiquette" and "consider buying N95 masks." Perhaps, not the strongest of warnings or the best of advice, in retrospect. Should we take the example of the *New York Times*, one of the world's leading mainstream newspapers, the media hasn't exactly showered the public with pandemic scare stuff, so that should not be the worry. As I'll show from the lackluster coverage of the few pandemic scenario studies that have been done over the years, it's quite the opposite.

The WHO R&D Blueprint's Disease X (2018)

Disease X is a placeholder name that was adopted by the World Health Organization (WHO) in February 2018 on their shortlist of blueprint priority diseases, called the WHO R&D Blueprint. The first list of prioritized diseases was released in December 2015. "Disease X represents the knowledge that a serious international epidemic could be caused by a pathogen currently unknown to cause human disease, and so the R&D Blueprint explicitly seeks to enable cross-cutting R&D preparedness that is also relevant for an unknown "Disease X" as far as possible." In October 2019 in New York, the WHO's Health Emergencies Programme took part in a "Disease X dummy run" with Johns Hopkins Center for Health Security, the World Economic Forum, and the Gates Foundation to simulate a global pandemic by a Disease X. The 150 participants from various world health agencies and public health systems were supposed to learn how to better prepare and share ideas and observations for combatting such an eventuality (see Event 201 a bit further along in this chapter).

While the notion of a Disease X is very powerful, in retrospect, there are a plethora of emerging pathogens that could have been modeled in highly specific ways in order to create a set of scenarios that would be specific enough to spur action. Instead, politicians seem locked into only responding to what is immediately in front of us. We just had a pandemic influenza so let's make the next scenario about pandemic influenza also.

The Global Preparedness Monitoring Board (GPMB)'s Report (2019)

The Global Preparedness Monitoring Board (GPMB), an independent monitoring and accountability body to ensure preparedness for global health crises composed of "political leaders, agency principals and world-class experts," co-convened by the World Health Organization and the World Bank Group, launched in 2018 to address "gaps, weaknesses and inefficiencies" in global health response to pandemics.

GPMB lists 18 media as having covered their report. Two US media (CNN and Fox News), a few British media (BBC, *The Guardian*, *The Daily Mail*, and *The Telegraph*), a few US specialty magazines (*Christian Science Monitor*, *Fortune*, *Fast Company*, *Business Insider*), a few online news sites (Quartz, Gizmodo, Vox), one German (Deutsche Welle), as well as a few individual papers (*Irish Times*, *Global News Canada*). Let's just say it didn't reach Asia or South America, two crucial continents for pandemic spread.

But did the GPMB's report deserve wider coverage? The GPMB's 2019 report of where the world stands in its ability to "prevent and contain" a global health threat concluded that *neither* the recommendations from previous high-level panels and commissions following the 2009 H1N1 influenza pandemic and the 2014–2016 Ebola outbreak, *nor* the previous recommendations from GPMB were implemented, and that "serious gaps persist." In fact, "For too long, we have allowed a cycle of panic and neglect when it comes to pandemics: we ramp up efforts when there is a serious threat, then quickly forget about them when the threat subsides. It is well past time to act." What GPMB means by acting seems to be to improve most countries' health systems, which is a laudable, yet unspecific, goal in the context of pandemic. Improve what exactly?

Furthermore, when looking at the GPMB's specific recommendations, they contain the same mumbo-jumbo that jars international reports of this kind. In fact, little indicates that there is a particular urgency. Recommendations are not particularly specific ("All countries must build strong systems") and the evidence is not alarmist enough to spur immediate action. The "worst" scenario they can come up with involves a terrorist spreading a lethal pathogen that causes a 0.2–2.0% of global GDP loss, "on par with climate change." There is a lot of talk about influenza preparedness, nothing on coronavirus, very little on stockpiles (beyond influenza vaccines), nothing on stockpiling personal protective equipment (PPE) or ventilators.

I'm forced to conclude that even if countries implemented this report to the letter, we would be roughly in the same situation as we are today as regards coronavirus response on a global level. Instead, the report wastes time discussing whether the UN or the WHO should be in charge. As we now know, in the current pandemic, most countries want to be in charge of their own response and few, if any, international institutions, whether they be the UN system or trade blocs like the EU, were in any way prepared to take this coordinating role. Whether they should is an important debate for the future, but likely not for the present.

The CSIS small-scale pandemic exercise (2019)

The Center for Strategic and International Studies (CSIS) is a think tank based in Washington, DC, which originally spun out of Georgetown University in 1962. The CSIS Commission on Strengthening America's Health Security delivered a report on November 18, 2019, arguing it is time to end the "complacency in U.S. Global Health Security" and recommending a new doctrine of "doctrine of continuous prevention, protection, and resilience." Their main point was recommending to "restore health security leadership at the White House National Security Council." Their findings were based on long-standing work in the area as well as a small scenario exercise.

Their exercise was truly small scale: "For our fictional pandemic, we assembled about 20 experts in global health, the biosciences, national security, emergency response and economics at our Washington, D.C., headquarters." How gathering a few people in a room was going to sound any kind of alarm is beyond me. What their scenario did was assume a "research laboratory-created virus first released in Europe," although they did pick a coronavirus with a 3.125% lethality rate, so the conditions were interesting.

In the scenario, three months since its first human-to-human transmission at Tegel Airport, the virus spread rapidly across Europe, North America, Northeast Asia, and the Middle East. Most interestingly, their discussion pointed out that international tensions inhibited information sharing and that the private sector will be vital to managing the outbreak because they hold the keys to unlocking technological innovation. Well, that may or may not be true, given the considerable pockets of the US National Institutes of Health and the National Science Foundation's funding of biological research both in the private sector, and in public and private universities. Finally, CSIS pointed out that health doesn't historically rise to the top of national security agenda (which may now perhaps change, we shall see).

The Kaiser Family Foundation on pandemics (2020)

The Kaiser Family Foundation (kff.org) started writing about the pandemic after it occurred. They have a sanguine analysis of disease models, stating that while models can be "important tools" for understanding the disease and policy responses, their approaches and assumptions "vary widely" and can give widely "divergent results." They have also written a very sanguine analysis of the relationship between the US and the WHO, pointing out that the "scope of responsibility that has grown" over time while its "budget has remained flat or been reduced" and with "greater reliance on voluntary, often earmarked, contributions," a cumbersome, "decentralized, and bureaucratic governance structure" and a "dual mandate" of being both a technical agency with health expertise and a political body where states debate and negotiate on sometimes divisive health issues.

KFF also runs a Health Tracking poll, with some emerging results on how Americans see the impact of coronavirus on their lives. I don't report the findings, because despite being nicely done, these statistics are highly volatile and will change from month to month and week to week, given the evolving situation. KFF also has a "policy watch" (kff.org/Coronavirus-policy-watch/). Finally, they have their "own" coronavirus tracker, lifting data from Johns Hopkins, which presumably means they have an agreement in place.

A Kaiser Family Foundation issue brief assessing global health policy 1 year after President Trump took office finds that half of Americans (54%) say they want the US to play a major or leading role in improving health for people in developing countries, though support for such engagement is strongest among Democrats (73%) and lower among independents (47%) and Republicans (49%). Fifty-three percent say the Trump Administration has made global health a lower priority than previous administrations.

Schools of public health on pandemics

Schools of public health have had some level of pandemic awareness for a while. Most notably, the Johns Hopkins Center for Health Security gathered public health experts many times, in 2001, 2005, 2017, 2018, and 2019 to be exact. I'll look at these three efforts in some detail because they are each quite unique.

Operation Dark Winter (2001)

The 2001 effort was called Operation Dark Winter and was a bioterrorist attack simulation conducted from June 22–23, 2001. The day-and-a-half-long simulation of a smallpox attack on Oklahoma City was created by Johns Hopkins Center for Civilian Biodefense Strategies (now Johns Hopkins Center for Health Security) in collaboration with the Washington-based Center for Strategic and International Studies (CSIS) and Analytic Services, Inc. (ANSER), a not-for-profit corporation with scientific, technical, and analytical expertise on national policy and security issues.

Dark Winter predicted massive misinformation about cures, inability to act by leaders who were shocked and surprised by the event, limited stockpiles of vaccines, a healthcare system with lack of surge capacity, tensions between state and federal authorities, domestic turmoil including assaults on grocery stores that had to be quelled by the National Guard.

In a poignant scene that gave the scenario its name, the CDC is informing the president that there will be a shortage of vaccines, asking him to see the following video clip dialogue. Lead Scientist: "We don't have sufficient stocks to protect the people of Oklahoma, Pennsylvania, and Georgia, much less the entire US population." News Anchor: "What does that mean?" Scientist: "It means this could be a very dark winter in America."

According to Staresinic (2014), Dick Cheney ordered 300

million doses of the smallpox vaccine within a week of watching the scenario.

The Atlantic Storm smallpox pandemic scenario (2005)

In 2005, "Atlantic Storm," a tabletop exercise convened at Andrews Air Force Base, Maryland, US, on January 14, 2005, by the Center for Biosecurity of the University of Pittsburgh Medical Center (UPMC), the Center for Transatlantic Relations of the Johns Hopkins University, and the Transatlantic Biosecurity Network organized by the Center for Biosecurity at the University of Pittsburgh Medical Center, simulated an international outbreak of a smallpox pandemic.

The conclusions from Atlantic Storm (2005) included that diplomatic and political preparation was key, although it "will not matter" if appropriate medicines, vaccines, and medical and public health "capacity" are lacking, that "homeland security must look abroad," pointed out that the WHO has "serious budgetary, political, and organizational limits," worried about losing the public's "acceptance and trust when they need it most," forecasted that "border closures...could be socially, politically, and economically destabilizing and serve to turn a crisis into a catastrophe," and stated that "biosecurity is one of the great global security challenges of the 21st century."

The SPARS Pandemic 2025–2028 (2017)

"The SPARS Pandemic 2025–2028," conducted in 2017 as a self-guided exercise scenario for public health communicators and risk communication researchers (meaning it was a piece of paper not a tabletop seminar), tested medical responses to the outbreak of a novel coronavirus in St. Paul, Minnesota, US. The St. Paul Acute Respiratory Syndrome (SPARS) coronavirus was imagined causing a mild "flu-like" disease in most instances and hospitalization only in a "small minority" of cases. The scenario offers 19 specific storylines, and an associated 23 communication dilemmas for readers to consider. The most interesting aspect of this scenario is the "vaccine injury" issue skewed toward African American children caused by a faulty vaccine and perhaps the observation that "as with many public health interventions, successful efforts to reduce the impact of the pandemic created the illusion that the event was not nearly as serious as experts suggested it would be." Beyond that, SPARS is presented as a scenario for health professionals, and its narrative, supporting materials, and somewhat cumbersome style reflects that goal.

The Clade X simulation (2018)
In 2018, the Clade X simulation was a bioterrorism scenario and it showed how vulnerable the world is to the spread of a pandemic virus. Please note that this description is largely based on the scenario description as well as press clippings such as Loria's (2018) *Business Insider* article about Clade X.

The setup was a day-long series of simulated National Security Council–convened meetings of 10 US government leaders. The scenario was conducted in front of a live audience of government officials, academics, and members of the health security community. The executive committee was supposed to advice the President meets to discuss Clade X, a moderately contagious disease, that, if left unmitigated, would kill 150 million in 20 months, and in the absence of a vaccine, would kill 10% of the world's population or 900 million people.

Outbreaks of disease first appear in Frankfurt, Germany, and Caracas, Venezuela, and are spreading person-to-person. The disease is spread primarily by coughing and causes severe symptoms requiring hospitalization and intensive care in about half of the people infected. Overall, 20% of the severely ill patients die.

During the four meetings that, according to the scenario, would occur over the course of several months, the players are faced with ten difficult policy questions for which they must make recommendations to the president. Information is provided to the players via preproduced news clips, staff briefings, and updates from each player's respective agency.

One month into the disease, as the committee met, they struggled to identify the exact pathogen, a "parainfluenza." There had been more than 400 cases and 50 deaths so far, mostly split between Frankfurt, Germany, and Caracas, Venezuela. There were *only nine players*, but they included former Senate Majority Leader Tom Daschle, Indiana Representative Susan Brooks (R), former CDC Director Julie Gerberding.

In the simulation, the virus was bioengineered and released by a group known as A Brighter Dawn, with the intention of reducing the world's population back to preindustrial levels. The group was largely modeled after the cult Aum Shinrikyo, which released the chemical weapon sarin on the Tokyo subway in 1995.

As a result of the Clade X scenario exercise, Johns Hopkins Center for Health Security recommends the United States commit to six strategic policy goals: (1) Develop capability to produce new vaccines and drugs for novel pathogens within months, not years (*could you imagine if that work had begun in 2018 not in 2020?*); (2) Pioneer a strong and sustainable global health security system (*that's a crucial goal that would take decades even with global commitment*); (3) Build a robust, highly capable national public health system that can manage the challenges of pandemic response (*that would take healthcare reform, among other things*); (4) Develop a national plan to effectively harness all US healthcare assets in a catastrophic pandemic (*this one is being done haphazardly in 2020 because of necessity*); (5) Implement an international strategy for addressing research that increases pandemic risks (*this is a likely but not evident outcome of the current crisis—and could mean many things—which aspects does Johns Hopkins think are most important?*); and (6) Ensure the national security community is well prepared to prevent, detect, and respond to infectious disease emergencies (*it clearly wasn't, as even US aircraft carriers got major outbreaks*). The recommendations reveal what seems to have been an expert-driven, elitist process with little concern for the important social dynamics that would also play out in a massive outbreak.

Interestingly, I'd say the recommendations that stem from Clade X are great, so it's a bit disappointing that few of them were acted upon. Could it be because the exercise, while widely reported in US nation media (PBS, *Washington Post*, NPR, Fox News), niche business publications (*Business Insider*), online magazines (Vox), specialty media and blogs (MIT Tech Review, Global Health Now), it didn't reach an international audience (apart from the *Toronto Sun* and a few UK and Australian papers) or indeed widespread awareness in the US population?

By the way, the 362-word Fox News article borrowed *heavily* from the *Business Insider* article (in fact the article mainly consisted of reprinting three quotes from the original story), so they evidently didn't have a reporter in the room.

Event 201 (2019)

On October 19, 2019, Johns Hopkins hosted a 1-day pandemic tabletop exercise called "Event 201" with partners, the World Economic Forum and the Bill & Melinda Gates Foundation. The scenario format was a fictional Global News Network (GNN) anchor setting the scene, followed by a panel, followed by a 3-hour discussion.

The Event 201 model simulates an outbreak of a "moderately transmissible pathogen" (modeled on SARS but more transmissible), a novel zoonotic coronavirus transmitted from bats to pigs to people, which "in a fully susceptible population" and "in the absence of adequate control measures," leads to "a severe pandemic." The scenario then charts global spread following "an initial spillover event in a large city in South America (and specifically "densely packed neighborhoods of some of the megacities in South America"), exported by air travel to Portugal, the United States, and China and then to many other countries.

Furthermore, the scenario stochastically seeds 300 cities around the world (and 300 cities in the US) with contagion "spread through international travel" with the number of imported cases "ranging from 1 to 4." The scenario ends at the 18-month point, with 65 million deaths, but points out that the likely outcome would be that the "pandemic will continue at some rate until there is an effective vaccine or until 80–90% of the global population has been exposed" and would likely end as an endemic childhood disease.

What's immediately shocking to me is the relative lack of contextual detail in the Event 201 scenario. It was as if the scientifically "constant" rate of spread is the only thing that matters (and the 1–4 they operated with is an incredibly low spread more matching the Ebola situation). In contrast, with the COVID-19 pandemic, we have seen how much local political and cultural factors such as the relative readiness of a city population to self-quarantine, for instance, impact the model, or local transmission factors that create superspreader events. The model was clearly built with a technocratic mindset, not taking in the full complexity of political economy or social dynamics realities.

Worry number two with the approach is that the players were a mere 15 individuals from "global business, government, and public health." The problem with that is that, as we have seen, the impacts can be felt (and influenced) among a myriad of much more specific personas, including mayors, superintendents of schools, grocery chain owners, mass event organizers, logistics company CEOs and airline CEOs, to mention a few.

According to *The Telegraph* (2019), Avril Haines, the

former CIA deputy director said something important during the event: "Having a trusted source, and really guiding everyone to that for information, is incredibly important." She added that survivors of the virus, faith leaders, and multinational agencies all had a role to play. This time around, take deep note of the fact that US mainstream national media did not cover the event at all!

Other media that covered the event included business media (*Bloomberg*, *Forbes*), online magazines (Gizmodo), and very few international media organizations (BBC Radio).

In fact, the coverage of Event 201 seems to have fallen *far short* of even the coverage of Clade X the year before, as if the "saturation" for such stories had been met in journalists' minds.

However, the recommendations that came out of the event were more bland and included the following: "plan to utilize corporate capabilities" (e.g., logistics, social media, distribution systems), "enhance stockpiles" (i.e., vaccines and therapeutics), "maintain international trade," "support surge manufacturing" (again, vaccines), "global business should engage," "reduce economic impact" (through international organizations), and "combat disinformation."

It is interesting that given the strong focus on vaccines, nothing in this exercise led them to believe there would be a shortage of ventilators or PPE. Also, given the way some have characterized that exercise, they have now come out with this statement: "Although our tabletop exercise included a mock novel coronavirus, the inputs we used for modeling the potential impact of that fictional virus are not similar to nCoV-2019."

All in all, I'd say the most important outcome of Event 201 was the calculation made in the brief one-pager on economic bailouts, where they pointed out that a pandemic might lead to national health system budget collapse and subsequent need for bailouts. However, that was a paper calculation that didn't require the exercise itself. Their $14 trillion amount represents the GDP of all low- and middle-income countries (excluding China, India, and Russia), but they only foresee a bailout for half of annual healthcare spending, which would be $400 billion. These numbers, which will be far superseded by the COVID-19 crisis, at least put a figure on the table, which is always instructive to guiding policy response.

The "medical countermeasures" one-pager is also instructive in that it admits that vaccine development typically takes a decade and openly admits the business-model challenges in vaccine development, for example, "competing interests, the cost of establishing or repurposing manufacturing facilities, regulatory barriers, and the lack of a consistent market."

However, Event 201 did not "warn" the world in any meaningful, effective way, given its small size, the relatively short time allotted (4+hours), insignificant political participation, and finally its lack of cultural awareness.

I'd hope that future scenario exercises involve deeply researched scenarios (not just one—since the world does not proceed in linear ways), a longer time frame for the scenario duration (allowing the debate to play out over several phases, not just several "topics"), wider participation (mayors, patients, startups, etc.) and top-level political participation.

Fictional accounts of plagues and pandemics (1722–2019)

Fiction can help us run through the myriad of emotions that pandemics evoke and perhaps also clarify what the human choices are during a pandemic.

A plethora of fictional books on plagues are in print, according to Carrol (2020), including *A Journal of the Plague Year* by Daniel Defoe (1722), *Pale Horse, Pale Rider* by Katherine Anne Porter (1939), *The Plague* by Albert Camus (1947), *The Andromeda Strain* by Michael Crichton (1969), *The Stand* by Stephen King (1978), *Love in the Time of Cholera* by Gabriel García Márquez (1985), *Journals of the Plague Years* by Norman Spinrad (1988), *The Child Garden* by Geoff Ryman (1989), *Ammonite* by Nicola Griffith (1992), *Beauty Salon* by Mario Bellatín (1994), *Blindness* by José Saramago (1995), *The Years of Rice and Salt* by Kim Stanley Robinson (2002), *Oryx and Crake* by Margaret Atwood (2003), *The Children's Hospital* by Chris Adrian (2006), *The Transmigration of Bodies* by Yuri Herrera (2013), *Station Eleven* by Emily St. John Mandel (2014), *Find Me* by Laura van den Berg (2015), *Severance* by Ling Ma (2018), *The Book of M* by Peng Shepherd (2018), and *The Old Drift* by Namwali Serpell (2019).

Given that pandemics is a more recent obsession of mine, I've only read a few of those books, but the ones I've read are definitely captivating and show the intense pain and suffering involved but also demonstrate that life itself, luckily, sneaks back in and people can still love, work, and even enjoy life.

Nonfiction accounts of pandemics

As for nonfiction, there have been a dozen or so notable books on pandemics published over the last 20 years (see Appendix). *The Coming Plague*, a New York Times bestseller in 1994-5, by science journalist Laurie Garrett is perhaps closest to having entered the public consciousness. She was awarded the Pulitzer Prize for Explanatory Journalism in 1996 chronicling the Ebola virus outbreak in Zaire. Since 2004, she has been on the think tank staff of the Council on Foreign Relations in New York. Another notable book was *The Hot Zone: The Terrifying True Story of the Origins of the Ebola Virus*, a best-selling 1994 nonfiction thriller by Richard Preston, also about Ebola. Lastly, John M. Barry's 2004 book *The Great Influenza* about the 1918 disease, was also a New York Times Best Seller, and won the 2005 Keck Communication Award from the United States National Academies of Science for the year's outstanding book on science or medicine. Arguably the definitive account of the 1918 Flu Epidemic, it is now being read across the world in light of the coronavirus pandemic.

Finally, *The End of Epidemics* (2018) by Dr. Jonathan D. Quick & Bronwyn Fryer attempts to both provide a deep historical perspective by analyzing ancient text for clues on the geopolitical, economic, social, and psychological effects of a pandemic and relate it to contemporary geopolitical configurations and technology. Quick and Fryer offer advice on pandemic prevention action including “spend prudently to prevent disease before an epidemic strikes” and “Ensure prompt, open, and accurate communication between nations and aid agencies, instead of secrecy and territorial disputes” and “fight disease and prevent panic with innovation and good science,” all of which are true but completely insufficient to prepare for or handle a huge pandemic like the one we are faced with in 2020.

Several sources report that pandemic books are selling well during the COVID-19 pandemic, which is a curious fact. We seem obsessed with our own fate, even as one might have thought that fiction would be a source of refuge where we sought to escape rather than dwell in our sorrows. What does that mean? For me, it’s not so strange. When something encompasses your reality, you start seeing it and looking for it everywhere. In the spring of 2020, that phenomenon happens to be a pandemic. Let’s hope reading these books make us just a little bit more compassionate, wise, and knowledgeable about what’s happening now and what is to come, which is the focus on the book you have in your hand.

The ‘Silent Spring’ criteria for a book to be a warning

As for “warning,” I’d say that books on pandemics, whether fiction or nonfiction, generally can create general awareness but that they rarely constitute a cross-societal warning. Notable exceptions to this rule would be *Silent Spring* (1962), the environmental science book by Rachel Carson. Documenting the adverse environmental effects caused by the indiscriminate use of pesticides, it changed many people's ideas about the environment and spurred President Kennedy into action. The year after, in 1963, the US Science Advisory Committee, released a report called "The Uses of Pesticides," and by 1964 vendors had to prove that their product "does no harm" and by 1972 activists managed to ban DDT, the pesticide Carson warned about.

The conclusion from this literature review is that none of these books have risen to the status of a Silent Spring or constitute any kind of uniform "warning" that could have spun up major international pandemic preparedness to the tune of billions of dollars.

The strength of the human imagination combined with the realism of projecting trends that we already can see around us is what I've chosen to do in crafting scenarios. They won't be as elaborate as the plotlines in these books, but they will approximate the fictional reality through small vignettes with personalities that could have lived, could have felt and could have done what they did.

We will see, but to my mind, bringing in a keen sense of humanity as well as a complex set of forces of disruption is the minimum the world needs in order to start imagining the kind of future we might want to see a decade from now.

Scattered futurists (2020-)

Whilst there weren't that many futurists that wrote on pandemics before COVID-19 (we did find some), plenty have voiced something now.

DW (2020) interviewed several futurists, let's look at a few. British astronomer and futurist, Sir Martin Rees prophesizes that 'bad actors' will engineer and release more virulent and transmissible variants.

Susan Schneider, director of the AI, Mind and Society Group at The University of Connecticut, predicts more automation as well as technologies to support remote work, but is afraid of the consequences of losing a human touch.

David Chaum, a pioneering cryptographer, says we now, more than ever need protection of our meta data, the social graph of who talks to whom and when.

Tobias Gantner, CEO at HealthCare Futurists, feels we need to say goodbye to our concepts of data security, since that was only a concern for "healthy people," but the unexpected benefit, he says, might be that our technologies evolve to encompass more of the inherent complexities and realities of living lives as relational, human beings.

University of British Columbia urban design professor Patrick Condon predicts that, as a result of the pandemic, the wealthy will retreat into their private homes, behind doormen and gated communities, fearful of public contact and with sanitized cars and drivers on call, abandoning public transit, interfering with the smooth functioning of a city, according to a university press release.

Futurist Amy Zalman (2020) muses that given that "the unimaginable is everywhere," we have to counter that with imagination, too. She imagines these potential outcomes: "Families and communities are creating joyful new rituals that will keep them connected long after this moment has passed, Business leaders are seizing this mother-of-all-disruptions to learn agility, reinvent, and transform their organizations to meet the future. Politicians look forward to presiding over a country so healthy so resilient, so productive that we all stand fearless and united, whatever lies ahead."

Digital health futurist Maneesh Juneja said something interesting in a recent interview in Sifted (2020): "When it comes to decision making and sharing of data, if suddenly the National Health Service can behave like a startup, in terms of the speed of decision making, such as building a new COVID-19 app or converting a conference centre in London to a 4,000-bed hospital, why can't it behave like that after the pandemic is over?"

National disease control, pandemic plans and studies

Most, if not all, nation-states have some type of "center for disease control." A few of them stand out because of their historical excellence in the domain or because of their handling of the current coronavirus crisis. Many times, these centers were either established or re-shaped by a an epidemic or pandemic, whether it be a national or a global outbreak.

The Robert Koch Institute—the German 'ordnung muss zein'

The Robert Koch Institute (RKI), the German federal government agency and research institute responsible for disease control and prevention was founded as early as 1891 and currently has a staff of around 1,080 including approximately 450 scientists.

Modi-SARS (2012)

In 2012, RKI published a risk analysis painting the scenario of a worldwide spread of a new pathogen originating from Asia, a hypothetical virus with 10 percent mortality rate called Modi-SARS. In the simulation, the virus spreads in Germany over a period of three years (until RKI assumes a vaccine should be available). After the first wave of illness with 29 million infected subsides, two more weak waves with 23 and 26 million sufferers follow, and 7.5 million deaths, although those already affected develop temporary immunity. Crucially, the scenario forecasts bottlenecks arise for pharmaceuticals, medical devices, protective equipment and disinfectants, as well as temporary food shortages. This is the first time I have encountered a scenario that includes the pain points currently experienced with COVID-19 and might explain the extraordinary difference in outcomes between Germany and other countries in Europe.

NIPH in Norway (1929) and PHAS (2014) in Sweden–the nimble North

The Norwegian Institute of Public Health (NIPH) was founded in 1929 and currently has 1400 employees, which is interesting in contrast with the Public Health Agency of Sweden which was founded as recently as in 2014 by a merger of the Swedish National Institute of Public Health (Folkhälsoinstitutet) and the Swedish Institute for Communicable Disease Control (Smittskyddsinstitutet), and only has 450 employees. However, it runs the only biosafety level 4 laboratory in the Nordic region – one of only six in Europe. Note that Sweden, with 10.23 million inhabitants, near double Norway's 5.37 million, is the country that continues the highly risky, yet modern and certainly less invasive on the economy in the short term, "herd immunity" strategy.

CDC in the US (1946)–the national giant makes a misstep

The CDC in the US was founded in 1946 and currently has a total of 10,639 on staff, which makes them the biggest such institution in the world, by a factor of five. Historically, countries around the world has looked to the CDC for guidance and their website is often referred to in the media. However, despite this size advantage, impact and media savvy legacy, the CDC committed a tragic error in the production of coronavirus test kits, which have made situational awareness impossible for US federal and state decision makers, and have been, largely, silenced by the US executive branch.

World Health Organization (1948)–the global dinosaur shows its age

Soon thereafter, the WHO was founded in 1948. The WHO has a staff of 7000 spread on 150 offices. US provided 15% of its 2018-19 budget - with more than $400m. The Bill and Melinda

Gates Foundation is the second-largest funder of the WHO. The UK gives most of any country apart from the US. China gave about $86m in 2018-19.

The WHO shares the bureaucratic weaknesses of any intergovernmental organization and has undergone many changes throughout the years. Its major strength was shown during the years Ms. Gro Harlem Brundtland led the charge (1998-2003), but she took liberties far beyond the organization's mandate, already in her acceptance speech she saw the organization as "the moral voice and the technical leader in improving health of the people of the world," notably challenging China on its handling of SARS. The current leadership has a much more diplomatic approach which may have backfired. Interestingly, there seems to be only two paths for the WHO in the next decade—upping their game or getting out of it.

NCDC (1963)—India's response to Malaria and plague

The National Centre for Disease Control in India was established in 1963, initially from the departure point of countering Malaria, but India radically revamped its efforts as recently as in 2009 with a US$110 million upgrade over three years, citing its 1994 domestic pneumonic plague outbreak as the main reason.

CCDC—the Chinese unorthodoxy

The Chinese Center for Disease Control and Prevention (CCDC) was established in 1983 and currently has a staff of 2120. Their methods are somewhat unorthodox. On 20 April, Gao Fu, Director of CCDC said that if the epidemic worsens, Chinese medics would be injected with coronavirus vaccines by end of the year, before these vaccines are fully tested, according to Global Times (2020). Head of CCDC, George Gao said something else interesting in an interview with Science (2020): "no one in any country could have predicted that the virus would cause a pandemic. This is the first noninfluenza pandemic ever."

KCDCP (2003)–fixing Korea's shame over MERS

Korea Centers for Disease Control and Prevention was founded in 2003, but it was its poor performance around MERS that spurred it into action. Determined not to repeat their mistakes, they acted swiftly on COVID-19 testing, with military precision and the speed of a highly efficient business unit.

CHP (2004)-Hong Kong's revenge on SARS

The Centre for Health Protection (CHP) of Hong Kong was created in 2004 based on assessing its weak response to SARS. Hong Kong was relatively successful in mitigating transmission early in the outbreak of coronavirus disease (COVID-19). A study by Kwok et al (2020) indicates that early action combined with high level of civil engagement toward disease control enables most business to continue as usual, which reduces the economic toll from strict quarantine measures.

ECPC (2004)–EU's tiny, late bloom

The fact that the European Centre for Disease Prevention and Control was only created in 2004 is shocking. It's also only charged with surveillance, not with coordination, unlike a traditional CDC effort. Despite this, already by 2016, Europe was actively assessing neighboring institutions (enlargement candidate countries like Albania, the former Yugoslav Republic of Macedonia, Montenegro, Serbia, and Turkey) and recommending improvements. Laudable work, but perhaps the EU should get their own disease control efforts in check first?

NCID (2019)–Singapore's response to SARS

Singapore opened its National Centre for Infectious Diseases (www.ncid.sg) in 2019, in a building that also houses Singapore's first high-level isolation unit, s 330-bed purpose-built facility designed to strengthen Singapore's capabilities in infectious disease management and prevention, building on the experience from the SARS epidemic.

TCDC (1999) and its ad-hoc command center–Taiwan's secret weapon

Taiwan Centers for Disease Control was established in 1999. Taiwan, with a 23 million population, is an exception in many respects. For one, it is excluded from the World Health Organization and its information channels due to political objections from China. After the SARS epidemic which killed 181 on the island, Taiwan implemented a whole-of-society approach (Schwartz & Yen, 2017), enshrined in regulation by the 2009 Communicable Disease Control Act.

Should an outbreak occur, a Central Epidemic Command Center (CECC) may be mobilized to execute actions without bureaucratic delay. The CECC was activated on 20 January 2020 based on the COVID-19 news from China.

Importantly, local governance structures *also* have the right to enact their own versions of a CECC. There's even a "neighborhood warden," an unpaid resource that only receives a monthly 'subsidy', a community resident elected by the community itself. The warden, typically monitoring 5800 people then selects 10-20 "block leaders," who is responsible for 100 to 300 people. Wardens keep track of who might be contagious, coordinate community recreational activities, and gather residents for vaccinations, assist residents in applying for government services and legal claims, even organize elections. The warden system provides a key link between the state and local levels. Equivalents to the neighborhood warden system exist in many other parts of East and Southeast Asia.

There are also six regional CDC centers on the island. Despite that, mistrust in government significantly curtailed their H1N1 influenza pandemic response over the past few years, which shows that this kind of work never is completed and that one cannot become complacent.

Enhanced cooperation between state, local government and non-state institutions, particularly neighborhood committees, has resulted in a strengthened, holistic epidemic preparedness and response infrastructure.

National security officials have also been concerned about pandemics. Lisa Monaco (2020), Barack Obama's outgoing homeland-security adviser, gathered with Trump's incoming national-security officials on January 13, 2017, and conducted an exercise modeled on the administration's experiences with outbreaks of Swine flu, Ebola, and Zika. She now claims "The government's halting response to COVID-19 is the foreseeable result of neglect," despite the fact that the admits to CBS News Michael Morell in Intelligence Matters (2020) that the "nightmare scenario" presented to the Trump Administration was based on "the new strain of flu," and not on coronavirus.

A few magazine articles, e.g. Scientific American (2005) discussed the pandemic threat, too, but were, again focused on "a lethal strain of influenza" and completely missing the point by conflating incubation period with how much time public health workers had to respond: "people infected by the SARS coronavirus that emerged from China in 2003 took as long as 10 days to become infectious, giving health workers ample time to trace and isolate their contacts before they, too, could spread the disease."

Leaving aside SARS, we now know the exact opposite to be the case with COVID-19: precisely because of asymptomatic transmission, it is near impossible to start contact tracing (once the disease is in community spread).

There was also some pandemic work related to the WHO's Pandemic Influenza Preparedness (PIP) Framework (https://www.who.int/influenza/pip/en/).

In a March 2020 piece, Uri Friedmann of The Atlantic boastfully writes "we were warned." But were we? None of the above produces the kind of *massively compelling, scary, or quantitative evidence, ideally with macroeconomic arguments proving significant amounts of lives and top echelon public leadership careers could be on the line,* in near future, all of which would have been required to mount any kind of credible global defense against what we witnessed in 2020.

To take another impending catastrophe to compare this with, consider for a moment the environment. Those who have expressed serious concern (and have been able to influence some readiness actions on global level as a result) include: Former US Vice President Al Gore, The United Nations Climate Panel, most science academies around the world, and the EU, just to name some credible institutions and people.

That list is significantly more impressive, the concern is expressed at very high levels of government and in the private sector. Yet, arguably the actions don't amount to very much. And, this is not even an exhaustive list, given that the topic of this book needs to stay on Pandemic Aftermath. Having said that, there are many who argue that a pandemic and the environment are related in many ways. This may be the case. However, investigating this point in detail would take up another book altogether.

The verdict on government foresight and science

As we have seen, the pandemic awareness in media, among experts, scientists and specialist agencies is mixed. What about true government initiatives to understand pandemics through reports or scenario exercises?

Institute of Medicine (1992)—an early agenda setting report
The year is 1992, Bill Clinton was elected to the White House and the Hollywood movies The Bodyguard and Basic Instinct are released. Also, unbeknownst to some of us, a landmark public health report was published. It was called *Emerging Infections: Microbial Threats to Health in the United States* (1992) and was issued by the Institute of Medicine (US) Committee on Emerging Microbial Threats to Health and published by the National Academies Press. The report singlehandedly created *expert awareness* around Emerging Infectious Diseases (and the acronym EID), spurred the creation of academic journals, and led to policy decisions informing how to deal with a set of newly emerged infectious diseases such as HIV/AIDS. The summary states: "The emergence of HIV disease and AIDS, the reemergence of tuberculosis, and the increased opportunity for disease spread through international travel demonstrate the critical importance of global vigilance for infectious diseases."

Bush Administration (2001-2009)—
HIV/AIDS, PEPFAR and Pandemic Readiness
George W. Bush took a lot of heat during his Presidency but, for all his shortcomings in waging unjust wars, was an excellent actor in global health policy. In 2003, facing the continuing HIV/AIDS pandemic, President George W. Bush established the President's Emergency Plan for AIDS Relief (PEPFAR) as of today having provided $80 billion in cumulative funding for HIV/AIDS treatment, prevention, and research since its inception, making it the largest global health program focused on a single disease in history. The Bush administration also developed the Pandemic Influenza Preparedness plan that is still in use today. "One day many lives could be needlessly lost because we failed to act today," President Bush said in a 2005 speech as he launched a pandemic readiness effort. The 233-page National Strategy for

Pandemic Influenza Implementation plan (2006) is substantial. As part of the plan, the United States would stockpile vaccines and antiviral drugs such as Tamiflu (oseltamivir) and Relenza (zanamivir) and accelerate the development of new vaccine technologies.

National Institutes of Health (2012)—scientific over-optimism
Ten years after Institute of Medicine's (1992) agenda setting report, in 2012, the year the Mayan civilization's calendar supposedly ends according to folklore, scientists David M. Morens and Anthony S. Fauci from the National Institute of Allergy and Infectious Diseases, National Institutes of Health, Bethesda, Maryland, USA write that: "We have made far-reaching advances in the past 20 years since the original IOM report, and scientists are guardedly optimistic that further breakthroughs lie ahead." Paraphrasing Ronald Reagan's old saying about government slightly, it's a bit like saying: "We're from the scientific establishment. We're here to help."

Simultaneously, Whitney Houston sets a then-record with "I Will Always Love You" staying at no 1 on the Billboard Hot 100 for 14 weeks, which is all I remember from the fall of 1992, as I was an exchange student in Liege, staying at Home Ruhl (now called Avroy Student house) at 67 Boulevard d'Avroy, a treelined street and park which hosted a month-long traveling street fair and Tivoli that played Whitney Houston's song on constant repeat until midnight every night right outside my bedroom window. I don't think I was the only average person who missed this debate.

As we have seen, only Germany had created a significant pandemic scenario relevant to the current crisis. The Event 201 pandemic scenario effort in the US was run by Johns Hopkins, a private institution, in collaboration with the Gates Foundation, a private foundation. International organizations' scenario exercises or studies were mostly run over a decade ago and were not comprehensive efforts. As a result, stockpiling (beyond efforts limited to pandemic influenza preparedness) went out of fashion or was certainly insufficient.

A Wired article called "An Oral History of the Pandemic Warnings Trump Ignored" by Graff (2020) tries to make the case that the constant droplet of various articles and speeches on the threat of pandemics constituted "clear and present danger," but is unconvincing because you could have picked any global issue (global warming, poverty, cybersecurity) and you would have found a similar litany of concerns, equally warranted.

Policy action starts with getting on the agenda, then becoming a priority, and then surviving a set of bureaucratic tests, debates, votes, and decision steps. In order to be seen as a priority an issue must have a compelling avalanche of information, stakeholders, as well as a policy window, in order to emerge. Leaving aside the issue of whether this would have been justified, based on my analysis, that threat level simply wasn't established regarding the issue of a generic, severe pandemic threat in the decades leading up to 2020.

Exercise Cygnus (2014-2016)—
the UK government's swan song

In mid-October 2016, the UK held a 3-day national multiagency pandemic influenza exercise called Exercise Cygnus. *Cygnus* is the Latin word for swan. The exercise was set 7 weeks into a severe pandemic outbreak of the fictional "swan flu" ("H2N2 influenza virus") which is relatively unique among such pandemic exercises, which typically start much earlier in an outbreak. The epidemic modeling was done by the same Imperial College team that is currently tracking the COVID-19 outbreak.

Very little is known about this exercise. The only public source at the time, Dame Sally Davies, England's then chief medical officer, in December 2016 said this to *Express*: "The

NHS would be unable to cope if Britain suffered a major flu pandemic," the economic impact of such a pandemic was "very worrying" and hospitals were "not ready to deal with any severe outbreak." She warned of "overcrowding in emergency rooms," pointed out that family and friends would "not be allowed in," specifically mentioned "not enough ventilation," and finally, she said it was clear the UK "could not cope" with the extra bodies.

The report from Exercise Cygnus was never made public. The conservative UK daily, the *Telegraph* (2020) has reported that Cygnus's findings were deemed "too terrifying" to be made public, quoting a senior former Government source with direct involvement in the exercise. The *Telegraph* also implies that government austerity measures at the time, which entailed cutting NHS beds, was why the revealed significant caps in the NHS's surge capacity including a shortage of ICU beds and personal protective equipment (PPE), were never acted upon.

The *Observer* (2020), the social liberal paper, revealed that minutes of the government's 14-member-strong New and Emerging Respiratory Virus Threats Advisory Group (NERVTAG) suggested the report had included four key recommendations, including one that the department of health strengthen the surge capability, and capacity of hospitals to cope with a pandemic. Interestingly, however, NERVTAG's Annual Report for 2016, in my reading, makes *no mention* of Cygnus. In the same document, NERVTAG's mandate is cited as to "provide independent scientific risk assessments and advice to the Department of Health (DH) over a wide range of subjects relevant to the threats posed by new and emerging respiratory viruses" and with this interesting caveat: "Pandemic influenza is of course the predominant threat."

According to the UK tabloid newspaper *The Sun* (2020), a 57-page classified report revealed 22 key lessons to be learned, suggesting it challenged the NHS "to review its response to an overwhelmed service with reduced staff availability" and concluded UK pandemic capacity should be "critically reviewed."

The exercise was led by The Department of Health and Social Care under the Conservative government of Prime Minister Theresa May and with Jeremy Hunt, Secretary of State for Health, later Secretary of State for Health and Social Care, as well as Sir Christopher Wormald KCB, Permanent Secretary, at the helm. There was also strong engagement from Public Health England, the executive agency, The National Health Service, the publicly funded healthcare system of the United Kingdom and other stakeholders. Local authorities across Britain as well as the devolved administrations of Scotland, Wales, and Northern Ireland tested their component parts alongside the core exercise. Phase one took place in May 2014, phase two took place in October 2016.

The UK government is currently subject to a lawsuit from Dr. Moosa Qureshi, an NHS doctor, who is demanding the government publish its report into Exercise Cygnus. The government refused to release the report after a Freedom of Information request. Update: The original Exercise Cygnus document was leaked to *The Guardian* on 7 May and reveals that social care was a deep worry and warned of a social care crisis in case of a pandemic.

Crimson Contagion (2019)—the US code red that was ignored

In 2019, a pandemic-simulation drill scenario game called "Crimson Contagion" was acted out by CDC with participation from senior officials of the US central administration, according to the *New York Times*. Note that the scenario was based on a *flu*, a hypothetical H7N9 strain.

According to NBC Chicago (2020), the drill involved 19 federal agencies, 12 states, 74 local health departments, and

87 hospitals responding to a scenario in which a pandemic flu that began in China was spread by international tourists. The states taking part included Idaho, Arizona, New Mexico, Colorado, Nebraska, Illinois, Pennsylvania, South Carolina, New York, Connecticut, Massachusetts, and New Hampshire.

In the drill's scenario, the flu became called a pandemic 47 days after the first outbreak, but by then, 110 million Americans were expected to become ill, 7.7 million would be hospitalized, and 586,000 would have died in the US alone. The experience revealed significant shortcomings in the governmental response, including confusion between HHS, FEMA, and the Department of Homeland Security on which federal agency would take the lead in the crisis, as well as confusion on how to apply the Defense Production Act. The HHS draft report concluded:

> *The U.S. also lacks domestic manufacturing capacity for the production of sufficient quantities of personal protective equipment, needles, and syringes. Domestic supplies of on-hand stock of antiviral medications, needles, syringes, N95 respirators, ventilators, and other ancillary medical supplies are limited and difficult to restock, because they are often manufactured overseas.* (Crimson Contagion Report, 2019, p.39)

Although a few local administrations put in place some changes, at least in Chicago, where the drill was held, few if any federal actions were taken as a result. The draft Crimson Contagion report (2019), marked "not to be disclosed," was recently put online by the *New York Times*. To add to the confusion about this drill, the Times says the drill consisted of a "series of exercises that ran from last January to August," while Wikipedia says it lasted for 4 months and NBC Chicago says it lasted for 4 days (from August 13). I'm not sure which is correct, although the draft report says it lasted for 4 days, but the duration matters little for this analysis (although the confusion gives food for thought). Interestingly, that report points out that the exercise also revealed "several strengths" related to collaboration with private partners as well as the ability to "conduct a crisis action planning session" and was a "valuable opportunity to learn."

Foresight in Fact and Fiction

Pandemic scenarios already exist in widely available science fiction books, and a bunch of fictional accounts (as we saw earlier in this chapter), although few would call science fiction a credible "warning."

If we go into the features of the scenarios used by think tanks and governments, what characterizes most of them is that they either are more severe (operating with 20-40% mortality) or regional, not global and simultaneous. Few scenarios truly embrace the possibility that the whole world becomes affected by this without ability to help each other.

Which foresight studies mention pandemics? Beyond the studies already mentioned I'm aware of the CSIS scenario exercise although I feel that running a pandemic foresight exercise is not the same as having foreseen the current pandemic.

The post-COVID-19 society—emerging foresight

As I have pointed out, before the pandemic, no matter what critics might say, there was a *dearth* of true foresight on pandemic impact. However, foreseeably, as the pandemic started to appear, armchair epidemiologists, futurists, and economists dusted off their skills and studies started to emerge, attempting to document the impending impact in real time. The success is mixed because it tends to be too bombastic or too focused on single aspects of the crisis, be it the impact on public health, economics, the environment, the poor, or otherwise.

European Parliament study on pandemics (2020)

The Economic Impact of Epidemics and Pandemics (2020), commissioned by the European Parliament, and issued on February 27, quantifies the impact on the health, transportation, agricultural, and tourism sectors, pointing out that "rapid urbanisation, increasing international travel and climate change all render epidemic outbreaks a global and not simply a local phenomenon." We learn from this report that the European Centre for Disease Prevention and Control was only established as recently as in 2004. This early report is shockingly modest in its assessment of the economic scope that already in mid-spring 2020 cannot be described as anything but a global calamity of unprecedented proportion in recent times.

Brookings' 7 socioeconomic scenarios

The world's top think tank has been relatively silent on COVID-19 but did produce a paper on March 2 on the The Global Macroeconomic Impacts of COVID-19: Seven Scenarios (McKibbin & Fernando, 2020). Reading them now, only two months after they are written, the amounts in Billions will become Trillions, and the entire set of assumptions need to be reworked. However, at some point, they point out that a "more serious outbreak" similar to the Spanish flu "reduces global GDP by over $US 9 trillion in 2020". In fact, most scenarios that came out in March operated with a global economic effect in the low trillions. That is no longer the case even just looking at the US Fed which is to provide $2.3 trillion just in loans. By March 25, CNN reported the global bailout had reached $7 trillion, although a pair of University of Chicago researchers found that social distancing creates $8 trillion in economic benefits (Morris, 2020).

The approach is sound, trying to convert epidemiological features into economic effects. Their assumptions are, at times, antiquated, such as "70 percent of the female workers would be care givers to family members" (p.11) in the event of school closures.

Lowy Institute (2020)—an Australian view

On April 9, 2020, the influential Australian think tank, the Lowy Institute, provided their analysis on a broad range of topics, covering the United States; China, US-China competition; the international economy; globalization; multilateralism and the nation-state; Southeast Asia; the Pacific; developing nations; misinformation, truth, and trust; extremism; and diplomacy.
(https://interactives.lowyinstitute.org/features/covid19/)

Lowy was founded in 2003 to change the impression that Australia was just surfers, Kangaroos, and convicts and to grow the continent's impact in the world through independent ideas and a strong infrastructure.

I'll go through their main findings (opinions) because they are quite interesting both in substance (wide ranging) and tone (displaying a near total confidence about broad, sweeping generalizations about massive changes to the global political economy). These views, while somewhat bombastic, are refreshing given the tentative approach that most other think tanks have taken to the significant issues at play. I find it personally quite intriguing how the view from "down under" completely discounts that the world might either go on relatively unscathed or might change in much more dramatic ways than they envision, even strengthen global collaboration. Instead, they bank on the "relatively" extreme contraction and US isolationism scenario that may be washed away by an election or two.

In Lowy Institute's view, COVID-19 will lead to further self-isolation of the US, an opportunity for China, with zero-sum competition from the two continuing to batter each other. The virus will inflict a permanent shock on the world economy, hyperglobalization (casual overseas holidays for Australians and overreliance on instantly sourced foreign supplies) might end, and globalization will take a temporary hit as travel, tourism, international trade, and foreign students have all imploded or retreated.

They foresee a reformatting of international agencies, largely without the US playing a key role. China will still, in their view, take a huge part of exports and foreign capital will still flow although debt will soar, and income inequality will worsen. Southeast Asia will see increased authoritarianism, and Pacific rim countries will fare worse.

Developing countries will be the virus' real target as a combined health and economic cataclysm combined with slower global economic growth in general will ensure lower foreign aid and meaning fewer can be brought out of poverty. Truth and public trust will also be victims to the pandemic, say Lowry experts, as they feel misinformation will reach new levels as they also point to the accelerating rise of right-wing extremism and growing impact of conspiracy theorists. Finally, they say, as citizens will demand national bailouts wherever they are (COVID-19 repatriations are already unprecedented), there will for that reason be a resurgence of diplomacy and it will be "refinanced."

Richard Haas: accelerate rather than reshape

Other observers are more measured. Former advisor to Secretary of State Colin Powell and now President of the Council of Foreign Relations, Richard Haas (2020), argues in a Foreign Policy article entitled "The Pandemic Will Accelerate History Rather Than Reshape It" that "waning American leadership, faltering global cooperation, great-power discord: all of these characterized the international environment before the appearance of COVID-19." However, these words are written from the perspective of a person who already has suggested that "the world is in disarray," so he had already incorporated change in his worldview.

CSIS (2020)—geopolitical scenarios for the Post-COVID-19 future

In a brief piece on Geopolitical Scenarios for Asia after COVID-19, Michael J. Green of CSIS (2020) outlines three scenarios for the coming 5 years, presented in rank order of likelihood: (1) intensified Sino-US strategic competition but no major reorientation of major powers, (2) resurgent American leadership and multilateral institution building, (3) pax sinica, where regional powers consolidate their positions at the expense of the center: China in Asia, Russia in Central and Eastern Europe, and Iran in the Gulf. The last scenario borrows from Tom Wright's book, *All Measures Short of War* (2017). Green claims "the course of international relations is determined by multiple variables that remain unchanged," such as domestic economic and military assets. He also writes the US more successfully recovers from "recessions." Let's see about that.

CSIS's Morrison and Carrol (2020) also offer another set of scenarios specifically based on health policy. *Scenario 1: Best Case—Rapid Recovery* (US deaths do not exceed 240,000, safe and efficient vaccine by 2021, and things are back to normal in 2022); *Scenario 2: Mixed Case—Roller Coaster* (US deaths range between 500,000 and 1 million, multiple urban outbreaks [e.g., Detroit, New Orleans, Chicago, Miami, Boston, Washington DC, Dallas, and Atlanta], flattening the curve achieved by spring 2021, crisis over by 2023); *Scenario 3: Worst Case—Decline and Catastrophe* (US deaths range between 1.5 and 2.2 million by the end of 2021, national testing fails, contact tracing fails, sectors of the economy are nationalized, US borders are shut, vaccine takes 5–10 years, immunity is short lasting). They do not offer probabilities or likelihood, but their headline says, "Which scenario will we choose?" which implies this is largely a policy choice. Perhaps, but I find that unconvincing on many levels.

The CIDRAP report

In an April 30, 2020 report, the Center for Infectious Disease Research and Policy (CIDRAP), part of the University of Minnesota, predict two more years of pandemic misery since COVID-19 "likely won't be halted until 60% to 70% of the population is immune". Despite their three nifty scenarios, (1) first infection wave with a few smaller waves, (2) first wave followed by second, more severe wave coinciding with the flu season in the Western hemisphere, and (3) first wave, second wave and several smaller waves to follow, they are also stuck in the *pandemic flu paradigm* making constant parallels to a quite different pathogen.

IHME Washington studies

I'm not going to go through in too much detail the numbers and forecasts made in the various reports from Imperial College (2020), University of Washington (IHME, 2020) and others that have had a heavy amount of media coverage as well as political impact over the first four months of the pandemic. The reason is that for all their short-term political relevance, I consider them all *wrong* by a magnitude that render the numerical calculations null and void in terms of actionable insight going forward. They are only interesting inasmuch as they had impact on specific decisions to lock down or open up societies, not for what they say about the progression of the virus itself.

For example, on April 5, Dr. Christopher Murray at IHME forecasts 81,766 cumulative deaths nationally (USA), with a range between 49,431 and 136,401. Yet, as of May 2, in the middle of the pandemic, and with social distancing only being loosened in a few states as of that week, the US death toll already stands at 66,369, and already on May 11, a week after social distancing is relaxed in a few states only, has increased to 80,087 (JHU, 2020). Moreover, the subsequent April 27, 2020 release of the IHME predictions are based on a model that assumes "social distancing until infections are minimized and containment is implemented" without explicitly accounting for the various ways that social distancing is practiced, the efficiency drop of this strategy over time due to lack of follow-through in key population groups and other factors. Also, their model does not account for easing social distancing or quantify the risk of resurgence, which are the issues that really matters in terms of societal planning. I know they are trying to incorporate this element because without it, the data just doesn't say much. Lastly, their model is based on a countrywide prediction (statewide for the US), but the COVID-19 dynamic so far has been city and county specific, which is a whole other level of granularity. A quick example would be Georgia, which, according to IHME's April 29 estimates has no ICU or bed shortage issue at all and a descending slope, even though recent trends indicates that the reality could be more complex.

Imperial College COVID-19 studies

If we look at Imperial College, Neil Ferguson, the lead scientist who warned that the coronavirus would kill 500,000 people in the United Kingdom (and changed the country's herd immunity strategy as a result of this prediction), on March 26 thought that if current measures work as expected, the death toll would drop to roughly 20,000 people or fewer (Miller, 2020). This is all interesting, but as of May 2, the UK death toll is 28,205 (JHU Covid-19 Dashboard, 2020). I do understand that the interpretation could be that he now thinks the UK mitigation measures are not working as expected, but I think with such wildly varying predictions, it might have been better to stick with a bunch of scenarios and leave it to the decision makers to figure out how to interpret the data and which way to choose. The Imperial College model explicitly made the decision to ignore the impact of widespread testing and contact tracing and the model itself is based on pandemic flu.

One observation made by Imperial College's 16 March report (Ferguson et al. 2020:16) is definitely sound and deserves quoting: *"[it is] not at all certain that suppression will succeed long term; no public health intervention with such disruptive effects on society has been previously attempted for such a long duration of time. How populations and societies will respond remains unclear."*

The saying "Lies, damned lies, and statistics" is often attributed to Benjamin Disraeli and popularized in the U.S. by Mark Twain but is poorly understood by all of us, since we fall for it, time and time again. What was the confidence interval or in simpler terms: the margin of error on Imperial's studies? Or perhaps just give a range to begin with, how about "between 20,000 and 500,000 deaths", which, unfortunately would be code for "we really have no idea." That got lost in translation.

The "Oxford study" on Covid-19 scenarios

A March 24, a five-page "Oxford study" got massive coverage in the Financial Times who claim "coronavirus may have infected half of UK population – Oxford study" (Cookson, 2020) and argued the case for large-scale testing. The paper prepared by researchers affiliated with Oxford's Evolutionary Ecology of Infectious Disease group, was pre-published, not yet peer reviewed, and was focused on infection rates within the UK's herd immunity paradigm. It said coronavirus may have (already) infected half of UK population. To the authors this was a good thing and meant the mortality was much lower than earlier assumed given the next assumption made, that the epidemic wave in the UK and Italy in the absence of interventions “should have an approximate duration of 2-3 months”. According to the Oxford model, there should have been a steep drop in daily new UK deaths in early April, which did not happen. Clearly, the peak in the epidemic had not already passed. Also, the study relies heavily on the crucial assumption that only a very small proportion of those infected would experience disease severe enough to be hospitalized.

The importance of the Oxford study was that one started looking for an “earlier start” to the epidemic, an aspect which indeed seems to pan out. The Oxford research suggests that Covid-19 reached the UK by mid-January at the latest and perhaps as early as December. The first recorded UK death was on March 2 in a care home. Interestingly, on April 22, the Washington Post (Chiu & Armus, 2020) reported autopsies reveal two Californian coronavirus deaths on Feb 6 and Feb 17 already. Initially, the first US death was thought to have occurred on Feb 29—and opens the door for the possibility that the virus in fact traveled from the US to Europe, not just the other way around!

The Imperial model is based on individuals. The Oxford model is a Bayesian approach based on populations. They attempt to answer different questions and use different values for infectiousness (Ro)—Imperial initially used Ro =2.4 but adjusted to 3 whereas Oxford used Ro =2.25 or 2.75 for different scenarios—and fatality (CFR) of COVID-19, which inevitably generated different results (Panovska-Griffiths, 2020). This is not to say that epidemiological modeling is not important, just to say that, in my opinion, until one has numbers that are reliable and valid, the margin of error is so large that one should reason *without the use of numbers* not to mislead the public, the media and politicians.

Harvard study on intermittent social distancing

A Harvard study issued on March 24, 2020, pointed out that intermittent social distancing might be needed over time, perhaps until 2022 (Kissler et al. 2020). It pointed out that lessons from the Influenza epidemic of 1918 was that a second winter peak came as a surprise after the first autumn wave. Interestingly, this study points out that even with available vaccinations, which would take months to adopt across populations, another peak or two might happen, although there is some hope, since: *"New therapeutics, vaccines, or other interventions such as aggressive contact tracing and quarantine - impractical now in many places but more practical once case numbers have been reduced and testing scaled up could alleviate the need for stringent social distancing to maintain control of the epidemic"*.

Possible breakthrough in the study of disease emergence

Future epidemic predictions might soon improve based on a new mathematical model of how information mutates when spread from person to person (Eletreby et al., 2020). The analogy appears to be that of genes in that it self-replicates, mutates and responds to selective pressure. This might resonate with findings by Christakis & Fowler (2009) on contagion in social networks and might offer better understanding of network diffusion in light of both virus and information mutations. Current simulation models mostly ignore evolutionary adaptations.

Playable scenarios

Epidemiologist Marcel Salathe and Nicky Case, a Canadian indie game developer, have created playable simulations for COVID-19 Futures (https://ncase.me/covid-19/). This approach is incredibly didactic about complex epidemiological phenomena all of us have been forced to learn about over the past few months. You can literally hit play and watch The Last

Few Months (epidemiology 101, SEIR model, R & Ro), The Next Few Months (lockdowns, contact tracing, masks) or even The Next Few Years (loss of immunity? no vaccine?). It's quite visual and techy but says little about the social reactions we need to expect will interfere with each of the scenarios.

Is COVID-19 a scenario exercise replacement?

Before moving to a brief reflection on failures as fixes to set up the scenarios, I want to consider the following argument: the current coronavirus pandemic is, in itself, a sufficient scenario exercise and "we all know what to do now."

While it is true that government leaders will forever be able to look back at the years from 2020–2023 (let's just take the immediately obvious time frame for now) and reflect on the enormous developments that unfolded, (a) it is not clear that the reflection level will be as structured and focused as in regular scenario exercises, and (b) disease X (or whatever you want to call it) is not going to follow the exact COVID-19 trajectory. In fact, it may be significantly stealthier (even more asymptomatic transmission) or harsher (perhaps with more severe mortality than Ebola). Furthermore, even if there is a coronavirus 2.0 (say from one of the other 5000+ or more strains that yet have to make a zoonotic shift), that is an almost 1:1 blueprint of the current strain in terms of transmissibility and mortality, it will not unfold in exactly the same way. This is a subject for another book, but I could think of at least 10 ways the first 6 months of the next pandemic could play out. You could imagine everything from full containment the first month, to a regional outbreak, to a worldwide outbreak, just to take three of them. Similarly, there is no way to predict *exactly* how each country and culture would react the second time around, although we should certainly try.

The point is that every attempt at foresight always will hit new forces of disruption, which is why it cannot be done only every so often; it has to be a continuous process, always updating the parameters, bringing new actors in, imagining deep, realistic, emotionally powerful, and rationally consistent (or perhaps inconsistent, at times) scenarios.

Failures and fixes

The following five failures seem most pertinent to reflect upon and fix to improve pandemic readiness. In this chapter we will not attempt to sketch too many solutions, simply point to the challenges and sketch a way forward conceptually. The solutions will have to wait until our next book on that topic, which will be written in 2021 as the crisis has unfolded long enough to assess the early fixes already in place. Instead, we will try to sketch what to learn from these challenges on a more general basis.

Preventing outbreaks

The first failure was not to have prevented the COVID-19 outbreak itself. Scientists were initially fairly certain it started at a wet market in Wuhan, China, where wild animals were sold (and consumed). Not having stopped all such wet markets and the trade in wild animals in China and beyond would seem to be the first failure, although one found during the earlier SARS outbreak that attempting to ban such trade would simply move the market underground. However, even before that, there is (scant) ongoing research on zoonotic transmission (i.e., the transmission of disease from animals to humans). As of mid- to end April, the entire wet market origin theory is in doubt, but let's still consider the zoonotic transmission argument, which has so much folklore connected to it.

There are two main pathways zoonotic transmission can happen. In direct zoonosis, the disease is transmitted from other animals to humans through media such as air (influenza) or through bites and saliva (rabies). Indirect zoonosis, in contrast, can also occur by contact with places where the animal lives or roams or items that were contaminated. Alternatively, it can be a case where the transmission happens via an intermediate species (referred to as a *vector*), which may carry the disease pathogen without getting infected. Foodborne (e.g., raw or undercooked meat, eggs, fruits, vegetables) or waterborne disease (from animal feces) may also be forms of indirect zoonosis. In the case of coronavirus, one running theory is that it was indirect zoonosis from a bat to a pandolin (also known as an anteater) who acted as the vector. If this is the case, Patient 0 might have been an asymptomatic pandolin. Others claim the virus could have circulated among humans for years without an outbreak and that the genetic make-up has a unique mutation that is most likely to occur during repeated, small-cluster infections in humans and that doesn't fit what's required for the pandolin theory to pan out as an immediate cause (Andersen et al., 2020).

In the aftermath of COVID-19, increased attention on trying to prevent an outbreak is likely. However, no matter how much we study the origin of viruses, one will escape again. There are as many as 5,000 coronavirus strains waiting to be discovered in bats globally, according to disease ecologist Peter Daszak, president of EcoHealth Alliance, in New York City.

What we usually can do is contain the initial outbreak to Patient 0 and the immediate people that patient has infected using the true and tested method of contact tracing. During COVID-19, contact tracing broke down in most superspreader events where it was attempted. One reason for that was asymptomatic transmission but other reasons were lack of resources or technology (manual contact tracing at scale is highly inefficient).

What to learn about zoonotic outbreaks?

As a world community, we need to know much more about zoonotic transmission, not just in theory but in all cases where it has happened. We also need to carefully map all potential pathogens, sequence their DNA, and already have a shortcut to a potential vaccine at hand. A lot of this work should be done by computers and synthetic biology.

To state the obvious, preventing outbreaks is really the bread and butter of WHO and all national centers for disease control. China actually has a well-resourced center for disease control and is not at all like a smaller (or under-resourced) African nation that, understandably, would be overwhelmed by the tasks needed to contain an outbreak of this scale. Why China dropped the ball is a complicated question. Some would have it they dropped the ball on purpose. Others would say COVID-19 surprised most doctors and even most epidemiologists. Certainly, the fact that Western countries took so long to prepare would indicate they didn't fully grasp the potential risks—even all the way up to March 2020 in some cases.

The importance of national and international centers for disease control

A voice of reason would say that, going forward, every country needs to have an adequate center for disease control. In this business, experience matters, because knowledge about diseases only evolves over long periods of time. Relying on the CDC or the WHO is not going to cut it, especially as those two organizations exposed *major weaknesses* during the COVID-19 outbreak.

For instance, several months before the coronavirus pandemic began, the US administration eliminated a key American public health position in Beijing intended to help detect disease outbreaks in China, according to Reuters. Also, the CDC botched the rollout of test kits. The WHO's problems are well known after what I've discussed in previous sections.

These institutions need to be well funded, open minded, innovative, and connected to applied research, the major hospitals, and vaccine developers nationally and internationally. In addition, they need to be on speed dial to those sitting on the national stockpile. Those countries who realize that they don't have this should drop this book down right now and set aside budget before they finish reading. It's that important.

Judging from the history of the Asian centers for disease control, and how they rapidly learned from their failures, the learning curve in Europe, the US, and even at the WHO should be steep in the aftermath of COVID-19. Nobody is going to want to repeat what is unfolding now.

Upgrading health security

Judging from the Global Health Security Index (which itself needs an upgrade, given its misleading ranking of the US and UK at top of the health security and pandemic readiness foodchain), upgrading national health security (which goes way beyond disease control and into primary care reforms, doctors and nurses per 1000 citizens, ICU capacity, and ventilators) is going to take some time. Foreign aid is needed to spearhead this in at least the 50 countries that score the lowest on health security, at the bottom of which you'll find North Korea, Somalia, and Equatorial Guinea. That agency needs to have a hotline to the WHO and there needs to be full trust between these two parties.

There can be no national pride or political concerns limiting the information flow between the site of the outbreak and the WHO. In fact, going via national channels is a waste of time, the message should simultaneously go to WHO and the national center.

Tracking outbreaks

The second and most basic failure of the COVID-19 outbreak was the way it was (not) tracked, even once it escaped the immediate contact tracing efforts. China was slow to recognize the virus, slow to diagnose it, and slow to release accurate information about its properties and impact. Although the WHO was relatively quick on the scene and from there onward tracked it to the best of their ability, they were slow to declare COVID-19 a pandemic.

As for China, there is still some doubt on the official Chinese death toll and infected figures, and on April 16, 2020, Chinese state media said 1,300 deaths, or near half the total, had not been counted in death tolls because of lapses, as reported by Reuters.

Best practices for tracking outbreaks need to reach the local level, meaning each hospital, primary care doctor, pharmacy, or even community health organization that may be the first point of contact or concern of Patient 0. In Italy, for instance, it would appear that their Patient 0 went to at least three healthcare providers before he got tested and diagnosed.

The specialty of infectious diseases needs to be upgraded as a field of research, as a policy concern and specialty, as well as in primary care practice and at hospitals around the world, particularly in those regions of the world that have a track record of being a source of lethal pathogens in the past (Asia and Africa).

Responding to outbreaks

Arguably, there were severe shortcomings in the global, coordinated public health response. Even though WHO has been there all along with guidance, their role has been subdued, their recommendations have been good but not sufficient, and their voice has generally not been heard. Also, the WHO's power is not commensurate with the impact of a pandemic. The organization lacks power to implement public health measures at scale and depends on its member organizations' goodwill and own response teams and funding to a large degree.

There are as of May 2, 2020, no regular therapeutic treatments for COVID-19. Given that situation, it is simply striking that it took several months to kickstart clinical trials on existing drugs (Ebola drug Remdesivir; HIV/AIDS drugs ritonavir and lopanivir combined with the general antiviral drug ribavirin and a multiple sclerosis drug called beta interferon) or vaccines (B.C.G and others) that might be part of future treatment plans.

During a rapidly spreading global pandemic it is evident that speed, consistency, and simplicity of communication and measures are important. Global concerns need to trump local concerns. In the COVID-19 crisis, national concerns have overshadowed the global response both in the public health measures taken, the communication flow, and in the analysis of data as such. The relatively novel situation of having private and nonprofit actors provide "data on the side" tracking outbreaks has confused more than clarified the situation, which brings us to the next point.

Analyzing outbreaks

Analyzing the spread and impact of an outbreak is important in order to tailor the response adequately. Public health measures necessary during a pandemic are socioeconomically costly and disruptive to daily life. At the end of the day, strict measures like quarantines and stay-at-home orders also cause their own negative health effects, especially when long lasting.

The role of web-based dashboard services has been surprisingly ineffective and downright confusing at times during the COVID-19 pandemic. Instead of guiding public health response and public understanding of the risks, many of these dashboards seem to have been quickly overloaded with noise. For example, the Johns Hopkins infectious disease dashboard has been widely criticized for its messy layout—*MIT Tech Review* (Patel, 2020) pointed out that an earlier version used "poorly sized circles to illustrate the extent of outbreaks in specific locations," uses "gloom-and-doom colors," and has "no way to learn more about specific cases or the history of the virus in a certain location."

What should outbreak analysis do, at minimum? One, provide accurate testing, death toll, and infection figures. Two, provide a prediction on how, where, and how quickly the outbreak might spread. Three, use a transparent model where the data used is accessible on an open-source basis so any independent observer can check and recheck data and provide alternate ways of analyzing the data. Four, provide a one-stop-shop for sharing such data. Five, build an accurate epidemiological model that is also simple enough that national disease control agencies and public health researchers and labs around the world can build on and improve it. Six, be simple and intuitive enough that a lay person can work with it and derive practical insight that guides their life, work and whereabouts. Seven, take into account non-numerical and not-yet numerical arguments, complexities and inter-relationships, notably social phenomena, trust, emergence, politics, human psychology, and network effects.

The WHO's COVID-19 page is not sufficiently prominent among all the other data providers around COVID-19. People will quickly go to other sources where the data are presented better visually or even seem more up to date or locally tailored.

Communicating outbreaks

Communicating the actions needed from an outbreak is crisis management 101. Public health officials, and especially government political leaders, need to communicate clearly, consistently, and in simple terms, with no grounds for confusion and no mixed messages. Leaders need to not only talk the talk but walk the walk. The fact that female heads of state have been highly successful both at communicating clearly and warmly, with emotional depth and empathy, has been widely reported. Their approach has also yielded the best results, even just thinking about New Zealand, Germany, and Norway. This is not surprising, but interesting, and not something we should lose sight of. After this, I'll consider moving to a country with strong woman leaders again. We need both warmer and more efficient leaders who don't have time for games in a time of crisis. If women consistently can provide that, I think most people are in favor. Let's see if this pans out long term.

Economizing outbreaks

An outbreak that is not immediately contained and spreads beyond a local context, especially to an urban area, will rapidly become equally a health and an economic concern. Bringing in economic expertise in order to evaluate the economic impact of various public health measures from the get-go is crucial.

It is entirely possible that countries that win the health battle against COVID-19 will lose the economic battle and calamity that ensues. In that case, the health benefits might have been too costly to achieve. The ethical prerogative must be clarified. If the objective is to save the most lives, a myopic public health response may not be the best option. If the objective is to shield those local communities who are affected by the public health aspect as such, then the economic effects must be only considered after the fact. These are important debates that have only been theoretical for the past decades. Now they are very real.

Innovating pre/during/post outbreaks

As we have seen in the past, the years and decades following a big disaster (Black Death or the 1918 Influenza pandemic) led to significant innovations, as described in the Introduction. That will also happen with COVID-19. However, given the fact that the speed of innovation is much higher now, we also expect innovations to literally change the course of the current pandemic. In some cases, that expectation is overblown. Vaccines take years, and the 12–18 months that have been indicated by presidents, prime ministers, and even by some public health officials is dangerously optimistic given the 10+-years average for introducing a new vaccine (Pronker et al., 2013). Sometimes, vaccines never succeed. The HIV virus was identified in 1984, but four decades and 32 million deaths later, there is no HIV vaccine. Also, who gets the vaccine(s) if they arrive?

First, you have the countries that finance them or where the pharma company or organization that makes it are headquartered. Secondly, you have the countries that trialed the vaccine. Thirdly, the countries that can pay or that hold the most political sway. Fourthly, you have the countries with the most infections. Fifthly, within each country there is likely to be an order in which the vaccine is prioritized—health workers, elites, areas near top medical centers—or simply more available—near top medical centers, in big cities, in rich suburbs, etc. A variety of vaccines are likely needed to cover the world's population, both for production reasons and in terms of efficacy for different use cases and genetic and epidemiologic characteristics.

Innovation is a long game. Early wins may be promising but the true effects are likely to be more in the long term. Innovation also brings disappointments. The name of the game is a high failure rate.

The most likely path of innovation during an outbreak is that it will lead to useful innovations for the next outbreak.

Recovering from outbreaks

The COVID-19 outbreak has in its first 4 months caused a big discussion on public health but only a small discussion on long-term recovery of societal functions that currently are disrupted. There seems to have been no recognized scenarios for what might happen in the aftermath of a big outbreak.

The recovery phase of an outbreak may, depending on the severity, last anything from a year to a decade. COVID-19 will, for most countries, and indeed for the world as a whole, likely last for a decade, which is why the scenarios that follow in the next chapters use the next decade as the timeline.

What does it mean to recover? It doesn't simply mean to put things in place the way they were before. That is simply not good enough. Leaders need to be fully aware of all the vectors that need to be considered. They need to have a plan to use the crisis to improve upon society.

Regulating beyond emergency state

Once they enter the outbreak mentality, governments are all too quick to pass emergency legislation. The reason for that is that this makes them look strong and also gives an excuse to pass pet projects they have wanted to pass all along. Trump's announcement on April 20 to curb immigration is one such case in point.

One area that might need tight regulation going forward is mass events. It's one thing to have a social distancing policy in place and to forbid gatherings of a certain size temporarily. However, when such matters become a regular, perhaps recurrent and intermittent occurrence, real debate needs to be had. One likely outcome is that we will see some governments essentially regulate mass-event organizers as if they were utilities (e.g., sports, religion). What do I mean by that?

Clearly, the cost/benefits to society of mass events beyond 1,000 people will be in question for some time to come. It would not be unreasonable that the organizers would have to prove the societal value of going from 1,000 to 5,000 attendees (beyond larger revenues for the organizers). Events most likely affected by such regulation would be megachurches, stadium events, and congress and exhibition centers.

Learning from failure

Learning from failure, as I pointed out in my earlier book *Disruption Games* (2020), is a fruitful exercise. Those who are best at it will thrive, even on serial failure. Just like the scientific endeavor, which in some sense is mostly an exercise of failed experiments with only occasional breakthroughs, all failures have the potential seeds to providing great lessons. Those that are willing to deeply delve into their own shortcomings are likely to emerge the fastest and sustain the biggest gains. This brings us to the last issue we will consider, which is a more novel strategy: imagining outbreaks.

Imagining outbreaks

We have described a few relatively recent pandemic scenario exercises. The problem with many of them is that they either were smallish operational scenarios with only tactical challenges (how to contain a flight with a few infected patients) or location-specific responses (responding to an outbreak in a major metropolitan center). The COVID-19 outbreak is global, simultaneous, and contains the X factor of asymptomatic transmission. Each of these parameters seem missing from most past scenario work. This cannot go on, which is why I, in the next part of the book (Chapters 4–8), offer five scenarios that could be adapted for such use by citizens, thinkers, activists, innovators, social entrepreneurs, public health officials, government leaders, nonprofit leaders, and executives around the world.

However, we cannot even assume that the characteristics that played a role in this outbreak would play a similar role in the subsequent outbreak, whether it was caused by a zoonotic coronavirus or otherwise. Each outbreak is situated within a particular context with forces of disruption (policy, technology, business models, and social dynamics) operating in highly specific ways. Therefore, any scenario planning is fraught with uncertainty.

Recognizing that we failed to foresee the scale and impact of this pandemic—all of us *collectively* failed, from presidents to academic thinkers—in the next five chapters, I have charted a set of scenarios for the next decade so that this mistake is not repeated. It is now incredibly important that we work to minimize the long-term fallout, exploit the opportunities that have arisen, and prepare to predict future calamities, whether they be pandemics, terrorism, wars, or environmental cataclysms.

These scenarios attempt to map the unforeseen, and as such are works of pure fiction. On the other hand, they very much build on projecting what is already unfolding around us. If you are unused to scenario thinking, you might find them somewhat extreme. That's a normal feeling. It takes a certain amount of imagination to engage with the future. Embrace it—we need you on board. In fact, as you will discover in the last scenario, I'm not discounting that many things might conspire to keep us from lifting our perspective beyond short termism, once again. There are some benefits to that eventuality, too. For one, we will still recognize our world.

If I'm asked which of the five scenarios are more likely, here's my take: they are drafted to be *equally* probable. That does *not* mean that I expect them to happen exactly as written. Each scenario extrapolates a few distinct trends and takes them to the extreme. The course of the next decade will therefore be something in between. The challenge is to know which parameters we want to optimize for, which would require some sort of political agreement. Failing that, at the very least these scenarios can be used to prepare for a set of possible futures, no matter if we could affect which of the trends pan out.

Learning from failure: national centers of disease control

Which countries have the strongest centers for disease control?

If you were a public health official in one of the most affected countries (say China, Italy, Brazil, Russia, Spain, the UK, or the US), what would you say were your biggest single failure?

Pandemic warnings

What were some warnings that were given about future pandemics?

Who tried to warn us? Why was the warning not heeded?

What would it have taken to inspire action?

Simulating the next decade

What does a futurist do, to your best knowledge?

What is scenario thinking? How do decision makers use scenarios?

Five scenarios for our post-coronavirus future

The time has come to prepare for a discussion that could change the course of the future. Knowing what your options are might change what you aim for. Each of us can help shape the future. At least, we all have the power to try.

Good scenarios are specific enough to elicit emotions, spur concrete thoughts and ideas, and they could even make you angry. Before taking in these scenarios, try to imagine your own favorite scenario for the next decade.

What would you *like to happen* in the next 10 years?

What would you *think will happen* in the next 10 years?

CHAPTER 4

SCENARIO I: THE BORDERLESS WORLD

Enrico is building his worldview

In this scenario, we consider what it would look like if world leaders were able to make massive progress in science and technology, fully implement globalization, as well as solidarity and implementation strategies to fix the weakest links (e.g., health systems in Africa). But the trade-offs are not trivial, and something gets lost. *From now on, and throughout this chapter, you are entering the realm of fiction.*

Milan, Italy, December 5, 2021: "Come help me, grandpa," said Enrico. Enrico had just celebrated his 11th birthday in his home in Milan, Italy. He shouted at his grandfather, who had turned away. Enrico tried to get his kite up in the air. It was a gift from his grandfather, along with an expensive watch. Even his father had been surprised by this extravagant gift: a Patek Phillipe watch.

Enrico was precocious, smart. He shared his grandpa's silvery grey hair. Only then did Enrico see it: Grandpa was leaned toward the street corner. Enrico had just rushed by with his kite too quickly to notice Grandpa Eligio was no longer alive. He had taken his last breath, just then and there, on Piazza della Scala. Like many COVID-19 victims, his grandfather's death was sudden, with no warning, and few visible signs of illness.

As he looked back on this event many years later, Enrico wished he would have had the man behind the monument there with him; the center of the square was marked by a statue of Leonardo da Vinci by sculptor Pietro Magni (1872). If the world didn't identify such talent and do everything they could to save "young Leonardos," he thought to himself, there would be no future now. He teared up for a moment, thinking back to the month after Grandpa had died, when Enrico himself had been admitted to the hospital with coronavirus infection.

It had been a dreadful experience for an 11-year-old. So much death. But that wasn't what jarred his mind a decade later. No, it was knowing that the 10 other people in the room he was in were sacrificed so that he could be saved. They only had one respirator. He was the youngest; the others were 15, 29, 55, and 82 (and he couldn't remember the rest) and had been lower on the priority list. Except the grey-haired guy on his right side—he must have been wealthy, and without morals, ultimately, because he also got a respirator. Enrico had seen with his own eyes how a young child like himself, perhaps only a few years older, had been yanked off the breathing machine and had been left to gasp for air until he died. Why, Enrico had wondered, had he been saved and not this child? The answer would not make sense until later in life.

The dreadful consequences of the virus' mutations

So sudden was the onslaught of coronavirus, more precisely "SARS-CoV-2ff", the 11th mutation that had killed so many in Italy, Venezuela, and just an awful number in China and India—where 10% of the population had died in the third wave of the disease, which had coincided with a particularly severe flu season, making it a double whammy. Enrico had actually been lucky to be playing with his grandpa that morning. There were so few grandparents left in Italy now, in the second half of 2021. Had he not been on that square that day, Enrico might not have known how to survive.

Grandpa had said, "If anything happens to me, take my watch and carry it with you always. It will get you out of trouble one day." For the first time, Enrico looked at the brand. It said PATEK PHILIPPE - GENEVE. "Just like mine," Enrico thinks. Okay, he thought, I don't know what this means, but quickly took it off his grandpa's wrists before he ran away, crying for his loss and not knowing yet what he had gained.

The year 2030—peace in our time—again

We are in the year 2030. After a decade of widespread agreement on the goals for planet Earth, world leaders and civil society have just concluded a Global Summit for a World Without Borders. A new world government has been approved. This follows 5 years in which experts from around the world have been hard at work drafting a new world constitution, setting up rules for the election of a representative world government to be situated in Geneva and regional headquarters in Dar es Salaam, Tanzania and in Dhaka, Bangladesh. World leaders opted against New York, London, Shanghai, or Rio di Janeiro on the grounds that this is the time for the small nations to rule.

A decade of science and technology progress—and hygiene

There had been an enormous progress in science and technology throughout the decade; for example, 3D printing was now commonplace; you could print any product right out of your home, if you could afford it. Bigger projects could be done in the local 3D factory based on your specification, if you could afford it. Working remotely was the norm, mostly because of the augmented reality platforms that were launched already in 2025. Truly amazing, really—some people said it was better than being present in the office. The most loved feature was the virtual backgrounds that now had evolved so you could look like you were wearing a suit even though you were in your pajamas. There had to be some benefit to this COVID-19 situation that had created so much misery. After all, it wasn't like they had a choice. Nobody was allowed to commute anymore. After all those intermittent periods where the lockdowns were lifted only to be brought back there became no point.

Besides, how do you make public transit (subways, buses, and commuter trains) free of infectious disease risk? Even our greatest minds couldn't figure that one out. We tried limiting the number of passengers, but our transit owners went broke. We tried risking it with no change, but too many got sick. We tried to sanitize each compartment with a new superfast infrared disinfection machine (the UV BeamoLight Sterilizer XL) after every ride, but people got sick anyway. We tried everything. The problem was density. Everything about density is now our enemy. Now, there is a standing prize for any idea that could resurrect public transport. I'm jotting down ideas every day and so are all my friends. Nobody has found the answer.

Besides, most businesses couldn't afford commercial real estate anymore. The big five consulting firms shared one office building in downtown New York, for example. Given social distancing, they could only fit 25% of pre-COVID-19 capacity. The new building codes were very strict: only five people per room, no matter the size of the room; thermal sensors at every door, registering even small temperature anomalies; separate entry and exit so you don't run into people; touchless doors, elevators, screens, computers, everything was done to minimize contact. The HVAC systems were running on a hypercycle, exchanging all the building's air every 10 minutes.

The new disinfection culture was quite astonishing. We all did our part to create it. Kids, too. The world has never seen such clean kids. Dirt is abolished, basically. There is a mandatory disinfection and health routine we all have to follow every morning at 8:00 a.m., noon, 4:00 p.m., and 8:00 p.m. Wash your hands for 20 seconds. Mandatory mouthwash. Take your temperature, send it to the global system for comparison. Mandatory change of clothes every morning. If you go out in public, you need to wear the self-disinfecting uniform based on a lab coat design created by MIT's smart fabrics team. Every working individual who wanted to commute had to have one. They cost a month's salary. Most people took out a loan to afford one. On the bright side, the uniform came in 100 colors and all sizes. There's an upside to everything.

We also abolished extreme obesity, since a BMI 40 or more obesity is risk factor for COVID-19. How did we do it? We simply limited rations. If you eat more than 2500 calories a day, 2000 for women or 1500 for kids, it gets reported. Repeated offences are fined. Highly efficient. I cannot think of why we wouldn't have done that a decade ago.

Handshakes got abolished by global decree 25.C already back in 2022, after some discussion by the Germans who really have turned handshakes into an art form. The Italians had abolished kissing as a greeting already toward the end of 2020. Let's not even get into our love life. It has gotten ridiculous, given the no-contact regime. The sensors are installed in people's home. The slightest rise in body temperature and you're caught. Try having sex without raising your pulse. It's near impossible.

But without contact, all you had was your eyes. It was simply not enough to get excited about meeting your colleagues. It was worth it for highly important meetings, right before a project presentation, for instance. The application process was cumbersome. After getting a special permit, you could go straight to the office, conduct your business, and go back to your house.

No more nation-states

Truly, it has been an amazing decade, marked by enormous

progress in understanding between peoples, cultures, and territories. What was there to think about? The world had come together.

The world has finally decided to abolish nation-states. Throughout the decade, that unit of governance simply became too impractical and hampered by isolationist concerns, lack of resources, and lack of empathy for others outside its borders. In fact, the whole notion of borders is abolished. Gone are border controls, passports, national anthems, even the Olympics had to concede that we can still compete for medals, but the whole idea that a large country would take more medals just seems irrational now. After all, we are all in this together.

A lot has changed. We have also nearly gotten rid of cities. The distancing just became impractical. It took time, of course. We had cities for 5 years. We tried distancing. We tried outlawing mass events above 1,000 people, then we tried 500, then 100, then 50, but the superspreader events returned again and again. Instead, scientists have divided the globe into squares of 100 x 100 feet where families ideally should spend most of their time. Needless to say, all of these changes have brought the end of simple pleasures such as going to the movies. The end of the theater-chain system happened relatively rapidly throughout 2021. Then followed the collapse of the Hollywood studio system and the stars who lived in Los Angeles dispersed. Instead, we now have distributed production and online distribution.

A lot of civil liberties have been permanently curtailed. That seems to be one of the more significant trade-offs we are experiencing, that of safety versus freedom. The alternative, no safety, doesn't seem so appealing having lived through COVID-19's devastation.

One of the more radical strategies that became deployed, although I'm glad to say only to a limited degree, has been the practice of killing off certain categories of infected patients before the treatment starts in order to save hospital resources. After an ethical review it only happens in cases where doctors feel the patient will not benefit from the care, and we try to get patient consent. The potential to save enormous hospital resources is definitely there. An influential analysis claims that if a hypothetical even more deadly pathogen reaches us, this will be the default strategy if we are to avoid an extinction event. Seems to make sense, although the study is highly complex. The justification is written in 10,000 pages of legalese. I doubt anybody has read the whole thing.

Mending the environment by synthetic mandates

The environment is mending, too. The climate crisis got very serious in the first few years of the decade. It was a close call, but nation-states finally got together in 2022 and realized that if they did not act now, we might not have clean air anymore and, perhaps more visibly, the food shortages would become unbearable only 10 years ahead, as arable land would dry out and concede to pollution and urbanization. The synthetic mandates had been the salvation. Synthetic biology is commonplace now. We can recreate nature by engineering. The circuitry of plain old nature is so inefficient. With synthetics, if it breaks, you just recreate it. There are formulas for everything–if you can afford it.

Synthetic is so pure, so free of nature, even more perfect than nature, in fact. Beautiful. Perfecting nature by technology. A new era has begun.

Geneva, December 1, 2030: "Enrico Salerno, the stage is yours," says the voice through the loudspeaker. This is the day. Enrico is going to represent his slice of the world, not a territory, for territorial rights and responsibilities are no more. No, Enrico is going to represent the young scientist-innovators who are 21 years old today and who now are the critical cadre of young talent that inhabit most of the world's research labs. They all have PhDs; they all have 140-and-above

IQs; and, what truly bonds them together, they all have lived through coronavirus.

If the virus reappeared today, what would guarantee Enrico a respirator is not his wealth, but his intelligence. It is a great responsibility he shares with one scientist from each of the 1,000 labs the world has created to enable the progress of humankind, at all costs. Enrico briefly shutters before he starts his speech: "I'm here today," he says, "not as the proud son of my father, but as a son of humanity itself." He continues, with elegant hand gestures, "We live in a new decade, a new beginning, marked by scientific progress and technological marvels, and we will prevail, because we will prioritize life, in its purest forms." As he says this, Enrico tries to envision his grandfather in the auditorium clapping for him. But his memory is a haze, a blur of facial features now lost to him.

With these final words, Enrico retakes his seat. The loudspeaker crackles again. This seemed to be one of those things that simply would crackle until the end of time. "Will Elena Wozniewskaya please tell us about the environmental efforts she is leading?" Elena, a 44-year-old synthetic biologist and serial entrepreneur with two degrees from MIT and a law degree from Yale, smiles and clears her voice. "Of course, I will," she says. She approaches the microphone. "I'll be quick. We have managed to create synthetic crops for all known types of grains, we have picked 21 that will be synthesized, and we are working on sequencing the genome of all known vegetables so they can be 3D printed instead of grown. From now on, gardens will be strictly ornamental. It will be nice to know you'll only see lovely flowers in gardens, right? This will continue for 2 years, after which we must all, for the good of mankind, refrain from any biological activity. We must avoid contamination of any sort. Natural DNA is so polluted. As you will remember, when outside, we need to wear masks and gloves, at all times, to protect the environment. There can be no exceptions."

Elena had thought for a long time about the speech. She was conflicted. She thought of the roses she had gotten from her boyfriend just the year before. Their pungent fruity aroma had charmed her. It reminded her of spiced wine. One of them had broken off when he had rushed to the elevator. It was kind of cute. Eleven red roses and one broken one. He had been so embarrassed. Now, all they would do is print some roses on the newest Epsilon-Xylon 33 X-ray 3D printer. The roses came out perfect every time and smelled wonderful. How could they not? She had syntheticized the smell of a red rose herself. The trick was to get that musty after smell once the sweetness subsides after 2 seconds. She got it just right. But the imperfections were impossible to simulate. She had to admit, she would miss that uncertainty, the snapped stem that had enamored her.

A society of experts to achieve certainty

After a massive effort which is obviously still ongoing, the world was able to curb its emissions to a 1950 level, which is enough to return to normalcy within the next decade. Especially because Elok Dusk in the US together with Jim Drayson in the UK, brought together the world's leading innovators, and created a set of self-flying, autonomous vacuum cleaners that purify the air on a constant basis and rely on distributed sensors across the globe to handle poor air quality before it threatens humans, animals, or plants.

What comes out the other end of the vacuum is actually recycled into space fuel, based on a new hydro-oxygen space propulsion engine that Elok Dusk has designed. We are also on our way to becoming a true interplanetary species by now. SpaceWonder's first few missions to Mars are complete and the mission there will become permanent from next year. Traveling there is still expensive, but not more than a first-class ticket between New York and Tokyo. There is a lot of demand. People are so curious these days.

The only thing is, both Elok Dusk and Jim Drayson seem to be bored. They are waiting for the next crisis. Nothing seems to be impossible anymore, now that research budgets are virtually unlimited for the top 0.001% of scientists who are competing for the Nobel Prizes they have qualified for. Are experts always bored when they succeed? I don't know. We have a lot of boredom now. Not so easy to deal with that. The only remedy, experts say, is ignorance. And ignorance is costly, and real. But reality often means death. We don't want that. Most people want to live forever. Right now, that means they could theoretically live until they are 120. Not bad. We think with a little bit of effort we can push that another decade with a few more iterations of immunologic, personalized medicine. The trouble is the treatment is still costly, so only the experts can have it, and, the fact that the earth couldn't support that many living for so long. Choices have to be made.

An explosion of interest in science

The interest in science and technology has exploded. Every kid wants to be an innovator now, just like they all wanted to be astronauts in the 1960s as the first space age got underway. Now, of course, with everyone owning their own set of microsatellites, you can already explore space from your living room. Virtual reality has become so good that there really is no need to travel to space either, at least not regularly.

Vaccines were the first we started to improve, once we got our head above water after the initial onslaught of the pandemic. The first few vaccines didn't work. Public health officials first told us they would have a vaccine in 18 months. The US president, at the time, told us less than a year, perhaps 6 months, perhaps sooner. Nobody told anybody who was sick or afraid of being sick that the average timeline to develop a vaccine is over 10 years, and that each vaccine attempt has a 6% chance of success (Pronker et al, 2013).

So even if there were nearly 100 vaccines under

development, most of them failed the first few years. But then we had a breakthrough, related to synthetic biology. We finally managed to sequence all known biological DNA in a near instant. All we need is a biological sample. That solved everything. At least if we can gather the samples. So we started sending out people to all corners of the world to collect biological samples. But now we have asked Elok Dusk and Jim Drayson to figure it out. They are working on an autonomous drone that can identify any DNA we don't have and take a sample right away. They hope to have 100,000 drones in the air by next month. That should take care of the problem.

Now, we can develop vaccines in a few months. That really helps. The only problem is that people still must be willing to take the vaccine. Unbelievably, we still have the antivaxxers. They are growing more numerous, and they have isolated themselves in the countryside. They refuse to enter our cities, because they say the cities are too clean, but in a false way. They prefer natural remedies. Those folks only live until they are 90, not until they are 120 like us. It's deplorable. They will not know their great-grandchildren. But they seem to like it that way, so what can we do?

Midway through the decade, a revolutionary movement of the upper-middle classes of the whole world united in the cause of "trusting the experts." Mounting this effort was necessary, because after the 2020 coronavirus pandemic, the world's strongmen had started to talk about abolishing journalism, democracy, tolerance for ethnic minorities, the environmental regulations put in place over the past 50 years, and a host of other issues that most, if not all, experts agreed were all bad ideas.

The revolution was brief, nonviolent, and successful. In fact, it mostly happened through elections. Perhaps most strikingly, the candidates that started winning in national elections throughout the decade were all under 30 years old. The Greta Thunberg Prize for the youngest activist had been won by a 7-year-old girl this year who advocated for the release of all known, sequenced DNA to a council of the young, all because the future must be debated for at least 10 years before we make any more tough decisions. Only the young are young enough to debate these issues now, was her mantra. She won.

Gone were all the 70-year-old senators; even the "establishment" of the 55+ generation who controlled most of the resources in the past decade conceded their power and instead started growing tomatoes in their gardens (which they now also had to conceal because of the new antibiological decree just approved). Literally, the world has 1 billion personal gardens right now. You cannot go anywhere without hearing people brag about their roses and their harvest. The biology prohibition is not going to go down well.

The respect for experts was clearly visible throughout the political process to establish a world government. Experts from around the world were able to discuss online in so-called world caucuses that then drew issues to the forefront.

After a long, Habermasian public debate (after the German scholar) where all the arguments surfaced, everyone started supporting various issues and got together in small groups. The vote was easy, in the end. The democracy model is a hybrid of the US and the UN, but where instead of only three balancing powers, there are six: the executive, the judicial, the legislative, the scientific, the religious, and the environmental. All in the service of achieving certainty, the one thing missing in the previous society, and to avoid uncertainty, doubt, inexactitude, which are all false starts for a society wanting progress as a sure thing.

Yes, that's true. Both science and the environment have their own spokespersons. In the end, the religious got theirs, too. That was almost a fight. But after the bishops and leaders of all the world's main religions got together in a massive ecumenical council meeting in 2025, they agreed on a new common creed based in human values. As it turns out, God is, largely, the same in most religions. The prophets might be different, but even Buddhists now recognize the value in a sense of progress in the world we live in. Similarly, all Christian faiths have come to realize that the soul is eternal, which puts less pressure on infighting in the here and now, yet really motivates everyone to do their best both here and in the afterlives.

Another thing is that religious rituals can no longer be performed; there are no worship services with more than five people gathered, you cannot make a pilgrimage, and ritual healing happens through online means. The online worship sessions have changed a lot from the early days. Things are more immediate. When we sing, each of us has a small part that everyone can hear. Having voice is important. We are connected by sensors. We really feel the common core we are celebrating in our bones through electrical signals sent to our brains, hands, shoulders, even our legs. All of that contributes to a much more unifying experience, a sense that what remains of religion very much is a feeling of togetherness rather than the division of syncretic ritual that had been allowed to diversify and split the churches and religions apart for millennia.

What, if anything has not changed, you ask? Well, sex is still the same; this is the one drive this decade has not been able to curb. But the context is different. The rules are different, too. It cannot happen in the home—that's outlawed. We have hygiene facilities. They look nice. If you want to picture something, think of the spa at a five-star hotel. And, there's competition from the virtual personae. Both sex in virtual reality and sex with robots has taken off in a major way. Some people like androids, other still like humans, yet others seem to prefer non-android robots that look and feel very different from humans as you may know them today. Others, again, just like sex with other brains. It takes too long to explain, but it is very intense. The point is, there is something for everyone, although there is still competition for the highest prize—the attention of the chief scientist of each region.

In fact, scientists have become almost like demigods. Even experts in public sector have an aura that previously was almost only reserved for senators. The elders are definitely not old, that's for sure. The youngest senator is 20 and the oldest is 50.

The coronavirus legacy

Okay, it is time to talk about some of the challenges we faced during the coronavirus pandemic. Things were not so optimistic then. We were close to what some of our experts call *global collapse*. What do they mean? As it turns out, hospitals across the world, particularly in the world's megacities such as Delhi, Caracas, and Shanghai, were forced to make priorities in who they would save. In retrospect, what is the most damaging is that there was no public debate, no time to discuss all of these things beforehand.

Italy was the first country that faced the challenge of choosing who was going to live or die. Then Spain. Then the US. Then the entire set of megacities in Asia and Africa and South America. There was a second wave of the pandemic in China. It didn't go so well the second time. All the draconic measure didn't work as well as before. The virus had mutated. Now it was attacking kids the most and elderly second. For kids, it was the unfinished immune systems of the children under 5 that hit the hardest. Only 10% of the affected survived.

The new virus strain preyed on people with unhealthy lifestyles such as lack of exercise, bad diets, and tobacco smokers. That's basically a description of the male, elderly population in China. The comorbidity with noncommunicable diseases such as stroke, heart diseases, and cancer were already the leading causes of deaths and disabilities in China. The mortality among the 60+ neared 20% by some estimates. That is, not 20% of those admitted. No. We lost 20% of all who were 55 and over in 2020. That's a lot of people. That's a lot of parents. A lot of husbands and wives.

See, the problem in retrospect is not that millions are dead. That's incredibly sad. It will take years to get over. No, the true problem is that, millions or not, they are alive because of priorities that a doctor or a hospital administrator made during the crisis, either as a (sometimes) misguided policy or a spur of the moment decision because of a lack of ventilators. How did they decide? It was many things. Sometimes greed. Sometimes principle. Sometimes tiredness just meant they did whatever. Not that we want to blame them either. But still, the moral dilemma is how do we deal with the Quislings, the murderers, the ones who thought they could be God? Or, is the real dilemma how to deal with ourselves, who let all of this happen, who watched it happen without saying something? But what would we have said?

The ethical imperative goes against our nature

The discussion started as soon as all the temporary hospitals after coronavirus were closed. Initially, there were 16 such hospitals in the Chinese megacity of Wuhan. All told, 3 years after, as the crisis was finally ebbing out, there had been 100,000 such hospitals created, but even that was not enough. And, often, the hospitals were really just beds, and sometimes not even that. In Africa it was mostly just a small cross in the sand indicating where to put dying bodies.

In the beginning, each hospital practiced priorities differently. Then, governments struck down and created blanked priorities. In the US, they quickly settled on the principle that those who contributed the most to the economy would get first in line for treatment. In Scandinavian countries, it was the principle of how much gain the individual patient would have by the treatment. In India, there was no principle, or at least it was never spelled out; they were treating just 1% of those who arrived at the hospital anyway, and there was nobody left to prioritize or to write about what was prioritized.

Then, by some miracle, doctors started stepping up. They organized into a new type of global union and set out principles for themselves. At the end of the day, they said they would make the call, but in times of doubt, they would consult ethics committees. Only 10 countries still had national ethics committees for clinical practice decisions; they were overloaded and quickly had to stop promising individual feedback. Also, decisions had to be made on a minute-by-minute basis, so there was no time. The real question, which is why ethics committees were still quite useful, was what to do about other vulnerable groups and treating illnesses unrelated to the virus. And, what about uninsured? It was simple, really—without insurance, society (and the private hospitals which were not nationalized) could not bear the cost.

But these are digressions. We now have a global ethical guideline for cost/benefit, severity of the disease, and resource use in all the world's hospitals. These were just created. Can you believe it took 10 years? In some way, we have not come very far as a human race. But at least it is here now. And we all, mostly, agree. The dissenters have been isolated or jailed—this sounds harsh—but they started going rogue in our hospitals. They disturbed law and order. In short, it is all a trade-off, but it can be mathematically modeled. The people who will benefit society the most must survive at all costs. Healthy children will always be saved first. Then, the elite, the experts who take care of us, and anybody with a graduate degree. Those are the ones who are smart enough to help the rest of us in times of crisis. And we have to assume that a crisis will strike gain. It always does. They all follow only one guideline: should resources become limited, they all know what to do.

It's almost ironic that, two decades ago, when they thought about readiness for pandemics, they were thinking of stockpiling and coordination of relief efforts as well as how to provide emergency cash to companies that would go under. Turns out, the real lack of readiness is the ethical fiber that turns out to be such a brittle, small part of the human psyche. Some ethicists say it's not even a natural human instinct. The survival instinct is so much stronger. We have to *legislate* goodness. As Hannah Arendt (1951) had already reminded us in *The Origin of Totalitarianism* when she wrote about the Nazism of the 1930s, which feels long ago now, it was not "they" that were evil, it was always just ourselves, if only put into a systemic form, logically consistent on its own terms, so it was harder to recognize. The Nazis were terrifyingly normal. They belonged to a distinct type of political movement. They just applied a higher order belief system that superseded the doubts that come to us looking at their behavior after the fact.

Again, it's important to point out that "Borderless World," which is the slogan of the current world government that will last throughout the next decade, was not an easy decision. That is, it became easy as we suddenly realized what was happening to us as a human race. However, immediately before, it was as if we were facing humanity's darkest moment. Perhaps it can be like that sometimes. Times of crisis can be clarifying. They were for us. Family against family. Husband against wife. Old against young. American against Canadian.

We had started to act more like animals, our true nature, according to some experts. Instead, we should have embraced world solidarity immediately. It took us too long. So many lives were lost. So many of the wrong lives. Although, as we also realize, there was perhaps no right answer to the pandemic. We were not prepared. We had no defenses. But it was the moral rot that got us in the end. And that's also what took us so long. A decade is a long time to live in chaos. Entire generations of kids have only seen disagreement, death, and infighting. But now it's over. We look forward to facing whatever adversity nature (or dissenters) send our way.

Policy with no market in sight

Policy and regulations became highly problematic in the immediate aftermath of the pandemic. The problem was to identify clear principles for who should be helped first, given the limited resources. The welfare states of Scandinavia even began to shiver in their foundations. Norway, even, a country with a pension fund the size of a percentage of the world economy, had a shattered skeleton left to build from. The first few months seemed relatively easy to deal with, in retrospect. There was money to go around in all national governments' coffers. Record high rescue packages were signed off on in parliaments around the world.

The next year, however, became a long one. As prime ministers and presidents attempted to restart society again and again, the weight of over half the world being offline, caught up in quarantines, extreme social distancing, and miserable choices, meant that there was only so much to go around. Markets would start up again for a few weeks, only to descend into chaos the next. Getting true confidence back in the market was difficult. Where would it start first? Some said China. Others said Europe. Yet again others said the US. In the end, global economics had to be rewritten.

Learning transformed—the campus model was abandoned

Behavioral economics now is the dominant subject in the university. Well, we haven't really covered that yet. Education has changed in so many ways as well, it is hardly possible to remember what it meant to go to college in the early 2000s. Back then, you might go to your local college and stay at home or be lucky enough that your parents paid for 4 years on a campus somewhere. In 2030, all colleges are online. We briefly tried blended learning for a while, where there still was a physical campus to go to and people had a choice between the online and the campus experience. But it simply became too expensive.

Can you imagine an entire generation being unable to pay for college? Can you imagine 100,000 colleges and universities scrambling for resources, trying to protect their campuses from the terrible virus that was still raging in society? Yes, I haven't even covered this yet. We never got rid of the virus. It is still in community spread and can reappear at any time. In fact, there are outbreaks ongoing still now. Just that they are all in small pockets of development countries that don't matter so much. I should get to that. We have fixed health systems in Africa, for the most part. That was expensive. In the end, it was a public-private partnership. Jill Mates, the founder of Petasoft, got 100 billionaires to sign on together with 1,000 of the world's biggest corporations, and all world governments. We fixed it in 2 years. Can you believe that? That's all it took. All of these years, millions of people died of infectious diseases, but, really, pretty mundane diseases, too. Turns out, we could have fixed it.

The price of fixing healthcare was that a lot of people started saying this about everything. If we have a societal problem, why don't we fix it rather than let it rage on? We tried it. We even had some more early successes. We got rid of pollution. We simply prohibited companies from polluting and had them pay hefty fees. It took 3 months. That was easy. What was harder, and I'm getting to the problem, was poverty. Remember the UN's Sustainable Development Goals. There's 17 of them. Most of them were not that hard to do, but poverty, that's hard.

So, we got rid of disease in most major metropolitan areas for now. That's a huge achievement. There were 47 megacities with more than 10 million inhabitants in the world in 2020, and we fixed all those. Then, over the next decade, since so few people died and everyone started living so much longer, they all wanted to live in cities, so we ended up with another 100 megacities. That's 147 megacities. We fixed healthcare in all of them. Oh, and we all practice social distancing, so we are not even that close together anymore.

As of 2024, these cities were huge. Five times bigger footage than before. But then, we started passing all the required legislation we had been waiting on. We realized that we can't be less than 6 feet away from anybody, ever, in order to keep the virus in check. In fact, that's prohibited now. We have the corona wave, the corona walk, and we even the corona kiss. What we don't have is corona sex—distance doesn't work among humans, apart from the brain stuff I talked about. But I'm reminiscing. What happened is that we had to abandon the idea of living in cities. Yes, you heard me. The whole thing. That was an adjustment. But the decision was made quickly, and it was a mass exodus. Moses and Noah's Ark kind of stuff. We spread out.

We need to talk about sports. After COVID, there was a 3-year sports void. It got so bad that the working classes in the UK revolted. They wanted their Premier League soccer back. And they did. Players who agree first get quarantined for 40 days, then live in separate compounds away from the rest of the world. They all live alone in these hyperclean military barracks of sorts. But they cannot socialize. It is a weird existence. They become media stars even more than before. You can only join for 1 year at a time. The game is played in empty stadiums. The bright side is, the cameras are much better now; the sensors make it really exciting to watch.

What's the problem here? The countryside. Pre-2025, those who don't live near a big city had nothing. We had to prioritize. After all, resources are not unlimited. At first, we sacrificed the people who didn't urbanize. Can you believe it? As of 2024, there were still people who loved to be outside, who would rather be in a diseased nature than inside with a sanitized environment, and near-perfect health. Rural populations always tended to be older, poorer, and less healthy than the national average. Healthcare systems in rural areas lacked resources and were short on doctors and nurses even before the crisis. It got pretty bad. Besides, all the elites have stopped coming. Now, the rich are all congregating in special resort towns that have built extra hospital facilities, and where you need an access card, country clubs of sorts. But, as I said, we then changed course completely. This idea of spreading out people on an even grid, each with a parcel of land is very land-of-Eden-like. Remember John Locke: life, liberty and the pursuit of property. Happiness was achieved by giving every family unit a small plot of land. Very small.

Industry consequences in borderless conditions

As we got the new order in place, the healthcare industry thrived. There was nothing like a confidence boost to ensure growth, which lasted throughout the decade. After the initial stress of having to provide a massive amount of emergency medicine without much medical equipment, medical staff around the world successfully lobbied to build out stockpiles. Health security and overall health infrastructure was the number one priority throughout the decade.

All countries rose to an acceptable 50 score on the Global Health Security Index based on health bonds and massive investments, debt relief, and a whole host of infrastructure projects that reached all the poorest countries in the world. World government had to mean health security for all, everywhere. Never another devastating pandemic, was the policy they all agreed on and implemented.

Finance proved surprisingly resilient. The financial

burden of the first 3 years of the decade was considerable, even too much for some countries. In fact, that's even why world government gained traction. It wasn't just the impetus of global health as much as the fact that the world's richest nations were downright broke. Consolidation just started to make more and more sense. After most of the world's financial elite agreed to a sit-down and went through how it would affect markets, the political deal was much easier.

Education was the second most important sector in Borderless World. Universal education became what people of the world felt would prepare them best for the coming decades. There was the shared idea that there was no time to lose. They wanted to educate a new cadre of scientists capable of making scientific breakthroughs at age 15 and up on average. Talent was picked out of slums, private schools, homeschooled kids—the race was on.

Higher education, starting at 12, became a highly efficient sector with the establishment of 100 Ivy League–style schools worldwide, which were more selective than Harvard is today, and a plethora of feeding schools. The other schools were largely left to themselves, as the notion was that excellence was the only thing that counts.

The energy industry shifted toward producing only sustainable energy from renewables. The oil industry was phased out over a few crucial years from 2023 to 2025 and then refocused.

Technology progressed in so many ways that it was breathtaking. The most impressive feat was perhaps the fusion of AI with the neural link, so that humans could morph with their digital avatar and download their memory to an everlasting AI.

Transportation became a crucial enabler of the massive project of unifying the world. Ground transportation, air travel, underground travel, space travel—there were innovations needed in each in order to be able to satisfy

COVID-19 social distancing concerns, environmental sustainability, and massively increased expectations for proximity to the world's outposts. The announcement was made, echoing De Gaulle's declaration that Paris should have a high-speed TVG (*Train à Grande Vitesse*) to each corner of France, that there would be high-speed transit to all corners of the globe, from and between each of the world capitals, which by now became tiny administrative centers, by the way. Building out this infrastructure took 20% of the workforce 5 years' worth of work, but on January 1, 2030, the job was done.

Travel rebounded quickly after the new safe means of transportation were rolled out, even though the full global rollout took many years and only will ready at the end of the next decade. Mass transit, of course, never came back. The notion of sitting tightly squeezed in a subway car just couldn't be brought back, even in cities like Tokyo. We got that early on. Leisure travel also took years to rebound. Business travel, however, came back, but only at 20% of its pre-2020 peak. There's not the same incentive to travel when where you travel to you cannot meet large groups, you cannot sightsee, and you cannot go out on the town.

Consumer sentiment was extremely weak at the beginning of the decade, but rebounded once the financial elite had agreed to support a global political union, and rose to record levels once a world government was announced.

Commodities, whether it was coffee, copper, or water, were not really an issue of great worry anymore. Toward of the end of the decade, scientific progress had fostered new materials that made precious materials less precious. Efficient industry structures took care of supply based on hyper-efficient extraction technologies and refinement plants. Commodity prices were reasonable and adjusted to local needs based on a global algorithm of purchasing power. Commodities was a good place to be on the disruption pyramid. The biggest conglomerates had been broken up, but regional players could still make good money, and the many smaller, innovative suppliers and vendors enjoyed great conditions.

Services just kept improving throughout the decade. Public services were all e-enabled throughout the globe, using the same three systems that had overlapping redundancies just in case of a crisis. The services industry had been completely rebuilt after the crisis, top to bottom. Being a food service worker was now a respected position comparable to being a part of the police or firefighting force. Health worker was the top of the food chain. Even nurses enjoyed high respect and had an upper-middle-class lifestyle now. Transportation services were all considered critical infrastructure and had professionalized into a set of powerful regional unions which demanded safe and equitable conditions across each region and globally.

Governments, which had become hyper-efficient, but not as lean as expected, given all the tasks of rebuilding and resilience the world government demanded (and the world's global citizens demanded from them). Imagine that senior public officials were famous again just like Greek and Roman senators in the classical period of antiquity. Nobody would have predicted!

Manufacturing was a whole different ball game now. The distributed nature of it, enhanced by additive manufacturing techniques, meant that factories became the cleanest, most efficient laboratories you could think of. Soon, each city had their own manufacturing facilities; in fact, each street corner had their own large-scale printing facility. New types of materials emerged, which meant an expanded marketplace. Demand just wouldn't seem to have any end as the sky was the limit.

The aerospace industry took on a new meaning now that everyone had their own satellite and was saving up for space flight as the 2031 Mars mission edged near. Massive space ferries were constructed to handle the first tourist mission to the red planet which would also tour the moon and include a stopover on one of Mars' two moons, alternating between Phobos and Deimos.

Media can mean many things. The media industry had gone through a lot of changes throughout the decade, starting with the renewed fast-speed internet which was gearing up to allow particle transmission to prepare for quantum travel of objects and, quite possibly, of living things toward the end of the next decade. The newly emerged newspapers were little more than highly efficient blog networks. Strikingly creative writers had bubbled up from the former slums of Delhi, Caracas and perhaps especially from Lagos. The stories they came up with! They didn't miss a beat and provided this new creative undercurrent that provided such a comic relief for the science heavy megacities that were bubbling up with hygienic precision on each corner of the planet. It was really a bummer when we had to disperse away from that effervescence of the city!

Food industry developments included synthetic food that tasted fantastic as it was artificially enhanced by the new super enzymes that were developed in UK labs. The variety of foods was just thrilling. What a great idea it had been to start providing nutritional compounds inspired by every element in the periodic table. Likewise, the idea to use food trucks to solve the food distribution problem in slums across the world. Well, calling them slums was a misnomer toward 2030, as they were more like a futuristic version of the tiny-house movement, complete with designer living, anti-COVID-19 coatings, and powerful nanotech based cooling systems replacing traditional HVAC systems with 10,000X efficiency pouring clean air through the densest urban corners.

Conglomerates still thrived, but they were all collectively owned now, since large companies beyond 500 employees and

$7M revenue were automatically broken up, unless they were pharmaceutical companies or promising technology startups, which were given a 3-year grace period in the name of scientific progress and saving the planet, two worthwhile concerns.

Nonprofits were almost the engine of the economy. They were governed rather differently though, as they went through a managerial revolution and started operating more like businesses, just with an outright social target. The new aspect was that they were required to report progress on a transparent community contribution scale that was open for all to see. Needless to say, some nonprofits were never ready for this kind of scrutiny, but those who were, thrived.

Hospitality was an industry hit hard by the coronavirus. The travel industry rebounded very slowly, and one could honestly not really speak of a rebound until the end of the decade. But as confidence in public health measures on airplanes and in local accommodation grew, the tourists started coming back. Mass tourism, however, was outlawed. What happened was a redistribution of tourists evenly throughout every city in the world, based on a world-government-established quota system.

Marine industries thrived during the decade because of the high importance placed on extracting food and energy from the oceans. Our scientists were even able to save 1,000 marine species that were about to become extinct. Offshore oil, obviously, was scaled down and eventually phased out in a controlled way that allowed those businesses to pivot to worthier concerns and commercial opportunities related to aquaculture. The countries that had access to a major ocean extracted the major benefits, but even landlocked countries enjoyed the benefits of ocean-based industries through their shared ownership and peer-to-peer models.

Telecom was still a winning industry, but not in the way one might assume. Communications changed a lot in a decade.

People stopped using cell phones, but only because the telecommunications firms launched a new way of communicating through a neural link. What that meant was that there was no external device needed in order to communicate. You were simply wired to the network directly, or your brain was, anyway. You only had to think of somebody when you would be prompted to potentially get in touch with them. In fact, if two people thought positive thoughts about each other simultaneously, the connection would be made automatically, with the option to engage at a given level of emotion.

The only challenge was the multitude of signals that human beings emit, and the limited attention span we still struggle with. With computers it was easier, as their 1000-fold increased efficiencies throughout the decade enabled even home computers using clustered resources in the cloud to conduct a plethora of parallel tasks. The improvements in CPU, chips, and parallelizing through container-based virtualization was simply amazing. Toward the end of the century, Moore's Law was finally abandoned because the efficiencies of quantum computing skyrocketed.

Defense industry concerns were initially a worry, given that with one world government one would have to rethink the role of the military. There were two answers to this. First, the existing military was redeployed as a public health force as well as a civil defense force more generally, taking more the role that FEMA would have taken in the US, combined with a role as the global government's last resort police force for highly extreme circumstances. Beyond that, the global space command provided a focus on space defense against potential aggressive alien missions to our solar system, of which there had been none so far by 2030, as far as we know.

Population reduction coming

Lastly, I should point out, we are planning to reduce the

population by 10% every year over the next decade. We did some simulations in 2029. As it turns out, we cannot support any more people. Right now, the population is growing exponentially, and this is not sustainable. The irony is, the pandemic actually killed off exactly as many old people as we needed in order to achieve the savings required for a major push in science and technology. It worked out well. But now, we need another push. We are planning a big vote in world government next year to approve the measure. We are hoping to implement it through some sort of "natural departure." There's great tension, because some scientists are very proud that we've achieved a "possible" average life span of 120 years. What's now being proposed is to cut that back to 70 for unhealthy people and 100 for healthy, intelligent contributors.

I've read that, according to folklore, the Swedish Vikings practiced ritual senicide (ättestupa) during Nordic prehistoric times, whereby elderly people threw themselves, or were thrown, to their deaths. I'm hoping we come up with something more civilized. Euthanasia has come a long way since the Vikings. Simply stopping treatments of certain diseases at age 60 would be a strategy that could work. We have music, fantastic psychedelics, and counselors, too. I'm sure they will find a way to get volunteers for at least 20% of the reduction. One can at least hope so.

Imagining a borderless world

What feelings do you get around a borderless world? Is it appealing?

Each scenario has fault lines, for example, where people and interests clash. Name a few such aspects of a borderless world.

Preventing or fostering a borderless world

Decide whether you want this scenario to happen or not. Then take a different tack. Let's imagine you could pick two to three elements or remove two to three elements from the scenario.

Which aspects would you pick?

Which aspects would you remove?

Finally, it's also possible that there are so-called path dependencies. This means that if scenario A happens, then B, C, and D likely follow. Try to name a few such path dependencies in this scenario.

CHAPTER 5

SCENARIO II: NATION-STATE RENEWAL

The scenario considers a permanent situation where borders close down and people stop traveling huge distances, because of a principle of proximity where long-distance travel and contact with more than 50 people a week is discouraged, at times outlawed. *From now on, and throughout this chapter, you are entering the realm of fiction.*

We are in 2030, and it's been a tumultuous decade. Not so much because of the pandemic; we solved that one well although it took a few years to get back on track. No, the real challenges we had were about how to coordinate international relief efforts and how to move forward with international collaboration. But we had successes as well, mostly related to technological progress, which helped us stay together, alone.

Tech for everyone

3D Printing is everywhere. You can now print anything you need for the house at home as long as it is less than 10 cubic feet, at which point you simply go to the corner store and pick it up or have it delivered. The pandemic sped up the production of anything that would help us enjoy being at home more. 3D printing is a killer application. It is 100 times more transformative than the cell phone and so much more useful.

I know we were about to implement 5G mobile broadband in 2020 as the pandemic hit. Now, the richer nation-states like the Scandinavian countries, Singapore, Qatar, and Germany, all have 8G with near-unlimited broadband. Just to give you a sense, I can download Hollywood's entire catalog of films through the ages in a mere 5 minutes. What this does is it has made work-from-home work like a charm. Healthcare can also be received right in our home. They will even ship you a robotic surgical arm you can connect to a computer and it will perform simple surgeries with only an android nurse assisting.

Artificial intelligence just got approved for full autonomy, meaning we now trust it to make decisions on our behalf. That is to say, it's only available for the top 1% so far. It costs the same as buying a car every month. Not all of us can afford the monthly subscription. AI is highly useful for most things.

Augmented reality is a hit, too. I don't have to visit my grandmother anymore. She shows up as a hologram. That's a big savings in airline tickets. Not that anybody flies anymore. It's restricted and only available by permit. Politicians fly, of course, and corporate executives, but only one per row.

Autonomous driving is now fully put in place. It was needed to restart public transportation. We don't have buses, commuter trains, or subways anymore. Well, we have them. We just don't use them much. There is no maintenance of those kinds of facilities. Everything is personalized now. These drone taxis take you where you want to go—if you can afford it.

Blockchain is a game changer. It didn't look like much in 2020 or even in 2025. The killer application was when countries put their national budgets and all trading on the blockchain in 2027. Oh, and I almost forgot, blockchain is used to do personal shopping as well; we have basically reintroduced a barter economy. I should probably explain, blockchain is this transparent ledger technology that enables everyone to see every transaction that has been made, sort of like opening up the books, you know, without revealing the identity of those who have traded. By increasing transparency, you drop the fraud to zero. We gained back 30% of the global economy, which was informal and black market.

CRISPR, the gene-editing method, has proven very useful in re-jiggering small children's DNA so they won't get COVID-19. What we do is manipulate the most common genetic defects related to breathing under stress. Kids are able to increase their lung capacity by 40%, which is sufficient to survive COVID-19 without the need of a ventilator in most cases. For the rest, there's always the antibody cures, thanks to the top scientists in Europe and the US.

Cybersecurity, well that's a big challenge. Given that the trust is not so big now between the nations, there are cyberattacks daily. Each country wants to know what the other is up to, particularly regarding technology. There is a lot of theft of state secrets. Contrary to what everyone thought, there is less rather than more collaboration than before the virus.

Precision medicine has evolved, in Germany in particular. Scientists there have personalized treatments for most major diseases. It is not available for free, though. This is private health insurance territory, a shocker for Germany, but after the EU issues (I haven't gotten to those yet), it became too expensive.

Nanotechnology is only just starting for real. The first nanobots are now at work on construction sites. It's funny but the first-use case for nanotech is in cleaning. Turns out these tiny machines we made can clean biological matter very efficiently. They essentially devour it. Fascinating to watch, we have these trackers that follow the nanomachines at all times. We have to. Imagine losing them somewhere. You never know what might happen. We cannot control the technology so well yet.

Quantum computing didn't pan out. Turns out, the quantum simulators cannot do the job. The qubits seem impossible to stabilize. We can do some types of advanced computations, but the computers disintegrate afterward, and sometimes it's dangerous, at least that's what I've heard. We'll look to the future for that one. Governments are mostly happy. After COVID-19, they were so behind that coming up with quantum proof cryptography was the least of their concerns. But I've heard the Chinese have a prototype. We'll see.

Robotics is fun these days. The robots look nothing like we expected. Few of us have humanoid robots, or androids, I guess they were called a while back. Instead, they help us clean, carry stuff, and do the homework. They are also great at entertaining kids.

Smart fabrics, now that's a story. We use them for two things, hygienic self-cleaning clothes and to cover up nature when we are outside. We have had to become really careful with being outside. There are always viruses lurking. It's easy to become paranoid.

Synthetic biology is a true game changer. We've carefully regulated it so that it cannot change the germline of humans or any of the larger organisms in nature. However, printing synthetic medicine on demand is better than going to the pharmacy.

Virtual reality isn't really there yet, but augmented reality is pretty good, as I pointed out earlier.

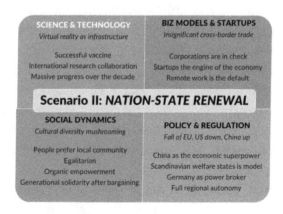

Figure 5.1. Nation-State Renewal

Resurrecting live mass event sports

Berlin, June 12, 2030: *"The Argentina-Brazil game in the 2030 world cup of soccer is just about to kick off," says the announcer on the radio. "We are coming in live from the Olympiastadion in Berlin where 5,000 people have been allowed to watch the game, in the first international mass sports event in a decade." The voice continues, "This is the first ever Class IV Public Hygiene-certified public venue with a capacity beyond 500 people. Obviously, everyone is sitting 6 feet apart, and there are strict rules for social distancing. No alcoholic beverages are sold, to the disappointment of all the German brewers who are left with advertising their online shopping options."*

The British announcer, Thomas Moorhead, continues, suddenly with a cracking voice: "I'm 60 years old. Before the age of the viruses, I had watched every soccer final since I was 5 years old. But I thought I might never see a live championship ever again. I'm sorry, I don't mean to be emotional." Over the radio, one can hear Moorhead quavering. It is a moment the audience will remember. Quickly recovering, he goes on to say: "It's a big day for Germany and a big day for the world. Ten years ago, on the day, Berlin was on its knees because of a virus, today the 200 flags of the world are again waving from the Olympiastadion. This is not just a victory for sports, but for humankind. May the best team win and the countries they represent be proud."

Over the past decade, sports had been severely curtailed. The first few years, there had been next to nothing. Then, intermittently, some games were played for empty stadiums. Seemed like a good idea at the time. That didn't catch on and the sports lost a lot of momentum and the sponsors disappeared. Then, toward mid-decade, there was a period of Augmented Reality, where sensors placed at all angles would give you a 360-degree view of how the players felt, their health, their blood sugar levels, even their adrenalin spikes, which Thomas didn't care much for. After a while, online sports were the only game allowed. The betting on virtual sports teams took off!

This was a big day in more than one way. It was the first game but also the first year Thomas was symptom free. COVID-19 had hit hard and then hit hard again. Thomas got it three times the last 7 years, having narrowly escaped the first outbreak. For the first time in nearly a decade, he felt free to breathe the air of this city where the anticipation of a great game seemed to crackle over the field.

The immediate aftermath—the best and the worst

It was the best of times. It was the worst of times. After the pandemic, which initially lasted about 2 years, with intermittent stay-at-home orders cascading through the world followed by months of near normalcy and open markets, stores, and schools, most countries decided to hunker down and build their own societies up almost from scratch.

What did intermittency mean in practice? Well, in Europe it meant 4 weeks off, 4 weeks on; the unions had even put it as a condition. That way, the workers couldn't be fired in the meantime. At the same time, employers needed relief. In welfare states, the government paid the difference at 50% salary. It was at least something. Each country had their own solution. It was frustrating, but better than the alternative.

The intermittency policy

The intermittency was key to fighting off the disease. It was also key to avoiding full societal breakdown. After months of stay-at-home, most people were tired of it. Some more than others. People living in small, one-bedroom apartments downtown could barely handle a lockdown or curfew. After a few weeks, some of them snapped. Those unemployed had little to do and resorted to drinking, pornography, and even a bit of playful violence in their surroundings.

Criminal networks had a field day. In the absence of government intervention, they were more than willing to provide "protection services" against eternal loyalty and 20%-a-month interest, sort of like the credit card companies, in fact.

Those in relationships who were not living together started to question whether they really loved the person they had spent so many weeks months apart from. People on the brink of divorce who were still living in the same household were at the point of bursting apart, some committed suicide or started domestic violence against their partner. It was a troubled time.

Elementary school children were tired of the endless, boring online assignments with little live action and all the teacher mistakes. The psychological toll was especially hard on the elderly, who in addition to the isolation now had to live with the very real and present danger of death right outside their doorstep.

Why was it also the best of times? Because surprising small pockets of gladness burst through the sadness and despair like green shoots up from dead earth in spring. The Spanish population had taken to thanking the first responders by going out on their verandas and clapping for them at 8:00 p.m. every night. People were volunteering like never before. They sewed face masks or ran their 3D printers to create transparent face shields needed as emergency protection in hospitals. People ran soup kitchens and volunteered at shelters at great risk to their own health, with only homemade protection, given the shortages.

Love was thriving, between couples who lived together, between friends, online, and among those quarantined together. Strong, near-unbreakable bonds were built. Deep experiences were shared. Those who spent years together became like the Israelites in captivity in Egypt—they became one.

Some wealthy people, and many companies, gave up their own medical supplies so the local hospital wouldn't run out. Others, it must be said, hoarded ventilators for themselves, even outbid governments for them and procured personal physicians doing house calls, taking them away from disaster duties. For the elite, this was a difficult time. Difficult to stand out as a good example. Difficult to be different. Difficult to navigate.

Singapore, May 16, 2024: "Tian, will you help me with the door?" His mom had gone out for groceries, even though the online delivery had already arrived. She wanted her special vegetables and the tea that could only be found in the corner shop. Tian knew what his mother really wanted: to remember what it was like to be able to go shopping. Tian was angry at her for risking going out; they lived in the Holland Road garden homes. They were part of an elite, but this did not shield them from the economic downturn. The virus had hit everyone, even with the improvements to their national center for infectious diseases. There was nowhere to go. Singapore had fared very well. But Malaysia had not, and they were neighboring countries. The causeway that links Malaysia and Singapore is one of the busiest land border crossings in the world, with 300,000 people crossing every day. The disease spread, again and again, but Singapore fought it back, seemingly endlessly. It had happened 10 times now, 10 smaller outbreaks, all quelled after a month.

But going back into lockdown all the time was tiring. The Singaporean government called it a period of intermittency. They would open up the city-state for business only to lock it down again after a month, or a week, or even a day; it became pretty erratic. It was all based on a mathematical model. More like terror, thought Tian. And no one seemed more terrified than his mother. His music business was near bankrupt. He depended on doing concerts and they all kept getting canceled.

Not that a lot of people could gather anyway. The limit was 50 people, 6 feet apart. The ticket prices for these kinds of events skyrocketed. Some people thrived on the risk. Where else could you listen to contemporary beats and have a slight sense of being a daredevil? This was perfect for Singaporean Millennials. But lately, he had experienced two delays and one cancellation due to the outbreaks. His friends had told him to turn to the online market, but how could he compete in that glutted environment? It was beyond frustrating. He wanted to scream, but instead he simply said, "Yes, Mom." "I love living with you again and thanks for bringing my favorite tea," he said. He was serious. The tea was good. His mom was great. And he was poor. It all worked out.

Economically, social distancing and shutdown of business-as-usual was a disaster. Unemployment was the highest since the war, and in some countries it was even higher.

The recovery took longer in Asia and Africa than elsewhere since the devastation was enormous in each of their megacities. These cities acted as incubators of superspreading events at mass scale. Enormous outbreaks happened in Delhi, Jakarta, and Tokyo, with combined death tolls of millions of people. Other megacities were not spared either and had sizeable outbreaks and big political fallout, economic crisis, and working-class populations at the brink of disaster.

The near loss of the EU

By 2022, Europe was back up again, although the EU had lost a lot of support. They really fell apart during the pandemic. First, the European Parliament was shut out of key discussions, so people started worrying even more about the democratic deficit, which steadily was an undercurrent of worry. European Union finance ministers failed, again and again, to agree on a strategy to mitigate the economic impact of the virus pandemic. Apart from an initial economic relief package and support to startups—both were great—they provided no medical supplies (although their procurement package included significant purchases of Chinese personal protective equipment), no support in terms of food or basic infrastructure support, and little political guidance to its member-states.

The response was bureaucratic and without heart, just like the critics of the EU always have said. The Prime Minister of Italy, the hardest hit country, said it best: "I never thought I would say this, but in the time of crisis, we were alone. There is no Europe." He was willing to test it out. In fact, Italy almost broke out of the EU, but in the end, the referendum tipped in the other direction and they voted to stay with 53–47%.

I don't know what people expected. The EU was set up as a regional trading block, not as a relief organization. Much of the criticism is unfair, which was something all political leaders across Europe realized, too, after a while. They came back together, united in a new way, but not with any expectations of a political project. Rather, it was now further clarified that the EU had an important role in furthering trade and coordinating policies toward the now weaker US, the stronger China, the resurgent Russia, the adamant Iran, and the emerging India.

<u>*European Commission, Brussels, Belgium, November 2, 2022:*</u> *"I just want to go for a quick beer," said Martin, a young, carefree bureaucrat working in the Foreign Affairs Cabinet. "Come with me to Ralphs on Place Lux?" "They closed Ralph's yesterday. The virus, remember?" said Denise. Place du Luxembourg in Ixelles was in the Middle of the European Quarter and up until the arrival of the virus, it had been the epicenter of young Eurocrats' political awakening, dating life, and socialization. This is where you became a true European, according to most young people working in Brussels throughout the 2000s. Now, it was a deserted zombie square in town, frequented only by those who had to cross it to get to the European Parliament, which was also near deserted these*

days. He couldn't have known it, but Martin's ability to forget was a privilege. He could push the virus from his mind. Denise couldn't. She had lost her mother to COVID-19 and could never forget. Anything. She was just trying to build herself back up.

A young, beautiful French stagiaire, *with her whole life ahead of her, Denise had been working at the European Parliament all along, the last 2 years remotely, even though her flat was just 3 minutes from the office. In a different world, she knew her life would be populated with dinners, dates, evenings with friends. But that world was more alien that Martin in this moment. It was surreal. The whole thing was surreal, felt Denise. But she was hanging in there. It was a miracle they hadn't sent all the stagiaires home. But the EU needed young working bees. There was still so much paperwork. Even more than before, it seemed. Well, it wasn't actually paper anymore, but it was piles of electronic pages on her laptop.*

America– the sick man of the new world order

The most surprising thing, to me, was what happened in America. The world's biggest economy really crumbled under the pressure. It probably didn't help that they had a president who showed few signs of being a "wartime" president throughout the crisis. Yet, his support stayed strong for the first 6 months. It even got him reelected, but then things fell apart from there. Most journalists attribute what happened to a toxic political culture where the infighting between the Republicans and the Democrats just didn't let up. In the end, the response was too little, too late. That is, the US actually went bankrupt. It couldn't fulfill its loan obligations and was declared bankrupt by the World Bank. Not that this was such a unique occurrence; it happened to 60% of the world's major economies, countries like France, the UK, India, Brazil, and Indonesia.

Why didn't the US handle the crisis well? It's not that mysterious. As Hans Rosling wrote in his book *Factfulness*

(2018), "The US is the sickest of the rich," even though they spend twice as much on healthcare than the other countries at a comparable standard of living—and even before the crisis lived 3 years shorter, on average. The absence of public basic health insurance had really hit them hard. The poorest part of the population got near decimated by COVID-19. With higher infection rates, many living in dense urban slums, black and other underprivileged folks had much higher death rates than the rest of the population.

The US economy took a big hit in the crisis. For many years, unemployment soared around 30%, which doesn't sound like much, after all that's the amount they have been dealing with in parts of southern Italy throughout the late 2000s. But for a US economy used to near-full employment it has been hard. People just don't trust the government so much, but that is slowly changing. There is nowhere else to turn, as we all realize that the private sector must take care of its own concerns. In times of crisis, government is the only thing you can lean on.

Mid-decade normalcy

Everyday life continued as usual throughout the middle of the decade. People got up in the morning, went to work, loved, went to church, got married, and divorced. The workplace hadn't changed much. It looked like it was going to the first few years, but as the virus fears subsided with the successful vaccine, the disease fell further and further back in people's daily consciousness. People stopped wearing face masks, cheated with social distancing, didn't care so much about the risks they were taking by going to restaurants, walking around shopping malls, or going to smaller sports events. The big events were already gone by 2021. In fact, Major League sports were all played for empty stadiums—which then prompted folks to suggest playing in much smaller venues optimized for camera angles not spectators.

Augmented reality really helped out. Watching baseball, basketball, football, rugby, and soccer became different experiences entirely. You could suddenly see the game from each player's perspective. You could switch mid-game, and you could even pretend to be a fan of the other team for a few minutes to really get the juices flowing. Immersion became the name of the game. People took it far. It was the only true entertainment we had had in years.

Cleveland, Ohio, 2028: As Sue's roommate put sunscreen on her, the young woman could not help but think about how exposure to sunshine seemed so trivial in comparison to what else they might be exposing themselves to. Not today, she thought, and pushed the idea from her mind. After much discussion, they had decided to take the risk. Each beach was allotted 100 hygiene slots, neatly arranged along the beach with markings and signage; they had won their lottery. How could they not take it? It wasn't exactly the roaring 2010s with thousands of drunk teens spilling into bars and restaurants.

What happened in 2020 when spring breakers caused a massive outbreak in southern US was still on everyone's mind. The data scientists tracking cell phone signals had uncovered a disturbing contagion pattern. Everywhere a spring breaker returned, an outbreak started. Each went exponential, not infecting five or 10 people, but, ultimately thousands.

All told, it was estimated that the Florida Spring Break massacre, as it was now called, prolonged the US exposure to coronavirus by 6 months. Estimates were not guaranteed, but of the 100,000 that died, half were attributed to the Spring Break outbreak. Well, it was history now. Sue was only 7 when the outbreak started. She was the youngest of a family of five in Cleveland, Ohio. In the very first months ensuing the coronavirus pandemic, she grew up. Fast. It was as if she went from 7 to 15 in an instant. She had started doing chores in the house, at first because her mother said so. Then, she started doing the laundry because nobody else had the energy to do it, since the weekly cleaning staff were on an indefinitely hold due to the contagion risk. Then, she took to making dinner twice a week. With only a little help she managed to put the dinner on the table and only with very few burns.

She had only one distinct memory from 2020. It was her mother crying. "Why are you crying, Mom?" she had asked. "Nothing," said her mom. "Just that 3 months ago you were playing in the garden. Now, you are doing chores I only started when I was a teenager. I'm so sorry that we can't offer you a proper childhood." That phrase had stuck: a proper childhood.

Her brother had almost gone on spring break that year, but her father, a heart surgeon at the esteemed Cleveland Clinic, had stopped him, looked him in the eye and said: "If I were your age, nothing would stop me from getting on the plane for Florida. I respect what you're giving up. That's why I'm offering you an out: you stay, and I'll get you a car." Her brother took the old Toyota. He needed to drive to the Cleveland Orchestra rehearsals where he played the viola. The Toyota and the viola, she was not sure which, had saved his life. Probably ours, too, Sue thought to herself. Not today, she reminded herself, and tried to consider nothing but the rays beating down on her, the waves crashing along the shore. The more familiar vista of Lake Erie suddenly seemed far away. She had grown up indeed, no question about it.

The rise of China as an internationally dominant economic actor

For China, the pandemic was a big boon. Economists say the pandemic accelerated China's rise to prominence by at least a decade. In the beginning, it was just propaganda. People kind of laughed it off. China started saying the virus hadn't been caused by them. Rather, the virus had started in northern Italy in October and November of 2019 and had been brought to

Wuhan by Italian expat Chinese. The Italian region of Lombardy (which includes the city of Milan) has the biggest Chinese expat populations in Italy.

Throughout 2020, however, the narrative took a different turn. Now it wasn't just a story. China was exporting its medical supplies the world over. In the beginning, they prioritized their "friends." Small countries such as Norway, which now were friends of China again, having been out in the cold for a few years after having given the Nobel Peace Prize to a Chinese dissenter Liu Xiaobo back in 2010 got a bunch of supplies. It was brokered by Jack Ma, the Internet billionaire.

Later, China reached out its big manufacturing hand to African nations. Billions of face masks were delivered in record time as state aid to ten chosen countries in Africa. As a result, China likely saved a million lives. But they were greatly rewarded. Chinatowns in Africa are a little different than Chinatowns elsewhere. They are now the financial districts in these 10 countries.

The Chinese quickly established a financial oversight authority for Africa, charged with building capitalism on Chinese terms. This was a term originally coined by MIT professor Yasheng Huang in his book, *Capitalism with Chinese Characteristics: Entrepreneurship and the State* (2008). What it meant in China in the 1990s and what they managed to push through in Africa was a weak financial sector, income disparity, rising illiteracy, productivity slowdowns, and reduced personal income growth. The advantage is to maintain state control and still rapidly develop the economy, a paradox that Western democracies never grasped nor fully understood (nor really wanted).

By 2030, they are the world's unrivaled economy, with influence around the world. Their Africa strategy has particularly paid off. It is estimated that China now owns 20% of real estate and 10% of businesses throughout Africa. But those statistics don't tell the whole story. China has been smart. Their investments are only in countries where they have the most combined economic and cultural impact. Chinese TV is the biggest station in Angola, Tanzania, and throughout Southern Africa, in fact.

China's influence in Asia is growing, too. After India crumbled during the pandemic, and Japan entered another decade of stagflation, they were the only Asian superpower left, if you disregard Russia.

A few words about Russia are perhaps warranted. Vladimir Putin is still at the helm in Kremlin; he enacted the new law already back in 2020, which gave him near lifetime rule. People appreciate a strongman in times of crisis. But the people are still suffering. Putin has set up a cordon sanitaire around Moscow. It lasts beyond the pandemic. What it means is that he has concentrated the wealth of Russia even further. He also likes Saint Petersburg, though, and has maintained one railway line that connects the two, although the roads have been cut off. Life in Moscow is as usual. People go out, they party, they drink, and they enjoy sports on TV.

Scandinavian welfare states reel but recover

In Scandinavia, the past decade has been quite interesting. The Nordic states, in particular, have fared quite well in the crisis. Initially, there was a major challenge surrounding maintaining the welfare state. The government's promises of salaries, pensions, and social security just couldn't be kept at the level as before. But people understand.

In Norway, the state pension fund, the biggest per capita in the world, was deployed aggressively to stem the depression. Estimates are they have spent near half of it this decade and they aim to spend it completely down by the next 5 years, after which they will simply be another country living year-to-year. What got Norway was its independent monetary policy as well as the complete collapse in the oil prize. With oil trading around $15/barrel throughout the decade, the government's main industry suffered greatly.

One consequence was that young Norwegians have stopped traveling. Before, you'd always see Norwegians in tourist spots around the world, and drunk on the Canary Islands. Now, because of the fall of the local currency, it was cheaper to vacation in Norway. However, only by car. The only flights that were affordable anymore were business flights to Brussels and London. The two domestic carriers went bankrupt already in the first 6 months of the crisis. The Scandinavian carrier made it through, but only after so many state subsidies that they had to increase prices by 300% to make it through the next decade.

Also, the EU put in a moratorium on using non-renewables. The EU calls it the Green Pandemic Shift, attempting to link the two crises the world has been facing this decade, the climate crisis and the pandemic.

Why do I feel this decade has been good to the nation-states? I think because most people had assumed that they would all fail to deliver on the basic promise of any state—that of securing the basic rights and responsibilities for its citizens. Moreover, nobody assumed that prosperity would return. But it has. In pockets of society, understandably, but it has returned, nevertheless.

Politicians are a bit different these days. The winning politicians all have nationalist platforms. Not that they all are strongmen, although they have also done very well. Countries that already were leaning toward the extreme right did predictably all establish governments, in some cases majority governments.

European Nations rebel against the European Commission

In Europe, this first happened in Austria before the crisis, and then in 2021 in The Netherlands, followed by France with National Front. Soon thereafter the big one, it happened in Germany, which everybody was watching.

It did happen again. Germany got a nationalist government. Nobody is calling it "Nazi government"; that would be too extreme a label. However, it isn't exactly the Christian Democrats. Let's look at their policies: full build-up of the military, which hasn't happened since 1945. The story is that they want to build an emergency response force that just happens to also have self-defense weapons. It kind of makes sense.

Germany was the most prepared country in Europe during the 2019–2021 pandemic. France doesn't like it, of course. Not sure if it's the fact that Germany has emerged as the new global superpower in the vacuum left from the US and given that China's economic superpower still hasn't produced the diplomatic finesse to navigate international waters in Europe and the US without friction. Germany is a bit of a powerbroker between Russia and a weakened EU and holds up clear boundaries (and requirements) against Turkey, which still hasn't made it into the EU.

The principle of proximity

The most important principle now is the principle of proximity. What does that entail? Let me explain. The governance principle we all, mostly, adhere to is that power can only be granted to somebody who is within 3 hour's drive. What it means is that regions have been granted more autonomy in some countries, so when I say nation-states, some of them have actually near broken apart and become more like federalist states.

This is the case in Spain, where Catalonia has near full autonomy now. The same has happened in Belgium, where Wallonia has broken apart from Flandern, and in Italy where the north, having been devastated by the crisis, refused to pay for the build-up of the south, which was similarly devastated, but has no chance of building back up in one decade. In Italy, the north is now openly calling itself Padania and is about to establish full independence from the rest of Italy. Siberia has broken away from Russia, Guangdong from China, Kashmir from India, Hokkaido from Japan, Khmers from Vietnam, Asir from Saudi-Arabia, and Bali from Indonesia.

Another facet of the proximity rule is that we are not allowed to gather more than 50 people at a time, so there is no point traveling for long distances for large meetings or sports events. Instead, we stay local, with some exceptions.

Technology helps with the proximity imperative. In fact, virtual reality has been especially helpful. It only took 3 years, and in 2023 the EU declared virtual reality part of critical infrastructure, and started regulating it, putting it in the same category as TV and electricity. Virtual reality (VR) is now so good that we can experience true emotions and act out scenarios with our hands and feet and all our senses without moving more than a few feet and using our headset and advanced sensors. We even perform operations in VR, we have sports in VR, and we let our elderly enter VR when they cannot walk anymore. It has become more than a hobby for the elderly—they depend on it for company and excitement.

People have generally found that they like their own kind. Not that they have a choice. Travel has become a nuisance—no, more than that, a chore. Business travel commands a premium salary, you literally get paid to take greater risk of viral exposure. The statistics are clear. Those who travel by air once a month have a 20% higher chance of contracting a serious infectious disease. Many find this is not worth it, even as healthcare has recovered and most doctors know what to do if you contract something serious.

Industry consequences in nation-state renewal

The healthcare industry changed drastically both during and after the crisis. During the crisis, healthcare workers became more highly appreciated. Their demands were taken seriously, even though governments couldn't immediately respond to the equipment shortages.

However, that was only a logistical setback and a year of full wartime production took care of the ventilator issues in the major countries, although it still was a massive issue in the lesser countries. The debate about universal healthcare raged wildly in every country. The Scandinavian countries became increasingly viewed as "honeypot" and got drastically increased immigration based on this fact. In the US, part of the political settlement after the crisis was a sort of national healthcare plan that stopped short of universal healthcare but at least afforded the right to free emergency care.

Finance is a resilient sector, but the nationalization of finance meant much lower margins. Only the biggest countries came up net positive when the markets readjusted. The smaller countries became poorer and goods were more limited.

Education became national priorities in every country. Nobody wanted to be left behind. However, building quality education takes time, is expensive, and is difficult to do. Not every country managed educational reform. Some countries completely failed at it. No country managed to keep their top-tier institutions unscathed from the nationalization wave. The world's top 100 universities declined in publication rates, rankings, and lost a lot of international faculty and students, some never regained their elite status. K-12 education rebounded based on national curricula, but largely had to go online because of the virus, which was not universally easy to do for teaching staff who had poor tech literacy to begin with.

The energy industry fared well with the national agenda, and simply retooled to slightly smaller markets. Some of the more innovative, experimental demand-response-based business models even thrived based on a more controllable market.

Technology developed relatively rapidly throughout the decade, but due to the lack of globalization, technologies took longer to get to market and some startups that would have become unicorns failed because they couldn't find talent fast enough.

Transportation was a priority, but the strain of catering to the COVID-19 restrictions upon social distancing killed off public transportation in most cities. Retooled business models and completely rebuilt buses and subways was the result, but some of that took years to implement.

Travel became highly reduced both as a priority and as a possibility. Businesses relying on travel largely went bankrupt. The exception was high end, "authentic" travel experiences where everything was preplanned, from destinations to each interaction. That process became quite complicated, given the permits and distancing rules that vary across even the same region and can change on a moment's notice.

Consumer confidence stayed at a steady low throughout the decade although there were a few bright spots in Germany and in Scandinavia where consumers continued to spend aggressively.

Commodities became largely nationalized. The production of metals (such as gold, silver, platinum, and copper) would happen locally and if any export was needed, the tariffs would amount to a significant percentage of the transaction. With regard to energy (such as crude oil, heating oil, natural gas, and gasoline), there was almost no trade of this precious resource across borders, as it was considered a critical infrastructure resource. Livestock and meat were similarly not exported anymore, but not just for national reasons, mostly for the food security risk it posed. Agricultural commodities (such as corn, soybeans, wheat, rice, cocoa, coffee, cotton, and sugar) were exported under significant tariffs and were only traded in kind for other similar commodities, in a modern-day barter system.

The services sector became a huge, and important part of

the national economies that surged after the COVID-19 pandemic. In fact, service workers got the same status as military service personnel and were granted full veteran status after ended service, given their increased exposure to the virus. For some countries, the cost of services spiraled near out of control, as the VAT on services grew to almost 50%.

Government services were obviously important in an era of nation-state resurgence. The sector itself didn't innovate much but ballooned in size. "I'm from the government, I'm here to help" became a standing joke even in countries that traditionally believed very much in their government, such as the Scandinavian welfare states. The government wasn't very well liked by the end of the decade, perhaps because the policy of intermittency and all the other regulations that became necessary gradually wore out the public.

The manufacturing industry built in numerous redundancies, grew in size, and each country made sure they manufactured not only most of their medical equipment but that they also had stockpiled even masks and gloves. The stockpile program grew so huge that the storage had to be built underground as well as under the sea, for the countries that had that option. As for the efficiencies, they were notable, but not earth shattering. The collapse of a working global supply chain reduced the incentive to build international conglomerates. Instead, manufacturers focused on cozying up to national and local governments in order to extract rents from as few customers as possible.

Aerospace was not a major factor this decade. The space program in the US was abandoned out of cost concerns, Russia had enough with staying afloat, and the Chinese refocused their efforts elsewhere, as nobody seemed to care about space anymore.

Media got reenergized under the national focus, which brought back the newspaper barons, strengthened TV's grip on the consumer, and brought e-commerce in all its forms to all screens in the house.

Food is always a major priority to any nation. Food security became number one priority in the middle of the decade and that lasted almost to the end. There was a strong emphasis on the main staples, and less emphasis on new ingredients, experimentation, and even synthetic options.

Conglomerates became nationalized again, lost their global character, but started to build powerful oligarchies in the larger nation-states. There seemed to be no alternative to having a few companies dominate most industries, given that some markets were rather small.

Nonprofit-sector players found new energy in building national specialties but were the only actors that at least had an incentive to continue international best practice exchange.

Hospitality rebounded as soon as intranational travel bans were lifted. There was an immense resurgence and interest in local tourism. People started to truly embrace their own heritage. The tourism industry became sustainable overnight. Given that there was little or no air travel, most people visited places less than a day's drive away, although trains were important in some countries.

The marine sector continued to be important for extraction of natural resources, which also meant that some types of aquaculture became quite taxing on the ocean environment. Given the lack of international norms, no nation could fully control another's use of the ocean resources. This coordination issue almost prompted a set of international marine regulations, but they were blocked last minute by the triad of Russia, China, and the US who, in a rare moment of unity, stood against Germany and were able to argue full freedom to exploit the ocean as a national right.

Telecoms were largely unchanged throughout the decade. National carriers simply continued extracting high rents from their infrastructures and built only incremental new capacity. The mantra was repair and replenish, not incessantly innovate for its own sake.

Defense became high priority as each nation-state inherently assumed that they neighbor envied them. Massive troop build-ups provided stable employment, but the raisons d'être of the forces were built on highly theoretical scenarios and little real action. Costs ballooned and at some point, the decision was typically made to redeploy the army to build infrastructure projects.

The next outbreak and our lucky strike

As we move into the next decade, people are quite optimistic. The pandemic is just about history, we have learned to live with a plethora of viruses out in community spread. (Did I not say that there was another virus, 5 years after the first coronavirus [first called COVID-19]?) Well, we had another outbreak. This time, the virus was equally contagious but more lethal. However, like COVID-19 and unlike Ebola, asymptomatic transmission was a huge factor, in fact the incubation period was up to 10 days. Had we not had the first crisis and started preparing national plans, we would have fared much worse. As it turned out, we caught it early.

The outbreak started in Africa, but by some strike of luck it was quickly discovered by a team of Gates Foundation researchers implementing work according to the US President's Emergency Plan for AIDS Relief (PEPFAR), the largest and most diverse HIV and AIDS prevention, care, and treatment initiative in the world. Those people were very smart and told Bill Gates right away, who started calling world leaders. We had a WHO crisis team of 100 people flown in from Germany on 3 days' notice. By the way, that's faster than a traditional military unit would mobilize for an international mission.

It was a bit lucky I must admit. There has been considerable resistance against building up a big international mission. Each country has been too proud to do so and feel they just need to protect their own borders. Germany stepped up, even though they have a nationalist, extreme-right government right now. They still feel they have a burden to carry from the two previous world wars. I think their conscience should be clear now. In any case, they finance most of the WHO's pandemic work now since the US stepped back from its role as the world's savior. Politics in the US is very isolationist these days.

The team was able to (almost) contain the outbreak to Sierra Leone, although it also spread to Addis Ababa, Ethiopia. There it didn't go so well. We had to abandon that city, but that is another story. The stories of a true cordon sanitaire is not rosy reading when the death rate is above 50% as it was in that city. We just couldn't go in to fetch the rest. In the end, only 20% survived inside since they ran out of food and water after 4 weeks.

Also, it must be said that 20% of the 100 health workers in the initial WHO team perished as well. They had taken an oath. They defended our world and won. These are the sacrifices we make. The team consisted of people from 20 nations, so the hit was spread out. We now remember them with a special Day of Remembrance. We all hope that day becomes more of a historical celebration soon, and doesn't accrue more casualties, but there is no way of knowing.

Most of us have learned to live with increased uncertainty. It is worst for the young. The kids are too young to remember anything else. The old are wise enough to reflect on it and they can recall the good old days. But Generation Z just cannot take this in. They still behave rather recklessly. But didn't we say that in the 1960s as well? The young will always be reckless, right?

Preventing or fostering nation-state renewal

Decide whether you want this scenario to happen or not. Then take a different tack. Let's imagine you could pick two to three elements or remove two to three elements from the scenario.

Which aspects would you pick? Which aspects would you remove?

Finally, it's also possible that there are so-called path dependencies. This means that if A happens, then B, C, and D likely follow. Try to name a few such path dependencies in this scenario.

Imagining a nation-state renewal

Nation-states haven't always been there—they are only a few hundred years old. Some think that nation-states will either go away or become less important as time goes by. What feelings do you get around a nation-state renewal? Is it appealing?

Each scenario has fault lines (e.g., where people and interests clash).
Name a few such aspects of nation-state renewal.

The COVID-19 pandemic challenges nation-states to help its citizens economically. This is going to be a high burden to bear for some of them. Will nation-states come out stronger or weaker from this crisis?

CHAPTER 6

SCENARIO III: TWO WORLDS APART

This scenario considers a radical acceleration of the separation of the top 0.01% of the population (8 million) from the 99.99% (8 billion). It foresees entire new cities purposefully constructed to avoid contagion, and filled with the world's most expensive real estate, governed by its own laws. *From now on, and throughout this chapter, you are entering the realm of fiction.*

It's the year 2030 and the world has split in half. There is really no other way to describe it. We have the rich half and we have the poor half. Except, that's a complete misnomer. There is no half and half. The rich don't take up that much room, that's true; they've not laid claim to the vast natural resources of the Yellowstone, to our national parks, or to the countryside. What they have done is secluded themselves. It happened gradually. They now live completely separated from everyone else, with strict quarantine restrictions between them and physical barriers. They have even retreated from our cities and never come out for air. Don't get me wrong, they still run businesses in our world, but only remotely through managers.

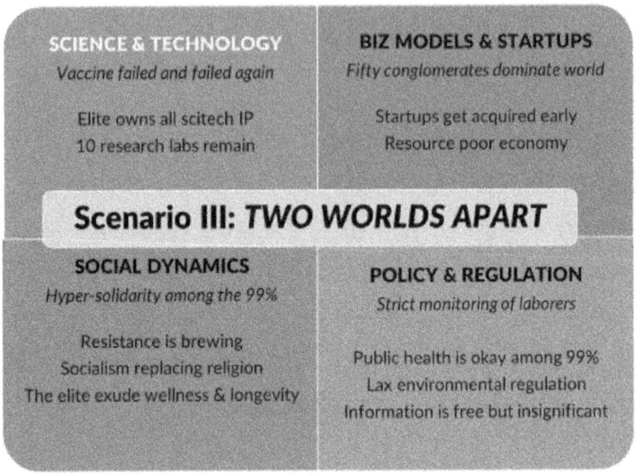

Figure 6.1. Two Worlds Apart

What I'm talking about is the fact that we, the 99.99%, have been left to deal with the world. Yes, really, that's what it is. The "1%," or to be more exact, the "0.01%," have isolated themselves in purpose-built enclaves, led and owned by the billionaires in the "0.001%." No, I don't mean gated communities and rich suburbs, like Beverly Hills, CA (90210); Upper East Side New York, NY (10065); Wellesley, MA (02482); Los Altos, CA (94022); Aspen, CO (81611); Oud-Zuid, Amsterdam (1059 and 1071 through 1075); or Gagnam (06000) in Seoul, Korea; Piper Point, Sydney (2027); Kensington, London (SW7, SW5, W8, and W14); 16th Arrondissement, or Paris (75016 and 75116). No, those who live there now are just the upper-middle class and the former broad upper class. In 2030, this is not a game of old zip codes, this is the post-corona zip codes. Let me explain.

The first thing to do is to is to explain the sequence of events. You will see how naturally this situation evolved. Now, it seems like it couldn't have happened otherwise.

Extreme elite isolationism

The first part of 2020 was a shock to everyone, rich and poor. However, as the super-rich retreated to their typical hideaways, New Yorkers to the Hamptons, Bostonians to Martha's Vineyard, and other east coast elites spending time in their villas on Harbour Island, Bahamas, or in their own or rented yachts, what they too quickly for comfort discovered was that those places were not fully isolated from the virus. They still needed groceries, they still wanted servants—chefs and drivers and cleaners. The problem was that they did not have the plans and physical infrastructure to fully isolate their staff from the disease. That's where the problem started.

As famous people still got sick, from rock stars to business tycoons to the government elite, either through their country clubs or through mysterious, unidentified routes, it became apparent that something had to be done. It even became a public policy priority at first. At least that's how the World Economic Forum, Bilderberg, the Trilateral Commission, and the other elite networks and top country clubs the world over saw it.

The US government were the first to publicly announce that they had put in place special procedures to protect Congress, the Supreme Court, and selected staff who were allowed to work from the White House and in the quarantined cordon sanitaire around the core of Washington DC. They even provided new housing for them, literally by vacating nearby hotels and apartments and turning them into permanent living quarters. Whatever space was not used became a ghost town, although it quickly got other uses as health clubs, restaurants, and all other functions a society needs.

That was the first post-corona enclave, right in the middle of Washington DC. What then happened was more extreme.

The government started building a wall around themselves. The wall was finished in record time. In less than 2 months, there was a 20-foot wall around the core of DC, in the style of the Middle Ages. They even started growing vegetables and holding cattle inside the wall. All core services were brought inside that wall. Powerful machine guns were mounted on top and guarded 24/7, including with sensor technology and ground-to-air defense.

The US experiment was so successful that others followed suit. Soon, there were walled city-like infrastructures built around the world. Paris. Tokyo. London. Sydney. Hong Kong. Beijing. Sao Paulo. All the financial centers in the world managed to wall themselves in by the end of 2020. In some cities, the financial elite were there together with the government; in others, the walled cities were filled with one or the other. You still don't believe it? Perhaps consider this: the first reports of failing vaccines came out already in the fall of 2020.

The failing vaccines

Of the 40 vaccines undergoing human trial, only three survived the early fall; the rest failed for all kinds of reasons. This was a big blow to the elite as it was to the rest of us. Even though some of us were aware that each vaccine has a 6% chance of success and on average takes 10.7 years to develop, we kind of all believed that with the massive effort, the vaccine track would succeed, and in record time (Pronker et al, 2013).

As it increasingly became clear that the vaccine track was risky at best and likely would fail in the short term, as in the next 3–5 years, the choice the elite made was easy. Make a huge bet on quarantining themselves, spending vast percentages of their fortunes on building fortresses in a completely new, pooled investment vehicle with a kind of real estate never before seen, or face the same risk as any other person in the regular "world." The choice for those who had the resources was quite easy, though not all took it. Some objected on ideological grounds, others couldn't afford it, or were worried about the friends or even the businesses they would be locked out of. We'll get to how they were able to run some of their existing businesses from the inside, but, as you can imagine, not all types of businesses were equally possible to run remotely.

What quickly happened as 2020 went downhill is that the world's super-rich almost simultaneously decided that they didn't want to have any part of this pandemic. Why would they have amassed such wealth only to be burdened with the same problems that we are? So what did they do in practical terms? The first projects were simply Band-Aids, for example, building a wall inside an already established city infrastructure. In a way, it wasn't that revolutionary. It was a historically proven strategy, it was quite intuitive, but the problem was it wasn't enough. Also, it was not the solution for the massive demand among the ultra-rich. The demand was enormous. Here's what then happened.

In early 2021, Kokooring, the high-end New York–headquartered real estate developer, was approached by the Saudi Royal Family as well as the 50 richest billionaires in the world, charged with mounting a few purpose built luxury developments and repurposing a few others to create hyper-elite enclaves where the wealthy would not only live but run their businesses, their entire lives from. The process did take a while. The whole global infrastructure took 5 years to build but was released in tranches. It was quite crowded on the first two resort cities in the first years, although everyone had to undergo a 40-day quarantine before being let on the property.

The financing was quickly in place. The first project had a $100 billion price tag, the second and third were so astronomical that it became near ridiculous. The smallest buy-in became around $100 million. Ultimately, the first wave of resorts catered to individuals with a total net worth value of

$9 trillion.

There are approximately 2,153 billionaires in the world. Many of them were concentrated in countries like the United States, China, Germany, Russia, and the United Kingdom, each of which got a time-share location. In addition, one vacation spot was built for each of those countries, but the time-share gave access to each of them. Very little existing infrastructure was kept. As it turns out, most resort towns are not very efficient at keeping viruses out. They had to put in place strict rules for nature, wildlife, and other contaminants, while maintaining the ability to grow food and have access to necessary natural resources as well as entertainment.

A debate quickly ensued as to whether there would be quotas for intelligence. They ended up accepting a 1% quota of folks with PhDs and IQs at 140 and above as long as they accepted a job in the research labs each compound was equipped with. And what about the extremely beautiful? Well, there was a quota for them as well, seeing as the elite needed eye candy. Based on how an AI evaluated people's looks, 5% of the inhabitants were screened for beauty as well as wealth.

What about those who already had a corona-passport, indicating they already had had the disease? The latter became the solution for all the waitstaff needed to operate these enclaves. The only way to apply for a "Golden Ticket" was if you already were immune. The applications were more popular than for a job at Disneyworld, which by the way might be the closest analogy to what they built: a hybrid of Disneyworld and Martha's Vineyard. In fact, Martha's Vineyard, the resort island outside Massachusetts, did get considered for one of the enclaves, but in the end, they chose the smaller island of Nantucket. More remote, easier to protect from intruders, and the exact size they could rapidly fill up. The only downside was the weather in winter, so Nantucket became more of a seasonal resort. The whole thing got worked out as they went along. Some obviously couldn't afford a global time share with five locations, which started at $500 million. Transportation was a bit tricky, since big planes cannot land on Nantucket. They built a bigger airport, which was costly.

Another resort was built on the island of Vis, a Croatian island in the Adriatic Sea, off the Dalmatian Coast. The farthest inhabited island off the Croatian mainland, Vis had a population of 3,617 before Kookoran bought the whole island and turned it into a resort with 1,000 luxury homes, cutting off the only way to access the island, which was by a 2-hours-and-20 minutes ferry crossing from the city of Split in Croatia. Instead, a major invisible fortress was built as an underwater belt protecting the island from the sea. The island of Vis was a secretive military fortress serving the Yugoslavian military throughout much of the 20th century and already had infrastructures that Kookoran could put to use in that regard, including coastal tunnels to hide submarines and a bomb shelter designed to help 200 people survive a nuclear war.

Given how well the island fared during the corona crisis, Kookoran had at one point contemplated buying the entire island of New Zealand and locking it down, but concluded it was too remote for the purposes of regular commutes between resorts (and too expensive even for them).

How did this go down in the rest of society? Initially not well. There were human rights protests, objections from the almost wealthy enough who were rejected and from various categories of elites who felt excluded, such as older popstars and the like. Overall, it was a uber wealthy, intelligent, and young lot that got the jobs at "Clean World," as the nickname became. Back in "Contaminated World" (also called "Dirty World"), it's not that things were necessarily tragic.

Differences escalate

Social differences remained within Dirty World. People were rich or poor, protected or not protected. The first wave of the

European outbreak in 2020 killed the elite who had been on ski vacations in the Alps, in France, Austria, Switzerland, and Italy. The second brief wave that year killed fairly indiscriminately across the board, as the contagion spread across the population at large. The third wave, however, visible in the second half of 2020 and in the years to follow, had a massive impact on the most vulnerable, the poor, the folks with preexisting conditions, and working-class people living in the densely populated outskirts of megacities. COVID-19 swept like a tsunami through slums. It affected those who had to go to work for fear of losing their job and couldn't self-isolate. It affected those without health insurance. It affected the elderly. It even disproportionately affected the severely obese.

Rural contagion shifts the focus

Then, in the fourth wave, it started affecting rural communities. That was the true shift. Rural communities don't have big hospitals. They have small grocery stores where contagion can roam wild. The local population all know each other and have a myriad of ties between each other. Ties that are hard to break apart just because of an outbreak where politicians you don't trust tell you to stay at home.

Additionally, there were the part-timers who owned vacation properties. They came in droves, hoping to escape the crowded cities, setting up and expecting to work remotely. However, there was limited broadband many places and there wasn't enough food supply. Delivery trucks started creating traffic chaos on small roads leading into the main arteries of smaller rural downtowns. The few doctors, ventilators, and the very scant personal protective equipment typically only lasted for a few months. After that, it was everyone for themselves.

The wealthy started bringing their own equipment when they got admitted to local hospitals. It just didn't work, though, because doctors and nurses refused to only use the equipment for the patients who had brought it in. Highly tense discussions ensued. Words were exchanged and the guns got out. In America this became a time to get a gun license. People who had never fired a gun, owned a gun, or thought about it, even some anti-gun activists, lined up at gun stores in droves. The notion was, if I don't protect my family, who will?

Technology helping us see that we're in it together

Futurists had hoped that technology would create a world without privilege or prejudice based on birth, race, economic power, military force, or any other external circumstance. They were right. The rest of us feel that way now. And we are making technologies, as best as we can, to help us do so.

3D printing is still expensive, but those who have it, and can afford to operate the printers and buy the expensive supplies for it, are helping others out. In some neighborhoods they share a printer. In others, volunteers bring them in and ask people to send them what they want printed. It's a great help. It can be hard to get anything mailed to you these days. Logistics are at times difficult. Private consumption has come to a halt. Whatever gets delivered has a hefty 50% delivery fee. Most people cannot afford that. The upside is that the printers gradually improved.

In 2020, the desktop versions mostly printed plastic spoons. In 2025, even though the most advanced 3D printers went to Clean World, the ones left for us could even print most basic food items, at least dry foods like pasta and synthetic beans and the kind of food that would previously have been considered military rations. They taste quite good, too. Toward the end of the decade, by 2029, we are even printing metal, just like Clean World had done for the past decade. We don't have access to any rare metals, but we can print aluminum. Besides, the plastics and carbon resins we are printing are very hardy. It works.

Kampala City, Uganda, March 15, 2023: Mukisa spent the day finishing the novel he had begun last week. After the quarantine, there were only three things to do: work, worry, relax. Mukisa, whose name means "good fortune," chose to relax. Uganda's tech ecosystem was surprisingly resilient and also quite advanced for that part of the world. Mukisa had an undergraduate degree in computer engineering from the University of Bath in the UK but was now pursuing his passion as an author back in Uganda. The crisis had given him time to pause. With the freedom to be able to read the online newspapers, be in touch with his friends over email, or even use his 3D printer to print out medical supplies for the local hospital, he didn't stress about it. Mukisa took it all in stride. After all, it was going to be a long game.

The Ugandan people as a whole were likely to suffer tremendously from COVID-19. He knew he could be the exception. Some days the guilt of that was so tangible that he could almost taste it. But this line of thought, he knew, was unproductive. He couldn't help anyone if he didn't keep himself healthy in every sense. In order to protect himself and build resilience, he had taken to daily meditation. Instead of immediately kicking off his morning writing session in front of his window that faced the jungle in the remote distance, he instead took out his yoga mat.

He recalled what Prisha, his instructor back in Bath, an attractive 27-year-old Indian-born student of performing arts, had said to him: "Slow down, Mukisa. Let your body's natural breath rhythm take you to places where your mind wants to go. Find your own mantra and make it count." At the time, his mind had only gotten to her cleavage and occasionally below that. He had loved the way she had touched him to adjust his positions. Even downward-facing dog became a joy that way.

The peace of this moment ran in stark contrast to his volunteering sessions at Mulago Hospital each day, the sick dying all around him. In these moments, it helped him to think of Prisha. Thanks to her, he was in shape, which was useful, as he also had to trek the 10 miles up Mulago Hill by foot, not being able to trust public transport anymore. On the way, Mukisa had to pass through the abandoned Kamwookya market, where only the surrounding slum area reminded him of what was to come on top of the hill.

Uganda had received a global top-25 score on pandemic readiness by the internationally recognized Global Health Security Index, nearly on par with Norway and South Africa and ahead of Germany and Japan. However, home to 1.4 million refugees, primarily from neighboring South Sudan and the Democratic Republic of the Congo, Uganda hosts the largest refugee population in Africa. It was when COVID-19 reached the Kiryandongo refugee settlement that things started breaking down. How were they to prioritize care? How to contain the spread?

In the end, it was the health workers, who lived across Kampala, who brought the virus to the city. Well, so much for a theoretical pandemic readiness score. COVID-19 shattered any such analysis. A pandemic among the refugee population was never part of the equation.

As the national reference hospital, Mulago was now overcrowded with ambulances every day. Patients had also started coming by foot. The narrow, unpaved sidewalks were crowded with fellow Ugandans, coughing, stumbling, sneezing their way up the hill toward what they thought was salvation. But what they could offer was simply nursing care on a metal frame bed, for those that even got that far.

It helped to think of Prisha and England. Now, a year later back in Kampala, looking out his window and seeing the familiar greenery of the jungle but also devastation if he looked down on the street, he suddenly was able to grasp what she meant. Find your own mantra. He knew what it would be. He was envisioning the world post-COVID-19, a world where everyone in Uganda was free to walk around, to create, to love, one where disease was conquered, and the spirit itself was, again, free.

He recalled a performance given by Spirit of Uganda, the dance troupe that usually traveled the world sharing East African dances at performing arts centers, before they traveled abroad for the first time. He saw the joy in their eyes more clearly now. Dance, music, and storytelling record our histories and instill values, remind us of the values we aspire to and those we want to instill in others. Drawing from the past, but not remaining in the past, their voices, rhythms, and movements were what he tried to include in his mantra.

Mukisa even developed his own Mudra, a personalized, symbolic gesture that he made into a pose that started and ended his daily yoga practice. The way he now could channel his energy flow and let go of all the stress—not think about the fact that 5,000 people died every day in Kampala city over the past month—it was almost unbelievable. Mukisa knew that Prana, which means breath or life force in Sanskrit, was among the most powerful Mudras. He developed his own version and performed his prana mudra by touching his ring and pinky fingers to the tip of his thumb, while keeping the other two fingers straight.

However, he incorporated a hand gesture from the Karimojong, his Ugandan family's tribe, waving first toward himself with the left hand, the servant hand in Ugandan tradition, and then with his right hand, the noble hand, as if welcoming strangers and greeting them with his breath of life, and ending with a motion as if he was rubbing foreheads with an invisible stranger, the most powerful of all greetings in Uganda. It was a powerful act of defiance against the outbreak, against everything that was happening. And it strengthened him for the day and for what was to come. His mantra was a sentence in Karimojong: "Iyai to?" (Do you exist?) "Ee, iyai ba iyong to?" (Yes, I do, and you?)

Back to technology, the mobile networks are lightning fast.

The 5G they rolled out in 2020 dwarfs in comparison, although poorer neighborhoods don't have the data capacity anymore. We had to reserve those for the business districts, after the tight restrictions our Clean World owners placed on unnecessary traffic.

Artificial intelligence has made some progress, although not as much as we would hope. The truly advanced AI is reserved for Clean World and the few labs they own scattered around Dirty World. What we mostly use it for is to estimate when we can expect the next virus lockdowns, area by area. Foresight is important. Planning ahead gives us a certain relief. At least we know what's coming. The grocery store closures, stay-at-home orders, and social distancing laws of the first part of the decade were draconian, but most of all, horribly disruptive because we didn't know they would arrive. Now, everyone can check the Covid-app on their phone and see what restrictions apply where they are going.

Augmented reality is extremely useful, too. The ability to really feel we are together with our friends even if we are apart or checking in with our family when we are on those rare business trips that require 2 week's quarantine on both legs of the trip. Yeah, I'd say AR is a lifesaver. All desktop computers come with the system, holograms and everything. Basically, we can touch and feel people who are apart, connected by advanced sensors wired to our head, hands, and even to our legs.

The emotional sensors are truly powerful. Basically, based on a face expression, the system tells us what the person on the other end is feeling. I've been surprised sometimes. Guess I never was any good at reading other people. It has been defined as a critical infrastructure technology in our legislation. I really wish everyone on the planet could have access, though. We still haven't solved basic access issues. But neighbors share with neighbors–it's wonderful to see.

Autonomous driving has kicked in as well. What that

means is that we have these computers assisting our driving, at least for taxis. They go slowly and in their own lanes on the road, but they'll get you where you need to go without having to be exposed to another human being in the driver seat. Those taxis are so small. Social distancing is impossible. Before we figured it out, in the first 3 years, about 90% of public transit personnel contracted COVID-19. That's a lot of people. There was no way they could protect themselves.

Basically, whatever is left of commuter trains, buses, and subways are operated remotely. The subways are barely operational. Six feet of distance doesn't work under ground. You have to wear masks at all times and special coats are recommended, but it's cumbersome.

Blockchain is now how we run our banks, our governments, and our barter economy amongst ourselves. The ability to have a transparent account, what they call a public ledger, which is a bookkeeping term, has enabled us to see when somebody is trying to be corrupt (although we still cannot always catch them due to the lack of police resources) and become highly efficient. We needed that.

The economy never got back on track, but blockchain got us to 30% of 2020 levels after only 3 years in operation. Thanks to all the startups as well as banks and governments who pushed for it, we now have open markets again. The barter economy is alive and thriving, too. Bartering for goods is interesting. Everything is on the market, even a virtual hug in augmented reality. It costs the same as renting a movie, basically, and you can often get a two-for-one.

CRISPR, the gene-editing method that was on the scene already before 2020, has now gotten optimized for COVID-19 prevention. It's reserved for kids, though, after they discovered kids with blood type A, which is 34% of kids, are 50% more susceptible to getting the disease. It was a defect on multiple genes, a complex disorder with spiraling mutations on genes IL-6 (a protein coding gene that induces cytokine in inflammations), TGFBI (a growth gene infected through the cornea) and MTHFR (an enzyme that plays a role in processing amino acids into the bloodstream).

CRISPR interventions resets all of that, but it costs a year's average salary in the Western world and takes 3 months to kick in. In 2027, 100 kids got it, in 2028, 1,000 kids did, and, thankfully, by 2029 we were able to help 10% of kids in the Western world through a fundraising effort led by the world's top musicians; most of those kids have blood type A.

Cybersecurity is a constant threat. Businesses report attacks 100 times a day. Small business has been hit the hardest, mostly because they cannot afford the top of the line software. It is estimated that 20% of small business is, to some degree, controlled by the black market by now, increasing manifold percent a year. If we don't do anything, estimates are small business will be completely controlled by various mafias and cybercriminals, including global syndicates. We're all in this fight together, though, so the remaining software engineers who are free riders, essentially all the 50+ engineers who cannot get approved for lab work in the Clean World, are all on it. I'm confident it will be solved.

Precision medicine is more than CRISPR, these days. Doctors, for those lucky enough to have an insurance plan (it is all privatized at this point, around the globe), can tailor medication to your social group, blood type, age, and specific disease. Genetic editing, beyond the kids' COVID-19 project effort, is reserved for Clean World engineers and top scientists working in their labs. It's not quite personalized medicine, is what I mean; the precision is still not where it should be. But for older diseases, we have decreased the mortality rate by 50% through the decade, which isn't bad.

Nanotechnology is only reserved for the Clean World labs as is quantum computing. Very little is released about the progress they are making. The big media is all owned by the billionaires, and they tightly control information. There are

1,000 bloggers left who can sustain themselves writing online through advertising and donations; those individuals are doing a great job.

An article that was out in 2024 described the progress in nanoscience this way: "Clean World is getting ready to use nanobots to do their dirty laundry, tackle cancer in the gut, and clean up all their waste, of which there is a lot generated, given their luxurious, lavish lifestyle on those resort islands. Who knew nanotech was so useful?" About quantum computing we know next to nothing, only that when it succeeds, it will break all known encryption. Our 50+ engineers are afraid it will break all of our cybersecurity defenses. Mounting a counterattack using quantum computing is the stuff of fiction for us who are on Dirty World resources.

Robotics have gone mainstream, at least in our factories, for deliveries, and in the home. They don't look that impressive, but they do the job. Still kind of clunky, but more efficient than humans, I'd say.

Smart fabrics have now replaced regular clothes, but they have an array of other uses. We now coat all of our surfaces with antimicrobial sheets that are mass printed in special facilities available only in the major cities. That way, we were able to reduce the amount of sanitizer we were using. It was getting completely crazy. Imagine having to refill sanitizer from the street's water truck that was converted to a sanitizer dispenser, every week. People got tired of carrying buckets of sanitizer. Their skin started turning yellow, too; our bodies couldn't take all the cleanliness. A lot of people got chronic allergies before we realized the problem.

Luckily, one of the 50+ engineers was much smarter than he had let on to the Clean World recruiters, he was also only 40 but had kept that a secret. He is now one of the secrets of the "science army" we are building up in Dirty World; those who are poised to defy the call to join Clean World labs even though they have an IQ of 140. The resistance, as we call it, is dying people's hair grey, artificially inducing wrinkles and falsifying birth certificates to create an army of smart people who don't get deployed to the labs. We need to preserve the chance to build a greater future for the 99.99%. It's a bit like I heard London was in 1944 before D-day: *Don't tell. Don't show. Do your part.*

Synthetic biology is, again, a bit of a mixed picture. We are mandated to stay away from nature as much as possible because of the contamination, but people are defying the orders. Synthetic nature is not the same, and they haven't built any true facilities in Dirty World yet. What we have is a way to regenerate the smell of almost anything. It is released on small bottles that you can buy online. I personally like the smell of fruit trees blooming from my childhood's orchards. A $500 bottle lasts me a month.

Virtual reality is mostly for games, still. But being able to play the top video games using an avatar that can change characteristics is one of the most popular past times. Imagine not just using a joystick, but actually experiencing joy. Needless to say, the sex is better, too. We actually use VR instead, because it's safer. We are practicing social distancing yet are able to induce feelings in the other person we didn't think possible. Isn't it great how far we've come?

Honolulu, Hawaii, March 23, 2023: Kookoran v. State of Hawaii: at stake is the legality of declaring the island of Kahoolawe part of the new global state of Futura Delight as part of a real estate development project. For the defendant, Mr. Springer, Esq. speaking on behalf of Futura. For the State of Hawaii, Ms. Nativa, representing the indigenous population of Hawaii. "We cannot accept the purchase of Kahoolawe island by Kookoran for the purposes of (a) building a resort on tribal land and (b) purchasing the territory from the State of Hawaii and declaring it a part of its own territorial state." Judge: "What does the defendant claim?"

Mr. Springer: "We have followed all legal protocol requirements. We have rightfully purchased the island and we will conduct only sustainable activities in full isolation from any other activity in the State of Hawaii. Judge: "The island is not inhabited because there is no clean water source on the island. How will you even build there?" "We have found a solution because of a new desalination technology owned by one of our future residents," says Mr. Springer. "We might even be able to export some to Hawaii for use to water your lilies on Maui."

Having made his deposition, Mr. Springer had to make a phone call. It was the last checkup before he was going into quarantine to get to Kahoolawe. It was all part of the compensation package he had received for taking on this case. He was one of the lucky ones, but didn't feel that way. He had unsuccessfully lobbied to have his family join him. The answer was no. He would have to tell his wife and kids they would never see him again. But they would simply have to understand. He would be the lead judge on the new island resort built by Kookoran. He would send money home to them. And, without the investment, there was simply no future for his family. The natural beauty of the island would not put food on the table. But for the good of the family, they would have to let him go. Kookoran and Co. would get what they wanted whether he stood in the way or not. So why not say yes? Make things easier for everyone. He was never one to stand in the way of progress.

What does the resort look like? Each of the smaller, purpose-built, 2-acre luxury properties has a spacious living quarter with a pool house, a wine cellar, outdoor kitchens, an Olympic-size pool, a bubble bath, ocean view, two tennis courts, a Japanese garden, a small fresh water pond, game and theater rooms, cigar room, three full-size offices, three spa bathrooms, massage rooms, exercise rooms, escape rooms, triple garage for golf carts and collectible cars, and individual desalination facilities producing enough drinking water as well as fresh water for the pools. The amenities for the high-end units is a state secret.

Any traffic in and out is subject to strict 40-day quarantines (after all, the venetian term *quarantine* means 40 for a reason). Inside, their new global state, the super-rich can now roam freely and safely, with no virus in sight.

There is a summer compound on a monastery island in northern France and a winter compound on the Cayman Islands. Each has an airport, helipads, casinos, and live entertainment, shopping, and everything. The brands allowed to open stores on the island, under strict conditions, include Ralph Lauren, Dior, Prada, Chanel, Hermes, Louis Vuitton, Gucci, and after a big debate, the newcomer Oscar de la Renta. On the larger resorts, where there are roads, expensive luxury cars have been brought in, although there are strict conditions under which residents can bring their own cars. For now, the only brands serviced by mechanics are: any Rolls Royce or Bentley, Maserati Quattroporte, BMW ALPINA B7, Mercedes-Benz AMG GT, Maserati GranTurismo, BMW i8, Jaguar XE SV, and after a long, drawn out discussion, Audi R8 Spyder, which is a favorite among Generation Z billionaires.

Fortuna has also chartered a few cruise lines and have created the cleanest ships in history. Only 100 people can be aboard these ships that were created for a 1,000 passengers, so they can observe “elite” social distancing, which is 10 feet, although they don’t do that, it’s just to show the outside world they care and for photos that are released to Dirty World tabloids.

This takes time and is not complete, but they are also building a new city. Origin Town, it’s called. Oh, and Elok Dusk is also building a spacecraft that can take them to a secure facility on Mars, should the entire earth be affected by some biological or other environmental disaster, like polluted air.

Fortuna Resort town, Little Cayman, Cayman Islands, February 4, 2024: "Carla, whatever happened to your Vuitton bag?" Kim was furious, she had wanted to sport that tonight. The expensive bag was not a real Vuitton, which only Carla knew because she used to work in the store. Carla was a transplant to the Caymans. She had come with the workers and had transitioned to a resident through marriage, not an uncommon route, but very uncomfortable socially. "Oh, I don't know," said Carla, "I might have lost it in the water when we were snorkeling." "You took your Vuitton bag snorkeling?" said Kim with a surprised look on her face. Carla said, "I had no other choice. All my other bags were being disinfected after that unfortunate episode with my staff contracting the flu." "Well, I'm glad you are okay," said Kim. "I cannot believe flu wasn't detected by your infrared scanner." "Oh, that scanner," said Carla, "I find it annoying. I turn it off on weekends." In fact, Carla found this entire conversation annoying. All she wanted was to go back to the mainland, where the real people were. But there was no way back. They wouldn't accept her now. She was contaminated with the rich people's bug. What a boring life, she thought. I wish I had stayed sober that night and perhaps I wouldn't have been married with kids in Fortuna Resort now.

Industry consequences of two worlds apart

After reeling from the initial shock of the coronavirus, the healthcare industry rapidly discovered it was serving two highly separate markets. One, a high-end market that demanded advanced, personalized medicine and gene editing and another than required mass market public health measures.

Finance was largely concentrated either within the Clean World enclaves or immediately serving the absentee landlords that represented their interests. Consumer finance, however, was a hugely lucrative business serving individual clients across Dirty World. These were people whose credit histories had been erased or drastically reduced by the crisis.

Education continued full force in Dirty World, but higher education was severely limited given that it was all feeder schools for the big research labs run by Clean World. At lower levels, however, online schooling continued apace.

The energy sector was largely geared toward extraction. The innovation that did ensue was all geared toward things like desalination for Clean World resorts, solar energy, as well as burning out all the oil before anybody in Dirty World could enrich themselves enough that they could mount a credible threat to Clean World's plan of eternal isolation.

Technology improved radically but mostly in personalized medicine, which was the largest concern. Other key technologies under development remained under the radar until they were tested on unknowing Dirty World populations and implemented in Clean World when it worked.

Transportation was not easy anymore. Coronavirus restrictions loomed for many years. Lack of financing stopped any major infrastructure upgrades. Personal transportation was kept to a minimum, and vehicles were aging.

Travel was not a major pastime anymore and even business travel was limited. Necessary travel continued but only after taking protective measures. Hotels were small.

Consumer confidence had taken a major dive never to fully recover, although the market was still huge. There was a lot of volume, but the quality went down.

Commodities like precious metals were brought into the hands of the Clean World billionaires who extracted enormous rents upon all who were willing to pay, mostly everyday consumers who wanted their everyday electronics. Other commodities were relatively freely exchanged on the market given the common interest in a working, frictionless market among the remaining citizens of Dirty World.

Services industries became divided into haves and have-nots, as Clean World took the high-end workforce and left the rest to Dirty World, who, largely, treated services as a commodity, much like it previously was in America. Service workers mostly lived on tips, although Dirty World attempted to collect a 5% toll based on the notion that they guaranteed a global marketplace. This was always unpopular but was still going on at the end of the decade, despite massive protest, televised to Clean World, although the footage was rarely, if ever shown.

Government was a highly efficient technocracy in Clean World, but more like an Italian bureaucracy in Dirty World, as it was widely regarded as a safe job amid all the uncertainty. Governments had little power on the upside but had plenty of responsibilities to fix people's troubles, which created tension.

Manufacturing was slow and steady, but there were few efficiencies introduced, beyond the high-end production lines which yielded only small amounts of custom products tailored for Clean World luxury consumption. There was little incentive to be innovative, given the low margins on either end.

Aerospace was not a major priority, in fact, Clean World actively discouraged it, in order to keep air dominance. Most of their facilities were only vulnerable from the air and they wouldn't have any of it. The space program was quickly abandoned due to cost concerns. In fact, life continued very much on the ground. Even drones were so stringently regulated, led by Clean World lobbyists who were afraid they would make their way to fetch luxury goods or take compromising pictures, that they only became play tools for teenagers.

Media was a tightly controlled affair where Clean World owned all the media houses and sent repeats of old shows. Hollywood had collapsed already in the first wave of COVID-19, as their entire business model was undercut when the theater system collapsed. Nobody could gather, so gathering around your TV or cell phone seemed a more rational pursuit.

Food was not a priority any longer. At least not in Dirty World. Focus was on survival, efficiency, and on staying safe. People ate what they could trust. It became a necessity, not a source of enjoyment. In Clean World, of course, it was the opposite, and all the top-ranked chefs were deployed there.

Conglomerates owned by Clean World began to emerge everywhere. It was a gradual process. It started with a few financial centers, then conglomerates owned by others were bought out on a systematic basis from the center and out.

Nonprofits were insignificant in this decade. Funding dried up. There were no international crises to focus on as all the emphasis was on staying alive locally. Some exceptions focused specifically on public health made notable contributions.

Hospitality rebounded but mass tourism was dead forever. The costs in the sector were such that most smaller establishments already went under and couldn't reopen under the new economic conditions. High-end tourism was simply nonexistent, as Clean World had taken the bottom out of the market.

Marine industry experts spoke of a possible resurgence based on aquaculture. However, Clean World's many resorts were located on islands and they wanted to control the amount of large boats that could interfere with their de facto jurisdictional control of the major oceans. International shipping routes were consolidated into the north-south route and the east-west route and only occurred under strict surveillance protocols. No vessels were allowed on the open sea without being tracked and slotted into a preestablished route.

Telecoms enjoyed a good first 5 years followed by a race to the bottom as prices had declined with the lack of purchasing power. Why have a phone when you don't have a house?

Defense contractors initially fared well with Clean World

business building their submarine fleets, ground-to-air defense systems, and police force, but after that, it completely dried up. There was ample need for law and order, but Dirty World culture emerged in such a way that police had to use much more peaceful methods of diplomacy that didn't fit the military system very well. Military technology made little sense, given that there weren't any major powers to defeat.

Life in the 99.99%

What do the 99.99% do? We go on with our lives. We have the rest of the world to ourselves. The only thing is, even as the remaining upper-middle class, which is my predicament, we don't have a lot of resources. The 0.001% have pulled everything in-house. They own most of the attractive real estate, even if they don't live there anymore. Instead, what we are is underpaid house-sitters. Granted, it's not bad to take care of mansions and turn-of-the-century Parisian apartments, but they don't feel the same when you cannot even hang a picture on the wall.

However, we still have most of the cultural and professional elite, so we are doing okay. The only thing is that these highly educated people are being exploited beyond belief. A doctor has the same respect as a cleaner, and academics are eating scraps. Physical labor has become the new capital, because those willing to expose themselves to contagion can command an enormous hazard pay.

Life is still good if you are savvy. Entrepreneurs have a privileged position in everyday society in Dirty World. If you can come up with something new, rally a team and obtain funding, you can do almost anything in Dirty World. Free initiative is unbound. Ideas that have been implemented recently include frictionless transportation pods, decontamination suits, and miniaturized virus sensors.

A further benefit of social distancing over time was that it has led to a culture of close friendships instead of the looser networks that were forming pre-2020.

London, June 14, 2028, Dirty World: Jeremy had snuck out of Clean World City of London to have a night out in Dirty World with his buddies, both young heirs. Their mission was risky. If they got caught, they would be thrown into a 40-day quarantine, and if they developed COVID-19, best case, they would remain in a Dirty World hospital facility until they recovered. It was a rite of passage. All his friends had already been out.

When you are a Gen Z and have unlimited financial wealth, being on one side of a wall almost compels you to see the other side. "Be careful," said his brother, Stew, who was a bit more anxious about their night out at a London nightclub. He almost got caught once, and did catch a cold (e.g. a mild coronavirus), which is extremely rare in Clean World City. He couldn't go to the country club for a month; the infrared scanners would have detected an anomaly and put him through testing. Stew wasn't as brave as his brother, and he wasn't as happy about the thrill.

Stew recalled all his friends who were not able to make it to the inside of City. Where were they now? He didn't dare to think. Also, he was simply trying to make do in Clean World City. It was hard enough. Why take all this additional risk? He simply didn't understand Jeremy, but as the dutiful thing to do, he followed him wherever he went. That was the very least he could do for his younger brother, he thought to himself as they jumped the fence, temporarily disabling the electronic sensor barrier with a clever hack.

In contrast, apart from the corona-restrictions, there are few other restrictions in Dirty World. Not having free universities anymore is a bit of a bummer. All the truly smart folks get offered jobs in research labs owned by Clean World. The rest of us are stuck with online learning from good, but not exceptional professors and teachers. Sort of like going to a state school, not Ivy League, not much worse. I've gotten over it.

We have become an Amsterdam of sorts, free will, free sex, free everything—but reined in by the virus. That means we don't do the free sex thing anymore. So the government didn't have to outlaw it anymore. Free will isn't all that attractive either. What is there to protest about? We mostly have what we need, apart from the uncertainty of whether we will die any given year, and we cannot access Clean World, anyway. But who knew when their hour would come before the virus? None of us. It was all just an illusion of safety. I say, good riddance.

Life with the virus spikes

The disease is pretty bad, though. We still haven't fully eradicated that nasty coronavirus. About 30% of us are immune at this point, but the immunity only lasts for 3 years. Then, it's at it again. Doctors have gotten pretty good about the treatment. In fact, there are a few therapeutic treatments now, including antibody therapy, plus the new antibiotics work very well for the bacterial pneumonia that typically follows serious COVID-19, but we still have people who die. There is some talk about a possible RNA vaccine to be rolled out among the Fortuna population in the next decade. After that, they say it may be available in Dirty World. Maybe so, maybe not. The cost would be exorbitant, and likely only for the 0.001%, anyway. I know the Clean World folks don't want overpopulation on earth. In any case, it's been tested on some of us right now. My son is part of that experiment. He says it feels nice to be in the test population. Gives a glimmer of hope, I guess.

We literally don't have people above 60 on the globe anymore. We also don't have people who are immunocompromised. The benefit is that we also don't have people who smoke, who don't exercise, or who are overweight. In fact, everyone has started taking care of their health. For people in perfect health, they have found that the mortality rate is only 1% a year. We can all live with that, even though with a population of 8 billion that means 80 million of us die each year, roughly comparable to half of the population of Russia.

But again, eat right, work out every day, don't smoke, take your vitamins, don't shake hands, wear a mask, social distance by 10 feet (the earlier recommendation of 6 feet was found to be insufficient), and abide by the frequent quarantines. We also have massive testing for the virus, tracing contacts occurs seamlessly and is tracked online and through a barcode on your arm. We have reduced human interactions by stopping most mass gatherings. We mostly work from home and travel is curbed. Life is entirely possible, just a little cumbersome, and at times, sad.

Religion is another escape. There are no restrictions apart from the fact that we cannot gather in person anymore. There are no services, everything is online. In fact, religion has changed a bit. I think we all realize that religion as we knew it before the virus was a bit old-fashioned. All that stuff about Paradise and salvation, all this time, we thought it was something fantastic. Turns out it is simply absence of the virus. That's all we dream about now.

The 0.001% ultra-wealthy have it, paradise I mean. They live in paradise. There is nothing special about it when you see it in the tabloids every day. I've also seen that since they live longer, there is no way of hiding that they are aging. In Clean World, they have people approaching a hundred years old by now. Those folks aren't very agile. In fact, they are probably quite boring, sitting in their wealth without ability to do much. Is that a better life? Well, since none of us here typically live beyond the age of 60, we just don't know. It's two different worlds, literally.

The only thing is that it would be nice to visit one day. We all apply for the Golden Tickets. I wouldn't mind working in one of the resorts. Friends of mine do. They chat about it online. In fact, that is my dream. I'm glad to have a dream again. I lived without one for several years. I had nightmares about not having dreams again, if you know what I mean.

As long as I am allowed to dream, I don't care about anything else. To some extent, I might be happier than those zombies in Fortuna. I saw some research that indicates they aren't that much happier than us on average, in fact only 2 percentage points more. That research was suppressed and never released in Clean World, could you imagine? They just wouldn't accept it. Quality of life is born in the mind!

Preventing or fostering two worlds apart

Decide whether you want this scenario to happen or not. Then take a different tack. Let's imagine you could pick two to three elements or remove two to three elements from the scenario.

Which aspects would you pick? Which aspects would you remove?

____

Finally, it's also possible that there are so-called path dependencies. This means that if A happens, then B, C, and D likely follow. Try to name a few such path dependencies in this scenario.

____

Imagining two worlds apart

There is a growing discrepancy between rich and poor. Some find it problematic.
What feelings do you get around two worlds apart? Is it appealing?

Each scenario has fault lines (e.g., where people and interests clash).
Name a few such aspects of having two worlds apart.

The COVID-19 pandemic may lead to even greater social and economic differences between individuals and specific social groups. What do you think should be done about it, if anything?

CHAPTER 7

SCENARIO IV: HOBBESIAN CHAOS

This scenario considers a possible next decade where survival of the fittest becomes an extreme reality. A set of partially independent set of "second" major events take place in the aftermath of the pandemic (wars, invasions, famines, major hurricanes, environmental disasters, grasshopper invasions, etc.). As a result, rule of law ceases to exist, and clans and ideological movements sweep through the earth with constant struggle and fight for scarce resources as a result. *From now on, and throughout this chapter, you are entering the realm of fiction.*

We are in 2030 and the world governance structures have just collapsed. They held up for a while, it is true, both the EU, the UN, and the big national governments. The smaller ones, obviously, succumbed first. Not the rich states, of course—Switzerland and Norway are still around although, as the world's honeypots, they are subject to looting from poorer nation's warlords as well as various international mafia organizations, mostly from southern Europe. Even Switzerland's war chest is not what it once was.

Norway was faring better. Except that Russia, hungry for an ice-free winter port from which to launch their ships to trade with Europe, invaded Norway toward the latter part of the decade. However, Russia's mainland also rapidly disintegrated into a weak, failed state, and have had to retreat to the coastline.

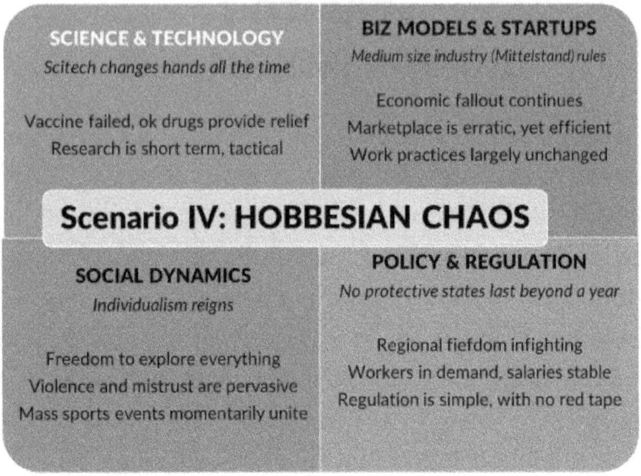
SCIENCE & TECHNOLOGY
Scitech changes hands all the time
Vaccine failed, ok drugs provide relief
Research is short term, tactical
BIZ MODELS & STARTUPS
Medium size industry (Mittelstand) rules
Economic fallout continues
Marketplace is erratic, yet efficient
Work practices largely unchanged
Scenario IV: HOBBESIAN CHAOS
SOCIAL DYNAMICS
Individualism reigns
Freedom to explore everything
Violence and mistrust are pervasive
Mass sports events momentarily unite
POLICY & REGULATION
No protective states last beyond a year
Regional fiefdom infighting
Workers in demand, salaries stable
Regulation is simple, with no red tape

Figure 7.1. Hobbesian Chaos

The Norwegian resistance, headquartered in the Dovre mountains, are starting to make a difference. Special forces, using high-tech gear including tactical suits and synthetic bioweapons, like tactical bacteria causing immediate overwhelming local inflammation that lasts 3 days and resourced from the UK, prove that guerrilla fighting can still be efficient. Other than that, life in the inland is almost unaffected.

<u>Hamar, Norway, February 10, 2030</u>: Norwegian Frøydis Hansen was only 3 when the virus hit. She is now 13 and is eagerly learning about world history before the virus. She completes applied math problems on how to plan how many potatoes one village needs each winter. She is eager to travel to neighboring villages with her new invention, a mechanical breathing machine that turns cold air into warm air. She has inherited the spirit of invention from her father, who was a petroleum engineer.

"Frøydis," says her mom angrily, "I've told you so many

times to turn down the music." "I know, I know," says Frøydis. "At least, local Norwegian music is the only thing left now that I cannot stream anymore. Aren't you happy about that?" "I don't know," said her mother, "I would rather you listened to Britpop. I used to love that when I was young. Are you sure we cannot find some of those old CDs in the attic?" "Oh, Mom, you are so nostalgic," says Frøydis. She pulled out an old Duran Duran album she had found a while back and started blasting "Hungry Like a Wolf." Soon, the house was filled with the familiar lyrics. Frøydis could hear her mom singing at the top of her lungs, which thankfully were healthy again: "I'm hungry like the wolf."

Well, thought Frøydis, I thought that was a love song, but here we are, I've been hungry for a decade, and our house is cold in winter now that we have to conserve heat. I'm freezing like a wolf, she thought, but then thought to herself, it's not that funny. Nothing was that funny anymore. Not to her.

Her father died last year, trying to rescue one of the smaller oil rigs outside Bergen that had been left there after the Russian submarine attack. She was glad the Russians had only decided to invade the coastline and not the inland where they lived. She had loved her father very much. Losing him had seemed like losing everything. Yet, life went on without him, just less joyful. Something had changed in her, though. Suddenly, the concerns of adults seemed more intimate and important to her. The world's problems were her own. But her mother's voice made her sound happy again, if only for a moment, and that was worth smiling for. As she glanced at the app that told her about the latest curfews and the grocery shopping guidelines, she noticed it was time for bed. Her first evening where she had felt at home. She felt like she could actually sleep.

The secondary events—wars, famines, and ecological catastrophes

I want to be clear. The pandemic was only one of many things we worried about in this tumultuous decade. Let me attempt to quickly summarize the seven plagues that hit us.

In the fall of 2021, the US experienced a major hurricane, aptly named Armageddon (after initially being called Alfred since it was the first of the season). Hurricane Katrina, in 2017, peaking at a Category-5 storm, caused $125 billion in damage, particularly in the city of New Orleans and the surrounding areas, and over 1,200 deaths. Armageddon, by contrast, had sustained winds by landfall in the Category 5, but peaked at unprecedented Category-6 winds on the Saffir-Simpson scale. With the entire city of New Orleans being overflowed by the tidal wave that ensued, there was no doubt that a new Category 6 was warranted. Given the already weakened Sun Belt infrastructure, the death toll was found to be in the 50,000s, but the infrastructure damage in five states was near total.

The real problem wasn't the initial death toll, but the fact that, because of the quarantine rules, reconstruction couldn't begin in the first 3 years. As a result, a generation of kids living in the coastal states stretching from Maine to Texas never went to school, as the Internet was also torn out by the storm. In fact, a third of the estimated 44.8% of the nation's population who live in these states didn't get back electricity until year 5, by which time half of them had migrated to other parts of the country. The surrounding states now found their infrastructure severely strained. It had been dubbed the "second main exodus" after the massive "first exodus" when people left US major cities for suburbia and the countryside in droves the first 3 years after the pandemic. The only people left in the cities were the financial elite and the poor, leading to severe clashes on the best of days.

In West Africa, just as the last case of Ebola in the Democratic Republic of the Congo (DRC), a 26-year-old electrician in the eastern city of Beni was found to have the disease. Just as that nation was going to declare victory of the disease, it broke out again. This time, it was to coincide with COVID-19. Early on, both Africa and public health experts had been quick to point out that West Africa's experience with successfully eradicating Ebola would serve it well when it came to COVID-19.

The problem was, they were, in fact, very different diseases. There was nothing in the past that could prepare West Africa for asymptomatic transmission. In fact, it worked the opposite way. Because they thought they knew how infectious diseases spread, they underestimated COVID-19, with devastating consequences.

Soon, Ebola again ravaged West Africa, and, this time, there was no way of keeping it out of the cities. Zaire Ebolavirus had earlier spread to Goma, a city of 2 million people, and then was subsequently contained. The second time around, Goma got hit with 10,000 cases and it soon spread to nearby Butembo, a city of 1 million people. That meant all three cities on the border of DRC, Rwanda, and Uganda had Ebola. A regional catastrophe ensued, and had it not been for the relative communication with the rest of the world due to COVID-19 restrictions, there is no telling where it would have ended. As it now was, a total of 100,000 people in West Africa died from the disease before they managed to contain it toward 2025, but not before a terrorist group managed to swoop up the virus and weaponize it.

On August 15, 2025, a mysterious disease started to appear among policy makers in France after a small bomblet went off in the Parliament. Initially thought to be an innocent smoke bomb, into which it had been camouflaged, the bomb had gone off during an important vote about COVID-19 economic relief to service workers affected by the crisis. Initially, only about 30 of them contracted the disease, but because they each were taken to different Parisian hospitals showing various signs of distress after the smoke attack, the Zaire Ebola strain of the virus spread to 1,000 others, many of them French parliamentarians or their families, plus three hospitals.

The incident stoked fear across Europe and took on a much different seriousness after it was discovered it was a resurgent Al-Qaeda who were responsible. A spokesperson from Al-Qaeda released a video streamed to Euronews stating that "we have unlimited amounts of virus, which we will release again, should it be necessary." No specific demands were made over the next few years, but the world now had to content not with another nuclear power, but with a new bioterror power.

In East Africa, the grasshopper storms that started appearing in the spring of 2020 had gained Biblical proportions; some would argue, far beyond. An estimated thousand billion locusts (a state of gregarious, swarming grasshoppers) were swarming vast territories from Somalia, via Ethiopia, to Kenya and Tanzania, and even into Zambia and Mozambique, essentially throughout the entire region, but also independently in Egypt and Iran, blackening the sky and devouring harvest from thousands of miles, decimating crops that were meant to last for the entire year.

The infestation, the worst in this century, caused a massive famine, 100 times the impact of the Ethiopian Great Famine that afflicted Ethiopia from 1888 to 1892, which cost it roughly one-third of its population. With the travel restrictions, none of the international relief organizations, not even Aid for Africa, Oxfam, Save the Children, and Care International's combined efforts, managed to get enough food to stem the tide.

Beyond the East African famine, the overall world food security system also took a major hit. Supply chain restrictions and years of downgrading of food storage facilities adjusting to the just-in-time principle where store shelves were only filled based on demand expressed by consumer choices 1–2 weeks ahead meant that the food algorithms we misleading, and global capacity could not reach around the world fast enough for the demand during the crisis.

What ensued was, predictably, national build-up of supply and attempts to build national food supply and vendors. The problem was that the costs were staggering. Several of the global food giants imploded as a combination of the renewed pressures, government regulation, and a lack of raw material. In the US, the availability of wheat became a problem. The leading agricultural wheat producers, the states of North Dakota, Kansas, and Montana, were locked down over COVID-19 concerns. Grain storage capacity in relative terms (to demand) had been in decline over the past decade. Even if the US had the third-largest grain storage in the world, stores ran out of flour as an estimated 50 million households turned to home-baking on a weekly basis.

The following year, in early 2021, the ozone layer over Antarctica weakened drastically, below 100 Dobson units, causing massively strengthened radiation rays over Argentina, Chile, and Brazil, as well as over Australia. Over the next decade, skin cancer rates skyrocketed to affect 50% of those populations, with melanoma, the most serious form of skin cancer, increasing to 20% of the total. The public health advice was to stay indoors or wear radiation suits, which proved to be expensive, uncomfortable, and incredibly hot to wear. Most people in those places took to spending most of their time indoors, leading to an increased risk of contracting COVID-19 indoors. Across the globe, skin cancer rates also increased, and children with vulnerable skin types similarly were advised to stay indoors.

In Italy, the Camorra mafia in Naples gained control of the southern part of Italy after it began capitalizing on the growing sympathy it had enjoyed during the first 5 years of the coronavirus crisis, as they emerged as a major local "relief organization," providing food and shelter to a growing number of the impoverished population in the Italian "Mezzogiorno" region.

The turning point was that the main mafia families joined a pact and even brought in the powerful Calabrian 'Ndrangheta as well as the Sicilian mafia. Ties extended to the US, where the New York–Chicago axis became a renewed stronghold.

Transnational organized crime, more generally, increasingly became a force to be reckoned with throughout the second part of the decade, as more and more countries experienced fragile and failing governance structures. In some cases, they co-opted state institutions; in others, they merely replaced them. Human trafficking increased exponentially because cheap labor was needed in the service industry as a lot of staff turnover became the norm because of the 50%-increased mortality rates among that segment of society.

On the other hand, those who worked in the service sector and did so of their own free will, enjoyed up to 100% salary increases compared to US minimum wage, and comparable increases in Europe and in cities in Asia.

Why technology didn't save us

Many put their faith in technology. After all, wasn't this the decade that supposedly was going to get us more progress than all other decades of this century combined? This was what the futurists had been saying before 2020. Now, the tune was different. Conditions have changed. Forecasts were revisited. Both the pandemic and the set of escalating regional events that we just experienced, particularly the famines, wars, and ecological disasters, slowed their growth and limited technology's impact to pockets of newly emerged elites.

What people wanted was to return to the way things were before. Technology became the means they deployed to make it so. Here's how it went.

3D printing got implemented quicker than expected. As a distributed technology, it was popular with everyone. The 3D-printing-service companies became the world's biggest, supplying everything you needed to print your own reality, your own version of perfection. Only, the devices were faulty, they were expensive, and the products they printed were mostly not edible, which means you could print a desk. But you cannot feed a happy family on printed pasta alone.

Internet speeds were soaring at the beginning of the decade. Then, it hit all the providers; people couldn't afford all the planned upgrades. Networks of 5G, 6G, 7G, 8G, they all got delayed and big cities were prioritized.

Artificial intelligence was available, but only to the highest bidder. What that meant was a huge discrepancy of what you could do with it. The poor could watch TV created by bots, which was something. The rich could outsource their life to the AI, essentially. Neither turned out to be ideal. But in the name of progress, governments around the world began testing the notion that everyone would have their own digital avatar, a persona that could stand in for them online. What it mostly was about was securing votes. This was the perfect scheme to ensure that everybody voted. Once your avatar was online, there was no excuse. Everybody would know that you didn't vote, and you could be punished. But it rarely happened. States were so weak these days. They had enough with fighting down rebellion.

Augmented reality first meant that business meetings, love at a distance, and computer games got extremely intense. That was the first few years of the decade. After that, AR shifted a bit. Developers were more excited about building up the various factions with facades that made them look more powerful. The middle of the decade was the age of deepfakes. It became impossible to figure out if whomever you were interacting with truly represented the country of Germany or simply was a hacker. How to tell? Entirely new actors appeared out of nowhere. Since the media was weak, and nobody knew whom to trust anymore; it wasn't possible to stop them.

Autonomous driving didn't pan out at all. That is to say, systems were launched but they were in an eternal test mode. The reason is that the cost of implementing a new traffic infrastructure couldn't be footed by failed or failing states, and there were few big companies willing to foot the bill. There were exceptions, of course. Germany managed to implement one through the combined efforts of their entire automotive industry in collaboration with the richest regions.

Blockchain became a good idea gone bad. Instead of fostering a transparent economy, it contributed to a collapse. The problem was that building a transparent ledger, at the end of the day, requires that a majority of actors have the self-interest of transparency. Failing that, the system requirements change, and the odds gradually tilt toward cheating. Anyway, that's what happened at first.

Then, governments, those that still had any power, tried to step in. But by then, most systems were so opaque, so entrenched, that little could be done. There was openness, but you had no idea who was behind each transaction. The principle of governance is very poorly thought out in blockchain. It relies on openness. But openness cannot survive when you don't have the tools to enforce it. For transaction after transaction, when corruption was exposed nothing happened. So, there you had it, a thousand open ledgers that displayed fully transparent corruption of the system that nobody were able to do anything about. The situation was quite ironic.

Additionally, the more central banks started printing money and buying a lot of government debt to hold interest rates down the way they did in the war years, the less efficient the blockchain became. Governments should have made the choice, blockchain or quantitative easing. When both were implemented at the same time, they became a bit like two parallel economies competing for attention. What the combined forces of the impact of COVID-19, a massive launch of a parallel economy through blockchain did, is to cause a big short-term economic decline followed by a much smaller rebound than expected, as people were putting their eggs in two separate baskets.

CRISPR, the gene editing tool, became a life saver for criminal networks who highjacked the top scientists and extorted them for the services of editing their genes so they would not contract COVID-19.

By altering just three genes, genes IL-6 (a protein-coding gene that induces cytokine in inflammations), TGFBI (a growth gene infected through the cornea), and MTHFR (an enzyme that plays a role in processing amino acids into the bloodstream), those thugs were able to secure a new extortion service which they made available to their highest echelon of supporters, those that owed them more than $100 million dollars each. That way, CRISPR came to fuel the largest criminal networks in the history of mankind.

Cybersecurity was a big concern, but not in the way one might think. The issue wasn't that cybercriminals would extort you. The real issue was that there was nobody who wasn't one. This creates a weird situation. If you can trust nobody, how to you practice endpoint security? Hence, that paradigm failed. Instead, corporations around the world had to implement a new system based on zero trust. The challenge with that paradigm is that it has enormous negative externalities, as economists would say. When you cannot trust your own employees to do the right thing, and the IT systems are the only monitoring tools, how can you trust your own IT systems or those that operate them. It becomes a vicious cycle.

Precision medicine requires a much different infrastructure than is available to us right now. The prospect of a major breakthrough whereby individuals can get meaningful, appropriate treatment is next to nil. Health systems have enough with treating emergencies. Any chronic diseases are left untreated. There are university hospitals still experimenting with it, but they treat very few patients. The field is left in an eternal state of limbo. Progress is made, but it never gets scaled up.

Nanotechnology and quantum computing are simply postponed to the next decade. All the researchers who were active in the field have been repurposed to more pressing matters. There's a time for everything and pie in the sky research is not something we can afford right now.

Robotics means vacuum cleaners and less factory workers, which means less jobs in the home services industry as well as in manufacturing. It took only 3 years before robots were blamed for the mass unemployment that was caused by an avalanche of factors related to COVID-19's economic fallout. Kind of a shame that it is so, but robots became a convenient vessel to put our blame upon. Robot shaming has become a thing. People are literally tormenting machines, if that makes any sense to you.

Smart fabrics was another pipedream of the early 2020s. Implementing clothes that incorporate advanced technology never became affordable. The prototypes are cool, though.

Synthetic biology is making quiet progress, but the few firms that managed to capitalize on the crisis were largely consumed with trying to develop a vaccine, which took their ball of their main R&D targets. As a result, the breakthroughs ceased to happen and investors largely lost interest. Perhaps the world is better for it. One report said that if synthetic biology had become one of the top-three industries, it would push us away from human nature, because synthetically produced "nature" is better. I'm glad this hasn't happened yet. I still enjoy my walks in the park, the occasional mountain hike, and my cruising down the slopes in winter.

Virtual reality—well—those masks are clunkier and more expensive than ever. But given the deepfake issue, I'm glad this is the case, we have enough trouble with AR. Can you imagine if virtual reality became indistinguishable from real life? I don't even want to think about how the mafia would exploit that.

The quiet first years of the decade

The first 3 years after coronavirus came down on us were relatively calm. Most of all, there was this lingering sense that things were unpleasant, and sad, sort of like a rainy day that is followed by another, and another, and.... Seeing the constant body bags was jarring at first, then we got used to it. Parents quickly started shielding their kids from any kind of live news. There became a watertight division between online learning for elementary school which was siphoned off from the regular Internet that contained news about the public health situation.

There were, of course, massive political discussions, but they were somewhat muted. Nobody had the energy to put up much of a fight in the early years. I think most of us, including politicians, expected the crisis to somehow miraculously end. First, the timeline was weeks, then we all adjusted to months, but as the months went by, we started thinking of it as an adjustment over several years. Nobody in their right mind really thought of this as the decade of corona, which is what it became, or worse.

The healthcare toll was enormous even the first year and cascaded into other sectors of society. We had all hoped to go back to some sort of economic normalcy, to open markets and go back to work. There was some of that, don't get me wrong. Different countries had staggered curves. Some weren't even affected the first 6 months but got it the latter part of the year. Then, the blockchain fiasco ensued, and money just got cut in half. It was an expensive experiment.

Minsk, Belarus, September 7 , 2021: Belarus, a landlocked country bordered by Lithuania and Latvia to the northwest, by Russia to the north and east, by Ukraine to the south, and by Poland to the west, had initially ignored coronavirus. The President initially called coronavirus a psychosis, and famously allowed the country's sports events to go on unhinged. In 2020, this was the only country where you could still watch soccer, so the players became as famous as the Spanish, English, and Italian league players for a few months. Then, it rapidly deteriorated. The outbreak came swiftly and without mercy. Now the memory of these events, once such a source of national pride, was a stain.

Natalia, the head of the infectious disease department at the City Clinical Hospital of Infectious Diseases in Minsk, the national center coordinating the clinical coronavirus epidemic response in Belarus, was tired. She had been up all night, all week, there were patients everywhere, and there were medical personnel gasping for air, and patients awaiting triage, and government officials wanting the updates, and TV teams, and everything was happening at the same time. And somewhere, in the back of her mind, all she could think of was her 5-month-old daughter at home with her mother. How long until her mother too was exposed? Darya was her only assistant now that they had to use all administrative staff as nurses. "Yes, Natalia, I'm working as fast as I can," said Darya, looking up through her eye protection with glazed eyes. "Did you know I just put on our last face mask?" That was the last Natalia heard from Darya. She never found out what happened, but her theory was that Darya ran away at the end of her shift, never to be seen again. Natalia didn't really blame her. Why would a 25-year-old administrative assistant want to die in a pandemic? She had lasted 6 months under unbearable pressure. Even trained military or medical personnel were caving. Darya had no such training, and Natalia blamed herself for putting her in the line of fire.

By the end of the year, 50,000 were dead from the virus and by the spring 2 million had perished. For a 9-million-person population, that means a 22% death toll, which was the highest of any country, save failed states. Even Italy, which got it hard and had no time to prepare, managed to keep their death toll much lower. Coronavirus isn't kind to countries without a functioning public health system, but that wasn't the issue for Belarus.

Belarus had a much better healthcare system that one would think. It is also free. That was the problem. They attempted to care for everyone, and the system simply broke down. Europe's last dictatorship, as it has been called, had another problem. Because they never implemented any mitigation strategies, they would have had a tragic outcome no matter what healthcare system they had, in a way quite akin to the US, which, surprisingly, also took a major hit with coronavirus.

Belarus shared its fate with other dictatorial states where the leadership either kept a lid on the true nature of the outbreaks or downright denied it existed. In fact, all the countries scoring the lowest on the Economist Intelligence Unit (EIU)'s *Democracy Index*, including Libya, Uzbekistan, Yemen, Turkmenistan, Chad, Syria, Central African Republic, Democratic Republic of Congo, and North Korea, had infection rates nearing 60% of the population and death tolls ranging from 20–30%, as the pandemic swept through over the first 5 years of the pandemic, in uneven waves depending on the attack path of the virus.

Failed states also suffered badly. Common indicators of

failing states, already problematic before the pandemic, quickly became staggering predictors of death toll. Central governments without practical control its territory lost all control or ceded it to criminal groups. Countries with few if any working public services had no independent capacity to stem the tide neither with public health measures nor with economic measures. Countries with widespread corruption and criminality became incubators of pan-regional terrorist groups, claiming huge territory, raping and pillaging already ravaged communities at a previously unseen scale. Countries with huge populations of refugees simply couldn't stop COVID-19 from raging through the camps or infecting near 100% of its health workers. Countries with sharp economic decline spiraled into further decline, further escalating death tolls in secondary problems such as famine, other community spread infectious diseases such as cholera and diphtheria. Those with high degree of failure on all of the above, understandably, completely collapsed.

Before 2020, the Fragile States Index (https://fragilestatesindex.org/) had only five countries listed under very high alert—Yemen, Somalia, South Sudan, Syria, and the Democratic Republic of the Congo. By end 2021, that list had expanded to the top-20 countries on that list, and by 2023 to each of the top-100 countries on that list, representing almost a billion people. The unraveling of Pakistan, with its 193 million people, and Nigeria, with its 174 million people, drastically increased the global death toll and spilled over into waves of smaller outbreaks in neighboring countries that had near contained the virus after the first 5 years, including Pakistan's neighbors India, Afghanistan, and Iran, and Nigeria's neighbors Benin, Niger, Chad, and Cameroon.

Other more remote locations didn't get coronavirus at all, or just had a small outbreak. Then, there were towns that deliberately isolated themselves. Each country had a few of those. But life there was miserable. They had to become self-sufficient. Moreover, once looters realized what those towns were, they raided them at night, sometimes bringing contagion with them.

Overall, the markets never reopened with the same effervescence as before. The mood was gloomy as if everyone was waiting for the shoe to drop.

Wall Street, New York, October 12, 2023: *Jeremy Ribbons burst through the door. "Edward, did you short all the virus manufacturers yesterday for $100 million? I hope not, because today they are up 200%. The FDA just scrapped human testing for any infectious disease. They found a way to create synthetic humans using a new approach to DNA sequencing."*

Jeremy Ribbons was the president of Shock Hedge Funds, LLC, a $10-billion player in the life science industry. Edward was his trading partner. That sector had been especially volatile over the last 3 years. All new technology was going up. People were shorting the big-five pharma players. However, governments were holding on because they had renationalized most of them. Government debt and holdings were not particularly attractive at the moment, which was good for hedge funds. It was easy to short a bond exchange-traded fund (ETF) and take the windfall.

Edward didn't answer, he was on the phone with his wife, the only other person he would take a bullet for. She said their son refused to come down from the roof. He said something about contamination of his room. It has been like this for months now. His son had watched too much news and read too many internet stories about corona. Now, everything was about corona for him. He couldn't think about anything else. They had a psychologist at the house every morning at 9:00 a.m., but by the time the shrink left at noon, the problem was back. It was frustrating. For the first time in nearly a decade, Edward was at a loss. At some point, he had hoped for his son to take over his hedge fund. Right now, he wasn't even sure if his son would be well enough to start school again anytime soon. He had lost all friends and had taken the death of his sister to coronavirus quite hard.

"Unfortunately, I did," said Edward. "But listen to this, I also found an early stage startup backed by five Nobel Prize winners and I took their whole scale-up round of $100 million. Then, this afternoon, the EU wanted in and bought my shares for $300 million. I went ahead and shorted the EU's new joint pension fund holdings with the money. We will earn a fortune by next month. Those guys are going down, I'm pretty sure."

Edward felt winded. Everything was coming apart so quickly these days. How long before he came apart? His son? And who would be left to help them then? Was he cutting off the last lines of assistance that his son might someday need? Too much to calculate in this moment, thought Edward, and returned to his monitor.

The volatility of oil prices spurs unrest

A main reason for the increasing unrest was the enormous volatility in the oil price throughout the decade. Initially, the crisis drove the price down from $60/barrel down to $20; this happened in the first 3 months of the crisis. Throughout that year, the price spiked back up to $50 for weeks on end, only to tumble back to around $15/barrel, at which point, extraction becomes less feasible for many of the world's oil producers, certainly in America, which relies heavily on shale oil, which has a costly extraction process. Several times, the oil price went negative, which was unprecedented. For US producers to generate profits, they need prices to exceed $45–$50 per barrel.

As a result of the oil crisis, petroleum facilities and subsequently the oil-producing countries became attractive targets for small proxy wars and then for regional terrorist groups such as Al-Qaeda in the Middle East and Boko Haram in Nigeria. Even in Texas, a patriot movement calling themselves the Real Texans emerged on the scene, effectively seizing the control over oil production in that state, which amounts to 40% of US oil production.

Corpus Christi, Texas, December 12, 2025: Church was a big deal in Texas. Texans are known worldwide for their love of big things: ranches, trucks, homes, vistas. The postwar era's reconstruction proved perfect breeding ground for taking that concept to religion, too. Throughout the 1980–1990s, megachurches took the suburban Sunbelt in Texas by storm. Highly mobile, consumer centric, well-educated, middle-class families flocked to them. By 2020, there were over 200 megachurches in Texas, each with a sustained attendance of over 2,000 people, and some beyond 20,000. Many of them were in the suburbs around Houston or Dallas.

Curtis and his big family had taken to the new megachurch that had come to Corpus Christi right before the crisis. Throughout the crisis, the services gathered about 3,000 people for worship, which was down from 8,000. The pastors were against social distancing; they said it was Satan's work. Curtis tended to concur. What was all the drama about? They even continued to shake hands, hug, and lay hands on each other and take communion. "What's a bit of physical contact?" he thought. A bit of Texas sunlight kills most bugs, why not viruses, too?

After church, as was his custom, Curtis stopped by his friend Joe Foster's before going to the monthly meeting at Texans for Vaccine Choice. Joe, that rascal, was sitting inside his old airplane, which he had turned into a living room of sorts, and he could hear Joe firing up the plane.

"I found some old jet fuel," said Joe. "Wanna go for a spin?" Curtis was thrilled. It had been 3 years since he had even been driving in one of his altogether 25 cars. He couldn't remember the last time he'd felt the thrum of the engine, something he always thought would be a part of him. "I dug up some fuel I'd squirreled away," said Joe and grinned widely. "The Texas Rangers came by to ask me for fuel for their trucks. I gave them

some, but I saved a little for one last ride."

This was going to be a great day, at least until somebody saw them. But burn that bridge when they come to it, right? In this moment, they remembered what it was to be free, to be their own men. As they got up in the air, they could see something strange. Along the roads, there were rows and rows with trucks that had red crosses on them. "What are those?" asked Curtis. "Oh, those are the morgues," said Joe. "I don't know why there are so many."

As much as religion fought back the government mandates not to gather in groups larger than 50, which was generally the case around the world, they also took major hits. Some megachurches kept it going until 2025, after which the jail sentences for pastors became too long to bear and many of them just closed down.

However, even regular organized religion suffered greatly during the period. I guess it is hard to keep a moral grasp of your parishioners when you cannot gather in person very much. Protestantism declined to a new low across America, that denomination's stronghold. Even Catholicism suffered greatly, from the double whammy of COVID-19 and continuing clergy abuse scandals, which didn't let up throughout the decade.

In the Muslim world, the prohibition of the pilgrimage proved detrimental to social support. Former religious strongholds across the Middle East secularized faster than you could say "mosque." There was also much consternation around the religious establishment's initial denial that there was a serious issue. Imams throughout the region continued to impose the same restrictions as before. Islamophobia continued in India as a billion people essentially took to the notion that the Muslim body was prone to COVID-19 infection and, as such, Jihad incarnated. This was only one version of hate speech that was echoed throughout the world, and taking different flavors among neo-Nazis in Germany (where both

Jews and Muslims were culprits, often in weird constellations), among the Taliban (any infidel), Islamic State (ISIS) who saw it as a Western plot to reduce the influence of Arab states, and Al-Shabaab in Somalia (arguing government is the problem).

Strongmen who at the beginning of the decade attempted to enrich themselves and profit from the chaos, in countries like the US, Argentina, the Philippines, and Venezuela, have long ago ceased to extract their population, although they did for several years. Now the problem is different. There was a revolution. Or, rather, there was an avalanche of smaller revolutions. Nothing too organized. Just a creeping feeling among the people, and among the military, and the private sector elite as well, that governments just weren't responding to the public health crisis. And, in the beginning, everyone agreed that the attacks on oil installations and transport routes had to stop. Several times a month, terrorists broke open pipelines.

The Yamal-Europe pipeline, which connects the natural gas reserves of Western Siberia in Russia to Austria and Germany, was now partially controlled by the Polish mafia who had intercepted the Jamal section that was supposed to reach Germany. The Trans-Saharan Pipeline from Nigeria to Algeria is being finalized by Boko Haram as we speak. The Eastern Siberia-Pacific Ocean Oil Pipeline linking Siberia to the Chinese border is being finalized by Siberian separatists, a newly emerged opportunistic group of former oligarchs. The Keystone pipeline running from Alberta to Illinois and now essentially down to Houston was initially controlled by the US government, then as the government weakened, was soon taken over by a consortium of US controlled oil interests. The Kazakhstan-China oil pipeline, the first oil import stream from Central Asia, was quickly seized by Uzbek separatists using it to extort the local government.

Germany initially took it upon themselves to defend the

4,000 km Druzhba Pipeline, one of the world's longest oil pipeline, running from Almetyevsk in central Russia to Schwedt in northern Germany, all on behalf of the EU. However, it quickly became clear that they had ulterior motives. After a far-right takeover of government, Germany effectively started charging the EU double, taking control of the petroleum market in Europe. This didn't go over well.

The EU attempted to intervene diplomatically, to no avail. Suffice to say, the French forces mounted an epic fight, and given that Germany's army after 1945 mostly has been a small defense force, they couldn't respond. With the French backed up by the EU forces now in control of the Druzhba Pipeline things calmed down for a few months. But in terms of European cohesion, this wasn't exactly a positive factor in Franco-German relations. For a while, the EU continued, and in Germany the Christian Democrats again took seat in Berlin, this time in leading a minority government. The world was watching and there was an eerie feeling this was too similar to the Weimar Republic, which consisted of a series of weak governments leading up to the world war. The Weimar Republic was Germany's government from 1919 to 1933, the period after World War I until the rise of Nazi Germany.

The Strait of Hormuz was historically the world's most important oil transit choke point. Located between Oman and Iran, it connects the Persian Gulf with the Gulf of Oman and the Arabian Sea. There are limited options to bypass the Strait of Hormuz. What happened there was that the US sent an aircraft carrier to control the strait. This worked well for a while, but because of a coronavirus outbreak on the carrier, likely planted by Middle Eastern spies of unknown origin, the ship's crew was much weakened, and couldn't perform their function over time. At some point, they also ran out of food and water and had to dock in Oman. While docked there, a series of bombs shelled the huge ship and it went down later that day. From that point onward, the US economy went into a tailspin and chaos ensued. The rest is history.

White House, July 3, 2025: "Mr. President, I have the King of Saudi Arabia on the line, he says it is important." The Chief of Staff was not usually answering the phone, but the last few months had been extreme. Morale was down. Press was bad. News was worse. What was it this time? "I report latest from Middle East," said a scratchy voice on the other end. "Oman says you must pay to clean up the Strait of Hormuz or they will go to war against the United States." "That's laughable," said the president. "Well," said the Saudi King, "they may be small, but they are now strong partners with Iran, and both agree this must have consequences. I tend to agree." The president was silent for a minute, and then said sternly, "Tell Iran we will go after them across the Middle East. And to you, I never liked you very much after you lot killed a journalist."

The president slammed down the phone. The shifting web of alliances was turning against him. Against the country? No. Against him. *Now, the Chinese, the Iranians, and the Saudis were ganging up on him.*

Pandemic death toll in Iran had spiraled out of control relatively quickly through the holy city of Qom, the seventh largest city in the country and home to the biggest China-Iran partnership since the Silk Road. Now that China has embarked on a modern version of the Silk Road, the so-called One Belt, One Road policy, Iran has been key to the effort. A total of 65 countries will build new roads, ports and airports on the Silk Road's modern route. In fact, the new China-Iran railroad is already built.

The geostrategic position of Iran, which is located both on the Caspian Sea and the Persian Gulf border, is important for China, who also is the largest importer of Iranian oil. Qom, 125 kilometers southwest of Tehran, is home to the Fatima Masumeh Shrine, which has a monumental gold dome and intricate blue tilework and draws pilgrims from all over the world. Qom also has major Shi'ite religious schools with

Chinese students. A Chinese company is finalizing the $2.7 billion railroad project linking up the two countries and more. China is also building a solar power plant in Qom. The outbreak coincided with two major milestones—the anniversary of Iran's revolution, on February 11th, and the parliamentary election, on February 21st.

"Give me the president of the European Commission," said the US president. "But Mr. President," said his Chief of Staff, "the EU is no longer in charge of its troops, so to speak. What good would that do?" "I want to speak to that woman," shrieked the president. "She loosened the sanctions, sent foreign aid, and convinced the IMF and the World Bank to agree major debt relief. She must be punished. I won't let China win!"

I should probably explain the human cost of the pandemic as well. As you can imagine, the coronavirus pandemic of 2020 had a devastating death toll. The final numbers were never published, but a good estimate would be that 2% of the world population perished in the first wave, and 4% in the next. I can imagine that doesn't sound like much to you. Perhaps not, but it spiraled into something bigger. The deaths weren't evenly spread out. What we previously called the "third world" was harder hit. Death tolls in Africa were closer to 30%.

The Asian industrial miracle

In Asia, it was uneven, but the megacities took a 20% hit for the most part. Beijing was spared because they had learned from the first outbreak. So was Hong Kong, Singapore, and Seoul, and a few other Chinese cities made out well, including Shenzhen, where the manufacturing revolution still was happening for a while.

International rebuilding efforts

The resource scarcity was a challenge, but the true problem was of another kind. When world leaders tried to deal with the crisis, there was a lot of debate about the repairs and rebuilding efforts. These were hampered by the fact that people were forced to debate these issues over (often) poor videoconferencing lines. Imagine the UN run from afar. It was chaos. At some point, the African Union countries rebelled and broke out of the EU. The situation there was starting to break down, anyway.

Lagos, Nigeria, May 10, 2023: "Kwame, can you fetch groceries today," his mom shouted from the kitchen. Kwame, 27, had come home from South Africa last year, almost a year before he was due to finish his bachelor's degree in Business from the University of Cape Town. He was home to take care of his family. He missed his girlfriend, who was South African and had to remain in Cape Town. No matter, it was the smallest of sacrifices, he thought to himself. No use getting married now, anyway.

To an outsider, it might have seemed shocking how quickly the infrastructure fell apart, how soon the relief planes stopped landing, the government officials openly worried only about themselves. Too few resources, scarcely any resources at all. And the HIV and malaria outbreak patients? They just fell by the wayside.

"No problem, Mom," he shouted from the backyard, where he had been trying to grow some vegetables in the baking heat. It was everyone for themselves now, and his family was lucky enough to have a fenced-in backyard in the attractive Lekki area of eastern suburban Lagos. The task was not just to grow the crops but to hide them from the many looters who frequented Lagos' suburban countryside homes.

This wasn't just a hobby and Kwame embraced gardening not just by necessity but also with intellectual satisfaction. Growing vegetables was literally how he would keep his large, extended family alive. They had all moved in here, all 10 cousins and uncles, a big happy family of 25 people, all hunkered down in a small townhouse with an enclosed garden patch. It was more than a mere family, though. They were a tribe now.

Everyone was contributing, and his younger sister Adaku had stepped up, providing education to all the children; she even gave a little course to the community through online learning. Kwame suddenly became the "head" of the family, as most male adults had perished in the second wave of the virus attack, either succumbing to the virus or because they had been killed in the riots for food and water.

They had gone from upper-middle class to being considered part of the "undeserving elite" of Nigeria, those who still had their own homes. Most days, Kwame did not feel like an elite. Kwame fetched his big wooden stick, reinforced with a metal tip, his homemade weapon, and started on the 10-mile hike to the only surviving open air market in that part of town. It was an arduous journey, not because of the distance but because on the way back he had to sneak around carefully not to be attacked by those who were less fortunate and had to steal food for a living.

He took his homemade face mask and a torn plastic bag that he would turn into an improvised set of gloves by the time he arrived and had to touch the groceries. He had already been attacked once and lost all the things he bought. This time, he put on raggedy clothes, showing his bulging muscles sticking out of a torn, black T-shirt. He was better prepared to hide his bounty. He had decided to only buy half as much stuff, so he could run away fast if needed.

As he walked, Kwame saw decomposed bodies simply lying in the street. Abandoned, burned-down homes, and looted cars with only the chassis left. It looked a bit like a Hollywood disaster movie, he thought to himself. What was once a slum and had become developed was reverting back. What would it become next? When he had first returned from South Africa, this lawlessness might have shocked him. But he had learned something at once new and simultaneously ancient. The cycle of life, Kwame thought and trudged onward.

Boko Haram extends its reign beyond Western Africa

The Nigerian terrorist group Boko Haram had been gaining foothold in that part of Africa for a while. Even before 2020, from their foothold in northeastern Nigeria, they were already active in Chad, Niger, and northern Cameroon. It only took them a few years to control most of West Africa and then they moved south.

With the pandemic, they literally took aim at southern Africa. Very quickly, South Africa succumbed as well. What this meant is that Boko Haram got access to all its mineral and other resources and could pool that together with all the Nigerian petroleum revenue. South Africa is rich in a variety of minerals. In addition to diamonds and gold, the country also contains reserves of iron ore, platinum, manganese, chromium, copper, uranium, silver, beryllium, and titanium.

By 2022, Boko Haram wasn't content with the south; they also moved on The Democratic Republic of Congo. DRC has one of the richest deposits of mineral resources in the world. Before the crisis the value of these untapped deposits of raw mineral was estimated to be worth some $24 trillion. The value after the crisis quickly rose tenfold, making Boko Haram the richest organization in the world. DRC is, by area, the largest country in sub-Saharan Africa. The prices of these precious minerals spiked rapidly the first 3 years of the decade, as there were oligopolies running most of the mines already.

In short, Africa quickly became run by various terrorist factions, and even the Chinese had to flee. You know it's serious when Chinese capital flees, because they will go anywhere to make a buck or a yen. The Chinese responded by expanding their Pacific Fleet and in as little as 5 years, they mounted a counterassault on Boko Haram, given that Chinese capital by the start of the crisis had taken aim at controlling

20% of the continent's real estate and didn't really want to give that up.

An epic battle ensued, but even though the Chinese "won" it was a bit like Afghanistan. You cannot really remove dispersed, networked warlords from a vast physical territory. The Chinese eventually gave up ruling Africa. They were resource stretched as it was, and toward the end of the decade they decided to shift strategies and rather consolidate a stronghold in their original territory, the vast Chinese territory as traditionally defined.

Growing unrest around the world

It wouldn't have been so bad had it only been southern Africa. But the same happened elsewhere. Wherever a faction already had some power, they weaponized and started capturing territory. The whole world quickly started to feel like the tabletop game Risk. Those of you who play, will recall that Africa is relatively easy to hold, but only for those that can avoid an assault from sea. Not so for Europe which has so many access points—the Middle East, Russia, and various ocean routes. The EU quickly lost control. Not so much by terrorists as by regional breakout groups like Catalunya, Scotland, Padania in northern Italy, Serbia, and a right-wing expansionist Austrian faction calling itself the Neo-Imperialists.

Industry consequences of chaos

The healthcare industry was initially near crushed under the burden of the virus, then it managed to deal with it and surged massively during the ensuing build-up as even nonstate warlords wanted to ensure their own kind survived the onslaught of the virus. Toward the end of the decade, the industry went into a massive downturn as warlord infighting made any structure break down. Financing had always been a problem, and even patchworks and volunteer contributions couldn't save the sector.

Finance was initially quite resilient to the crisis. The bigger countries had a lot of spending power and used all of it. The ones that survived build new empires for themselves which were nimbler. This turned out to be a good idea as the secondary disasters struck.

Higher education quickly shifted online, but that was not enough to save the middle market. Any college without a major endowment went broke by 2023, as student decline and local enrolment became steady trends. K-12 education was still needed, but there was a massive privatization as the public school systems were unable to respond to the crisis and the nation-states started folding one after another. Warlords don't care too much about education, although they also built some more ideological schools of their own to serve in the recruitment of future military leaders and troops capable of joint action.

Energy industry volatility began quite early in the decade as natural resources became inaccessible or were unsustainably tapped. All the major players went through a plethora of different ownership structures before they all consolidated into a few large players controlled by some of the larger terrorist networks.

Technology made some progress throughout the decade but because invention needs to be applied widely to have full impact, many good technologies died on the vine. Human inventiveness stays relatively constant but when the interesting application fields dry up there is little to do about it.

Transportation was the only sector that survived the period, although public transportation could no longer carry the same amount of people. Business models were quickly unsustainable, as buses could only take 20 people, not 100 people, and train cars could take 50, not 250.

Travel became a pure necessity. Business travel continued

throughout the decade, but the notion of business was different. The variety of tradeable goods shrunk considerably.

Consumer confidence sank to new lows, steadily throughout the decade. The consumer goods segment changed drastically as people increasingly consumed necessities as opposed to leisure and luxury goods.

Commodities simply weren't traded apart from in the barter economies of cartels. The markets were small, non-transparent, and highly localized. Smaller wars over natural resources were fought between various transnational criminal networks, but it never amounted to bigger things, as it was in each party's interest to conserve resources and make peace.

Services weren't really a thing. It was everyone for himself. If you wanted something done, you had to do it on your own. Even the terrorist organizations only had very insignificant networks of service delivery, for fear of creating too much communication between people. They realized that being informed fuels unrest.

Manufacturing was small, local, and inefficient, although the quality varied from okay to excellent, depending on who carried out the work. There was no quality control, so it was hard to know what you were getting. All the major industries had been crushed. The remaining mid-size firms produced things on-demand but couldn't afford any warehousing. As a result, the supply chain was extremely vulnerable to any disruption. This frustrated the warlords a lot since some of their plans depended on large scale production which was simply not available.

Aerospace simply was not a sector anymore. The few airplanes left were chartered by terrorists. Planes were poorly maintained, and without a working air traffic control system it was a bit like driving a car during the first era of the mass-produced car without a lane divider—lots of crashes, accidents, and misery.

Media was purely local. Anything larger was quickly

crushed. All communication was tightly controlled between the ruling networks, and those that feuded simply would shut down anything that attempted to communicate across criminal jurisdictions.

Food meant eating to survive the day-to-day. There was no industry to speak of, only agricultural production.

Conglomerates were all in the hands of various warlords. The oil resources were tightly controlled, although the powers at be shifted a bit, too. Larger organizations mostly focused on their role as "political" weapons, although politics was mostly the power of might and fear.

Nonprofits mushroomed in cities because it was the only place where they could operate slightly unseen. These organizations took on almost the form of mini governments, attempting to compensate for the loss of a centralized function carrying out essential functions.

Hospitality and travel industry concerns were never met, and the industry never came back. After all, what was there to see anyway? Roads were poor, monuments were destroyed, resorts were poorly maintained. The few hotels operating were purely hideouts for criminal activity.

The marine industry continued only in support of fisheries, which was still an important primary sector. Basic shipping vessels could still transverse oceans and did provide some amount of globalized trade.

Telecoms, perhaps the last of the industrial era's companies to survive, were all obviously on criminal hands. On the other hand, that meant that there was sufficient incentive to continue to provide services. However, Internet went down and was never brought back up, so you could talk, nothing more.

Defense industry contractors made it through the first 5 years, but not the 5 next. Instead, warlords traded internally and built up their own supplies, often produced in much simpler ways.

The outlook is grim

At the end of 2030, the outlook is grim at the macro level. All indicators point to continued hardship and slow economic growth worldwide. However, individual pockets of innovation ensure that societies and communities can thrive, even on relatively modest means. Technology has truly improved a lot of things, although not as much as many had hoped. The realization was that technology was no panacea. People still died. Public health still worsened. Technology can't bring together what humans tear apart.

Apart from the main conflict areas tied to natural resources and as well as technological labs, life could even be thought of as relatively quiet at times. Nobody knows how long this will last, but we are all enjoying the relief from daily worries.

Athens, Greece, April 9, 2027: "Only twice in more than 7 years has my company relied on the state—Greek, American, Chinese, Turkish, or any other—to settle our disputes, although there have been plenty," exclaimed Yiannis. His business lunch with a government liaison, Dimitris had turned a bit hostile. "We rely on direct conversations, industry standards, well-written contracts, third-party inspectors, insurance companies, and arbitration agencies to protect ourselves from bad business. Voluntary agreements typically serve our needs far more effectively than, to be frank, any coercive government. Being direct and knowing that we can retaliate helps, too. And, I very rarely pay bribes, and when I do, they are very small. But this time, I need you."

Dimitris looked at him with a strange expression in his face. "You cannot ask this of me. Not now. Not ever. Things are different now." Dimitris hadn't always been this way. This was not the first time his childhood friend Yiannis had come to him. But it was the first time he had been asked to do something clearly illegal.

It seems the crisis had changed everything, even the moral compass of good people. For a moment, Dimitris weighed the cost of honesty, the cost of doing what was right. It was a balance that he did not need to measure long. Nothing else mattered. Dimitris knew this was his moment. Dignity had to have a cost too, didn't it? The anarchy might be coming, but he was going to have no part of it, even if he was the only one. He hoped he wasn't.

The coming decade will likely offer more of the same. The hope among many of us, is that we can gradually rebuild governance structures from the ground up. There are some embryonic initiatives, mostly just local organizers at the town level, but we seldom hear about them because the Internet remains down after too many nodes and cables have been damaged. This was a system thought to withstand nuclear war. Well, it didn't survive the aftermath of a virus, although it wasn't technically the fault of the virus.

What has survived is the unbreakable human spirit. The spirit that stops us from our deepest, darkest urges, at the moments we most need it. There is a growing sentiment that this moment is coming.

Preventing or fostering Hobbesian chaos

Decide whether you want this scenario to happen or not. Then take a different tack. Let's imagine you could pick two to three elements or remove two to three elements from the scenario.

Which aspects would you pick? Which aspects would you remove?

Finally, it's also possible that there are so-called path dependencies. This means that if A happens, then B, C, and D likely follow. Try to name a few such path dependencies in this scenario.

Imagining Hobbesian chaos

People differ in their view of where the limits should be for asserting your individual strengths v. the interests of the community. The COVID-19 pandemic brings this conflict to light. There will be enormous opportunities but also matching challenges.

What feelings do you get around Hobbesian chaos? Is it appealing?

Each scenario has fault lines (e.g., where people and interests clash).
Name a few such aspects of Hobbesian chaos.

Who do you think gains the most if aspects of this scenario play out?

CHAPTER 8
SCENARIO V: STATUS QUO

This scenario considers the possibility that nothing much at all will be different as a result of COVID-19. That is, after a period of readjustment, society and the world economy, on most dimensions, will not be significantly altered by this pandemic experience. *From now on, and throughout this chapter, you are entering the realm of fiction.*

We are in 2030 and the world hasn't changed much from a decade ago. After a successful, worldwide COVID-19 vaccine was introduced by an international vaccine consortium exactly 18 months after the crisis hit US shores, and effectively administered to about 20% of the world population, the crisis blew over by the summer of 2021. By that time, the world's mobile population had either got immunity or the vaccine. Antibody therapy also started coming online throughout 2021, so there were treatment options for the limited outbreaks that still occurred in the Western world.

Governments operate as before; nation-states haven't changed, they keep jostling for positions, international organizations still battle for relevance. Politically, the world largely looks the same as a decade ago. The gradual weakening of the US vis-à-vis China and the EU continued, but the world was still in a tri-polar political order and hadn't completely shifted to the multipolar world of G7 countries' regional prowess that many political scientists had predicted in the years leading up to 2020.

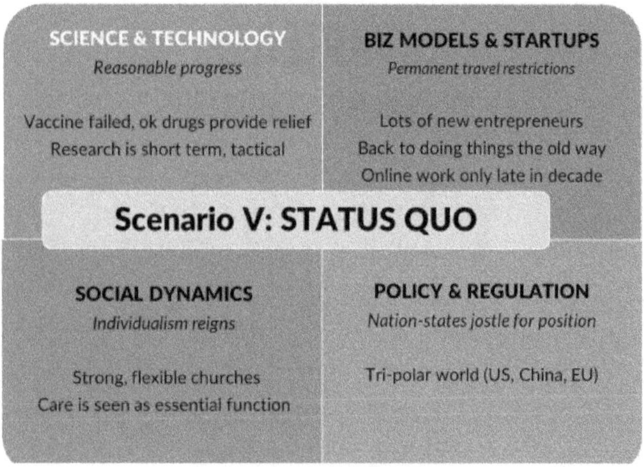

Figure 8.1. Status Quo

Countries like Russia, UK, Germany, Japan, and Canada had taken time to readjust and only in 2023 did their growth get back on track. Looking at the Morgan Stanley Capital International Emerging Market Index (MSCI)'s 23 countries, only Brazil, China, India, Korea, Russia, South Africa, South Korea, Taiwan, and United Arab Emirates were able to sustain rapid growth rates in the early parts of the decade, although most of them caught up by the next 5 years.

Science has largely continued as before, as a slow evolution most akin to the table game Chutes and Ladders, up and down, through triumphs and failures. We've had some triumphs, including major progress in life science, vaccines, and each of the basic sciences. However, these developments have been largely in line with what was accomplished in the past decade. The pandemic provided an impetus to seek bigger breakthroughs, but those didn't pan out yet.

Reasonable technology progress

Technology made progress in the same pace as before (nonlinearly and in surprising ways). As in the previous decade, many new products were launched on the basis of exciting technologies. On the other hand, as AI and a bunch of other technologies progressed, it became clear that the platforms that would transform society (e.g., AI, quantum tech, nanotech) needed more time to mature. There were some foreseen improvements in technology roughly according to the lines we saw becoming apparent at the beginning of 2020—although we probably lost momentum by about 2 years with most developments that were not COVID-19 related.

3D printing had already progressed enormously in the past decade. Already in 2020, 3D-printed medical supplies, particularly PPE like masks and plastic screens, were deployed across the world to stem equipment shortages. Throughout the decade, metal 3D printing moved from the prototype stage to full deployment across industry and even in the home, allowing those who could afford the top models to print nearly any commonly manufactured item.

The 5G network was the telecom standard that defined the early part of the decade, although the rollout got massively delayed by COVID-19, particularly in the developing world. Because of the delays, the next 6G standard, which entails 100 times faster speeds, originally slotted for a 2030 rollout, will only arrive in 2035.

Augmented reality became important as a supplement to online education technology as well as for group demonstrations in a business-to-business setting. There were no game changing applications beyond those two, which was a bit disappointing.

Autonomous driving hit major delays, but eventually brought increased efficiencies and convenience back into commercial transportation in cities and on highways. It took most of the decade to build out the infrastructure for autonomous trucks.

Blockchain had a tremendously positive impact on digital businesses, increased the value in stock markets, although it proved disruptive to those banks that didn't get on the bandwagon in the first years of the decade. Dramatically reducing the cost of transactions and information flows, it was exactly the boost the financial system needed to recover from the crisis, in fact adding trillions of dollars into the market by 2030 and boosting trade in excess of 30%.

CRISPR-based genome editing services hit a massive milestone in 2024, as a complex set of biological therapies enabled regenerative medicine products that increased longevity of life span by several years for most people who had private health insurance or were covered by welfare provisions. The more than 10,000 patents in the area tripled and generated significant revenue for the growing number of new biotech companies that had mushroomed in the venture capital funding spree in the first 3 years of the decade. In fact, from a base of around 100 companies, there were now 500 companies providing such services, mostly to hospital and to other biotech startups as well as corporations.

Cybersecurity proved to be a battleground in the first part of the decade as criminal activity surged. Toward the latter part of the century, governments and large businesses regained control and were able to introduce technologies with no major security breaches. The same could not be said for smaller companies, who suffered greatly. In private homes, data breeches were commonplace, and there was nothing much to do about it, given the increasing sophistication of cybercriminals. Governments mandated all software and hardware vendors to include a basic cybersecurity protection package in their software by 2029, which took care of 80% of the issues.

Precision medicine is relatively common, but personalized sequencing for cancers and regenerative diseases is only available on a pay-to-play basis and is not covered by insurance. One of the limiting factors is human germline experimentation, which remains a controversial issue ethically. The highly repetitive gene sequences, centromeres and telomeres, which particularly affect cancer and aging, respectively, are at the forefront of the experimentation and promising results are seen.

Nanotechnology made some progress through the decade, but some of the experimentation with nanobots in the brain which act like T-cells, the white blood cells that are so important to our immune defense, was slowed down due to the economical constrains of securing medical nanotech production at a sufficient level.

Quantum computing, which can massively parallel-compute numbers that classical computers cannot, was beginning to make inroads toward the specialty computing market such as large businesses and governments. The technology was still expensive and a bit unstable, so repairs would have to be made at the frequency of a veteran car, but the results were impressive. Distributed weather reports. Engineering calculations from the work site. The first experimental results of breaking traditional encryption algorithms began to show up toward 2029, but cryptographers devised a way to extend cybersecurity for another few years.

Robotics was mainstream in most factories by 2025, but the use cases were rather limited. Personal robotics hit a snag as the humanoid robots didn't catch on the way the manufacturers thought. People thought it was creepy.

Smart fabrics began to change regular surfaces, which all became interactive and embedded with inexpensive heat, motion, and chemical-composition sensors. The first truly virus-proof work outfits went mainstream by 2027 but didn't make it to all corners of the world because of the price of the raw materials.

Synthetic biology gained rapid adoption in the US, but was still prohibited in Europe, which meant that food production largely was kept within the borders of the Americas. Non-food applications of synthetic biology included fabrics, sensors, medical technology, and organic manufacturing.

Virtual reality didn't take off in the consumer market because the headsets were still clunky and the neural interface it depended on never materialized. Instead, gamers continued to embrace the technology and it was widely used in flight simulators and advanced construction projects.

Consumption patterns were massively disrupted for a year but quickly bounced back to what they were before, and consumer confidence grew from there. The world is always changing.

Caracas, Venezuela, July 10, 2023: In the early morning hours on Monday, July 10, US troops conducted a controlled raid of the Venezuelan capital in joint operation with the opposition forces. The president was captured without major bloodshed; the opposition was installed as a new temporary government until free elections were held in early fall. As the opposition leader declared in a televised statement: "After countless violations of human rights and misuse of Venezuela's petroleum resources by the president, we have seized power to return the wealth of this glorious, proud nation to its rightful owners, the people. We are thankful to the United States for its support in overthrowing the government. At the same time, we hope this will be the last time a western government has to assist in the democratic transition of a Latin American state. From now on, a new era begins."

A few months later, riots break out in Brazil, and world media starts talking about the potential of a revolution in that country. Nothing comes of it. The next year, Argentina's pesos edges dangerously close to 0 as the inflation rises 1,000%, once again. It seems that part of the world is back to normal.

Despite world leaders declaring "victory" over the virus after 18 months, a significant proportion of people across the world had lost working hours or jobs when this was over. Some would never again join the workforce due to psychological trauma, lack of skills, despair or even death.

At the start of the outbreak, COVID-19 was dubbed "the rich people's disease" because contagion spread at ski resorts, cruise ships, country clubs, and the like. At the end of it, the proportion of poor people to rich people who contracted the disease and who died from it was overwhelmingly poor or of poor health.

The correlation between poverty and quality of the health system one has access was quite definitive. It became clear that virus transmission is near optimized in a slum, for instance. Africa as a continent that got severely and disproportionately affected, just as it is with any other infectious disease. South America was also not spared. The timelines of the spread and the intensity of the spread differed across the world. The world was not all on one contagion cycle.

The new normal

Although eradicating the virus after 18 months was possible in Europe and the US, it still raged on other continents, notably in Africa and South America, and in pockets of Asia, particularly in China and India. There were also recurring, smaller outbreaks in a plethora of Asian megacities.

Only continued travel bans for travelers from those countries were sufficient to keep an outbreak at bay in the US or Europe until 2024. Especially after the travel bans were lifted in 2024, there were limited outbreaks and even a few large-scale, intermittent outbreaks. However, the severity of those outbreaks was somewhat under control due to the fact that there were no surprises, no medical equipment shortages, and the fact that the lockdowns became more surgical and efficient.

Throughout the decade, there was a running discussion of

what the "new normal" should be. Intermittent social distancing, stay-at-home orders, and surgical quarantines of affected groups was the consensus strategy to deal with this situation for years to come. But the question became how society should evolve to cope with such a situation. Answers differed in Washington, DC and Tokyo, in Paris and Tehran. Some countries adapted a 6-foot distancing, others simply said "try to keep sufficient distance," while others again wanted 12-foot distancing to be on the safe side. Some lockdowns were voluntary, while others were mandatory; some included all workers, others included only nonessential workers.

Living with that kind of uncertainty impacted the insurance market, consumer confidence, the severity of other diseases a patient might have (i.e., comorbidity) or even stress reactions to other life events that sometimes became more serious than the worry around coronavirus.

Many cities, and Millennial populations particularly, had challenges coping with having to institute both a regular vigilance whenever a large amount of people were gathered and emergency protocols that would efficiently shut society down and reopen it again without losing too much steam. Physical infrastructure changed in permanent ways.

Over 250,000 people commute through New York's Grand Central Station every day on Metro-North trains, on the subway, and on New York City buses. In 2020, as the virus took hold, New Yorkers wondered what Grand Central would look like when it reopened for true commuter traffic again. What would a social-distancing-compliant version look like? Would the alternative be to shut it down intermittently? It was hard to envision an in-between state, but that's what happened. The station gradually opened. Various experimental designs were tried. Working hours in New York flexed and the early shift started 5:00 a.m., the mid-shift started 7:00 a.m., and the late shift at 9; that's how they reduced commuter traffic significantly.

Early on in the crisis, stay-at-home orders and curfews were happening on a city-wide, county-wide, statewide, and countrywide basis. Already by 2021, given the market imperatives, governments became more sophisticated when implementing such measures. In order to protect economic life and avoid full shutdowns, we even saw "come into New York city by car only if your last name starts with A–H," which are measures we previously have seen in large cities trying to handle air pollution.

How did markets react to intermittent shutdowns? Surveying people did little good; the financial markets ended up giving an unequivocal response—as long as it was predictably open for trading at least 1 week every month. The market could take the disruption.

Early on, one thought that there was a lot to learn from China. However, China was not the best model for learning to cope with the aftermath of COVID-19 given its peculiar governance structure. Italy, Spain, and the UK were earlier in the curve and held better lessons for Europe.

Living with intermittent quarantines

Short of a cure or a vaccine, which both seemed several years away in the spring of 2020, the prospect of a miraculous return to full normalcy were but a pipedream. There were also seasonal spikes in addition to the regional outbreaks and occasional outbreaks in random locations with high concentrations of potential superspreaders.

The lesson from spring 2020 was that even a single superspreader event, such as a wedding where one person is contagious, could cause an entire cluster of COVID-19 for months to come. Such outbreaks were hard to contain unless detected immediately. Given some inevitable amount of asymptomatic transmission, these kinds of outbreaks occurred even in countries with particularly abundant testing, such as Korea and Iceland, all the way until 2024.

World Health Assembly, WHO Headquarters, Geneva, Switzerland, February 6, 2023: The 75th session of the World Health Assembly was a unique event. After the previous two assemblies were drastically reduced, the first was run online, and the second was canceled, the world was, finally, again gathered in Geneva to discuss the status of the WHO, financing the organization in the decade ahead, and future and emerging pandemic readiness. "We want to motion for a dissolution of the WHO, because of China bias and the fact that nations better learn to be prepared on their own," said the American delegate. "We have decided to pour most of our resources into the European Centre for Disease Prevention and Control and rather support the build-up of such centers in individual countries in greatest need, including in our neighborhood countries," said the representative from Belgium, also pointing out that he represented the EU in this context.

"We have made great progress in terms of transparency," said the WHO Secretary General. "The COVID-19 outbreak is now to a large extent under control, due to our international coordination efforts. I would also like to warn that further reducing our monitoring capability would increase the risk of another pandemic by 500%, according to an independent study we have commissioned from McKinsey." That study was countered by a study brought forth by the UK, showing that national centers of disease control had a 1,000% higher efficiency rate per dollar spent. The room broke out into a chaos rarely seen save in national parliaments where the tradition is to show dissent by arguing with the person next to you. "Order in the room, order," said the speaker.

After 3 day's negotiation, the end result was that the WHO continues to have a monitoring function based in Geneva but that all subject matter experts are pulled back to the member-states and financed from there directly. The budget shave amounted to a 90% reduction in real dollar terms but only a 50% staff reduction, given the strict travel restrictions and the reduction of wet lab activity which now would only be carried out locally.

The new everyday life

The rules for everyday life changed in various small ways. Birthday parties shrunk in size (perhaps a good thing). Dinner parties tended to be held only with people you trusted and considered to be in the "inner circle" (again, not a bad thing, but led to less serendipitous encounters).

Presence went from being a commodity to becoming precious. When will we ever go to a major public parade again? When will we feel comfortable in a crowd? (Some people never were for other reasons.)

Coronavirus anxiety was already hard to control among folks who hadn't even experienced any symptoms and who were only watching news of the crisis on TV and following social distancing. Virus-induced fear of crowds (enochlophobia) became commonplace. Other anxieties included financial anxiety, medical anxiety (around personal health or those of loved ones), unfamiliarity with the virus, frustrations with repeated leadership failures (from the WHO to national to regional leaders to employers), conflicting advice as well as a general sense of not being able to control our environment. Even separately, these anxieties became quite debilitating to some people, and as a whole, were major societal issues throughout the decade. Taken together, these anxieties at times brought even the most balanced person to the brink.

Superspreader places (tourist resorts, sports events, vacation towns, ski resorts, mega churches) needed a new business model. It was nearly unthinkable that those places would continue operating as they do. But what was their alternative? The proximity was almost baked into the infrastructure. For many such events, short of drastically limiting the allowed capacity of each facility they continued to pose the same risk when they reopened. As a result, mass events became few and far between and needed government permits to go ahead.

Mass surveillance

Overnight, the debate of privacy shifted to how we could enable our technology companies to help governments put in place wide-ranging mass surveillance in the name of virus vigilance.

The reevaluation of care as an essential function

Some social functions had been grossly undervalued in contemporary society. Caring for others was one of them. Food service was another. Logistics and transport were a third. Each of these professions saw a significant change of public respect, financial compensation, and societal acceptance, although it didn't last throughout the decade.

Going to a sports events became a high-risk activity. In countries with a legal system like the US, tickets became pricier due to added insurance. In another societal models, that risk was uninsured due to the organizer claiming a pandemic, or any infectious disease, was covered by force majeure principles and made them not liable.

The future of religion

Religious freedom is deeply ingrained in most societies. Yet, the ability to gather in large groups became questioned for years to come. Are mass gatherings essential to the practice of religion? The Friday prayer at the mosque, Saturday synagogue, and Sunday mass or worship couldn't continue in its current form. Each was temporarily or permanently scaled down and adapted to respect social distancing rules. This was despite a vaccine and various treatments being available.

The advantage of online church services was that you could now attend church many thousand miles away. It opened the possibility that suburban churches who lost a lot of their attendance during summers or other holidays, potentially could regain it online. The increasing sophistication of online tools and the experience churches were making with them became a lasting strength for religious congregations going forward.

Rise of social discrimination

Already back in 2020, some called for preexisting conditions listed on passports. The notion of a corona-passport was discussed in several countries and became implemented in many countries, including in the EU by 2023, as the question of how long immunity lasted got clarified (immunity varied between 6 months and 2 years at maximum). In China, a makeshift solution already existed from early 2020. The impetus came from the desire to find ways to return people quicker to the workforce.

Permanent or temporary travel restrictions

We saw the continuation of travel bans between certain continents and countries continue for some time. Countries that were low in the pecking order found that they were near permanently locked out. Forced or voluntary quarantines became a regular measure to take in all countries that had an active outbreak.

US Presidential Policy Directive 21 (PPD-21) defines 16 critical infrastructure sectors whose "assets, systems, and networks, whether physical or virtual, are considered so vital to the United States that their incapacitation or destruction would have a debilitating effect on security, national economic security, national public health or safety, or any combination thereof."

The role of startups

Early on in the crisis, funding froze up for many emerging or existing startups. But one thing we saw more of, was new entrepreneurs. Change presents new opportunities. Particularly because bringing large amounts of people together is more complicated, smaller, leaner organizational structures gained foothold. A startup is a perfect example of that, especially of the product or service provided could be provided at a distance.

Inequalities will widen

People with low incomes were hardest hit by social distancing measures, both in terms of purchasing power, overall choices in life, and health effects. The poor are (always) most likely to have the chronic health conditions that increase their risk of severe infections. Only, after the pandemic, there was less of a safety net from governments or nonprofits as they themselves were reeling and struggling to even take care of themselves.

Diseases have destabilized cities and societies before, and the overall story is always the same: some things change, and some things stay the same. The difficulty is figuring out which. The most lasting part of the coronavirus pandemic were the cultural shifts. Some parameters that changed included: psychological effects, since they are typically longer lasting than economic effects at similar magnitude (beyond the fact that the two are also closely related); the moral fallout (and integrity still mattered a lot); and power shifts.

Social dynamics did not change much. The same organizations are operating. Human psychology is the same as before. Culture continues to be a force for change but also a limiting factor as we cannot move too fast. Everyone needs to be able to catch up with change, so nobody is left behind.

Regression to the mean

I've studied another period of dramatic change due to the vision of nomadic work. In the first Internet wave around 1999–2000, businesses were (almost) convincing enterprises and workers that they would soon be able to "live, work, and play" remotely. Often, the advertising mentioned vacation hotspots, typically very remote locations where you could "check in with work" and then continue uninterrupted vacation life. This visionary talk went on for a few years until people suddenly realized that making decisions only based on online interactions wasn't as attractive as they had hoped. Making marriage proposals, business decisions, investment decisions, making love, all of these things are now possible, yet seldom taking place online.

Instead, a lot of maintenance activities are taking place online. We keep up with what happens. We update our staff. We check in with somebody.

Normal but more intensely so

There are reasons to believe that a similar effect will come in the aftermath of a coronavirus-induced remote-work spree. Once the restrictive measures are relaxed, the great majority would want to go straight back to what they are used to. They might even become more extreme at doing things "the old way" and may become increasingly passionate, as well. Change is hard. Regression to the mean is far more probable. Habits are hard to break.

What that might look like is hard to say exactly, but it's not inconceivable that travel would spike in the first months after the major "back to normal" orders have been put in place. The consequences of unleashing a world population to do what they please, having been curtailed for months or in some cases perhaps a year or more, is anybody's guess but they won't be pretty. We could be looking at spikes or even massive outbreaks that make the first outbreak dwindle in its consequences.

Also, at the end of the day, the quality of the interaction matters. If we still, as a company or as an individual worker, discover that we can better accomplish our job by commuting, we might still want to do so, regardless of the opportunity to work from home. If we discover our ideas are ignored if presented in an online call but accepted if we walk into somebody's office and present the same (which is often the case), we will of course make sure we present important ideas face-to-face.

The impact of this type of regression to the mean might be that a lot of the change we expect to happen around future of work changes will be reverted quite quickly. On the other hand, there is something to be said about seminal crisis events that are sustained over time. It may depend on how long these special restrictions are in place. It will also depend on how successful we are as companies, communities, groups and individuals under these new conditions. Those who thrive under them might be more likely to sustain the activity even when given the choice to go back to the way it was done before. It will all play out in interesting ways, and there is no way of fully predicting which way a particular social group will go.

Industry consequences of status quo

Businesses did undergo quite drastic adjustments but now operate in the same way as they did in the past decade. Most industries are back where they were before the crisis, some have even grown faster than the regular economy. Specific industries were each very differently affected, and the effects were not uniform across the globe. However, the big picture was the following:

The healthcare industry underwent quite significant

change in the years after the pandemic. First off, it got higher priority in most countries, as they realized the downsides of years of underinvestment as well as the lack of spare capacity and flexibility. It was not that capacity increased that much during the decade; it was more that, at least among the most developed nations, the basic system got much better at scaling up and down fast based on need.

Healthcare security didn't improve much in the poorer nations, despite everyone's best efforts. There was not willingness among international donors to upgrade the whole world's medical system to a minimum standard, it was each country for themselves.

Stockpiling medical supplies, which had been at an all-time low, got a boost, but it didn't get crazy either. All public health authorities had to ensure was that they had the right agreements with private sector manufacturing firms who would ramp up production on a month's notice.

The finance industry quickly bounced back. For instance, since the US economy is highly consumer based, once the crisis was over, consumers produced never-before-seen pent-up demand for traveling, eating at restaurants, going shopping, going to the movies, and beyond.

After the financial crisis a few years before 2020, the stress testing of banks had made them quite resilient, even to huge shocks, which now served them well. Toward the end of the decade, there was even a slight overheating, as finance became kingmaker again based on the growing wealth of second and third cities, and the real estate markets in smaller cities also followed suit. The megacity growth trend did not continue, in fact most megacities lost population throughout the decade. It didn't seem to make sense to pack everyone into the same densely spaced area when there were credible alternatives.

Higher education bounces back

Higher education had a bouncy year in both the 2019–2020

and the 2020–2021 academic years, which both got quite interrupted. After that, the situation went back to normal, with some minor adjustments and a greater emphasis on online learning. K–12 education became much more flexible, as teachers had learned new technology skills during the pandemic. In the US, snow days became a thing of the past, as they simply became online learning days.

The energy industry grew moderately throughout the decade, as oil continued to decline in importance and the proportion of renewables rose quite significantly. Most of all, the markets became more transparent as blockchain increasingly stimulated the market with an easy way for consumers to monitor energy prices. As a result, demand-response systems were introduced almost across the board, on all continents.

Travel industry shakeout

The travel industry had a major shakeout. Travel rebounded but the travel industry did change quite a bit. Mass tourism took a major hit in the first 3 years of the decade, as people struggled to make sense of the various travel advisories that varied regionally. Congestion at airports was a considerable nuisance as a minimal version of the emerging social distancing rules were continued in most international airports. Changes were about as notable as those after 9/11, where security tightened. Similarly, after the pandemic, temperature monitoring, health checks, distancing, and other minor inconveniences did put a damper on leisure travel. Major tourist destinations managed to offload some of their tourist traffic to second- and third-tier cities and destinations by offering incentive packages and by making travel to such destinations easier. Travel between capital cities incurred what became called the "COVID-tax" which essentially meant a 10% fee, which governments wanted to use for public health efforts in the travel industry and at airports.

Consumer confidence was low until 2021 but rebounded and stayed high after that.

The service industry got a boost immediately after the coronavirus crisis as service workers were highly appreciated for keeping society running during those trying times. However, fairly soon after the crisis was over, things went back to normal. Low-end service work was still compensated at minimum wage and high-end service work was still priced high.

Governments made it through the crisis in different ways. Generally, the wealthier governments fared better. Some nimble governments with female leadership, notably Germany, Norway, Finland, Iceland, and New Zealand, gained support through the crisis and managed to come out better for it. Though there were some public health consequences, they were all offset by the positive externalities due to reduced occurrence of other problems such as influenza and traffic accidents.

Public transportation in crisis–the death of commuting?

The environmentally sound solution to mobility is public transportation. Yet, the density of people required to defend a train commuter service often decried social distancing. Could we envision a commuter train maintaining 6 feet of separation between travelers?

Well, it took a while, but it happened. A typical train car that takes 200 people over would now only carry 50 or less. In a typical 2+2 seating arrangement, there was now only one person at each end of the row. What about the distance between rows? Most train operators increase it by 50% or more, and at a high cost to the consumer. Compartment cars have a side corridor to connect individual compartments along the body of the train, each with two rows of seats facing each other. That arrangement was made virus compliant, too. The real problem is the combustion in waiting areas and at the stations themselves. Interim solutions were found, but by the time the vaccine was distributed, nobody saw a reason to relax the measures. By now, the awareness was there that there could always be another outbreak, coronavirus, influenza, or some other disease.

Impact of remote work on commuting

A percentage of commuters either shifted to remote work or chose to drive their own modes of transportation, typically a car. The impact of that shift on local air pollution and on carbon emissions was initially a devastating toll on the already strained environment. As this became increasingly clear, government and city pollution mandates had to be introduced, and that brought online work back with a vengeance, just like it had been in the early days of COVID-19.

Major shifts in the real estate market

The real estate market was poised for one of the largest structural changes. Intuitively, one might think that the fact that infectious diseases are more prevalent with population density would lead to a mass exodus to the countryside. Upon closer consideration, this is not self-evident. There are fewer hospitals and healthcare services in remote areas. Already during the first year of the corona crisis, we saw tensions in local communities due to the influx of seasonal or part-time residents. The local argument, somewhat inconsistently presented, was that the local community "could not handle" the additional burden of the incoming residents. Those were the same residents that the local economy typically loved and appreciated for the additional consumption they provided during summer or winter vacations. On the other hand, accepting the part-timers meant the need to upgrade public health infrastructure.

In Norway, the government prohibited cottage owners from going to their legally owned cottages during the early stages of the corona crisis and that was one of the most unpopular measures and generated enormous discussion. The complexity is what to do after the crisis. Do you still maintain the position that you want to control the influx of "outsiders"? If not, do you then try to invest to scale up your emergency infrastructure? If so, will you tax the part-time residents at a higher rate than before? Tensions will ensue no matter what choices are made. In Norway the solution was a mix of government subsidies, higher cottage taxes, and a higher local tax burden.

Suburban real estate was another matter entirely. A plausible argument was that wealthy suburbs are the near paradise in the age of coronavirus. People live in their own houses have plenty of space and are typically also in proximity to hospitals and core city-like infrastructure and most such suburbs are within an hour's drive of a major city.

One would have thought that such communities would thrive. Those suburbs that are situated near major medical centers would likely benefit the most from the post-corona recovery. This panned out. To take the US example, the areas affected positively included the Boston Longwood area (and the Boston MetroWest area suburbs), Tucson Medical Center, Tucson, AZ; UCSF Health, the top hospital in San Francisco, they are surrounding the National Institutes of Health, Baltimore, Maryland; St. Louis, Missouri, the area near the Mayo Clinic in Rochester, Minnesota; the surroundings of the Cleveland Clinic, Cleveland, OH; The University of Pittsburgh Medical Center (UPMC), Pittsburgh, PA.

New York and Houston were a whole other discussion. Even though both cities have massive hospital systems, they dwarf the demand during a pandemic type scenario such as 2020's coronavirus. Similarly, Bumrungrad International Hospital, Bangkok, Thailand, a beacon of technology and innovation and Southeast Asia's biggest private hospital treating over a million patients annually, also crumbled under pandemic conditions. Bumrungrad had implemented thermal imaging cameras at their entrance points already at the start of the crisis, but that was not enough to stave off a loss of medical tourism, as people didn't travel across the world to get elective procedures any more.

Switzerland's record of a stellar public infrastructure with world leading healthcare and top hospitals meant increased pressure on real estate from wealthy foreigners and Swiss expats moving back in droves to seek safe haven. Similarly, German university towns with medical schools and top university hospitals (e.g., Heidelberg, Mainz, Tübingen) saw a similar influx of buyers.

Commercial real estate suffered. However, the larger, more resilient players who were able to upgrade their facilities to become somewhat "virus proofed" with social distancing measures and security, thrived in this new environment.

Impact of remote work on real estate

However, to the extent the future of work happened online, this altered the equation. Certainly, suburban communities were pushed farther out. However, truly rural areas did *not* receive an enormous lift from this crisis, given the relative lack of infrastructure. It is one thing to use a vacation home as a weekend getaway and another thing entirely to start using it as a permanent home. However, for the ultra-rich and even the higher end of the upper-middle class, the crisis led to upgrading their second homes to equip them to provide relief and "change of air" for their families over greater stretches of time.

Manufacturing rebounds

The manufacturing industry became much nimbler as a result of the crisis, partly because of government mandates, partly because of internal review of work practices, and also because technology truly began to make a difference. At the end of the decade, manufacturing was as technology intensive as any other industry and there was a strong emphasis on local production. Having said that, countries like Australia that previously depended a lot on international markets, continued to both import and export a lot.

Aerospace struggles and changes forever

Early in 2020, airlines were grounding a high percentage of flights. In some countries, carriers already went belly-up by the end of 2020. There were lingering effects on travel patterns for years to come. The aerospace industry did restructure, as many airlines had to be rescued by their respective governments. However, after some consolidation, at least two carriers survived in most major markets, so the competitive dynamic was maintained. Customer traffic rebounded slowly in the first 2 years, but business travel came back quite strong as they found ways to travel safely. Planes became smaller and people had to sit much further apart, so prices went up across the board. Temperature screening as well as instant result coronavirus testing was installed at many airports throughout the first part of the decade already.

Media continued to evolve during the decade, although freedom of the press continued to be under attack, both in the US and in a myriad of countries that had come under populist rule.

The food industry enjoyed a strong resurgence during and after the COVID-19 period. Meat consumption, which had spiked during the crisis, went back to normal levels and even leveled off as the vegetarian and Mediterranean diets gained ground. Restaurants were closing at a staggering rate, and those that couldn't reopen within months never opened again. Others took their place, but "eating out" looked significantly different given that some amount of social distancing continued throughout the decade and beyond.

Conglomerates grew moderately during the decade. Large

companies generally were better off than small companies, as long as they were capable of change. A few dinosaurs didn't manage the needed shifts in business models. In the end, the biggest shift was perhaps that people redrew their floor plans and spaced employees further apart.

Nonprofits continued to thrive and gained importance with their public health efforts, which were highly appreciated across the board. Donations were easy come by at least for half of the decade, but after 2025, it tightened again, as business as usual again took hold.

The hospitality industry struggled for a while. Hotels were empty for 2 years but after that, business travel rebounded. Leisure travel came online only a year later and continued to grow throughout the decade. People initially vacationed domestically but slowly ventured further and further. By the end of the decade, globalization of travel was even more prevalent than before, and going for a weekend trip to another country became commonplace.

The marine industry became an important way to maintain exploit the ocean's variety of resources. Business models related to aquaculture flourished.

Telecoms had already grown considerably during the crisis and continued their growth throughout the decade, as 5G became 6G, 7G, and 8G and speeds and content continued to amaze consumers and businesses alike. Telecom networks became crucial in the delivery of telehealth, which was widespread by 2027.

The defense industry, which was highly resilient to most societal developments, had only been strengthened by the uncertainty of the crisis. Military leaders in most countries successfully argued they could play an even more important role in public health and a significant emergency powers were transferred to the military as well as to NATO, which became a coordinator of public health for pandemics.

All in all, not much changed in a decade, but most leaders

realized that also meant they were unprepared for any possible future calamity—virus, climate or terror.

Preventing or fostering Status Quo

Decide whether you want this scenario to happen or not. Then take a different tack. Let's imagine you could pick two to three elements or remove two to three elements from the scenario.

Which aspects would you pick? Which aspects would you remove?

Finally, it's also possible that there are so-called path dependencies. This means that if A happens, then B, C, and D likely follow. Try to name a few such path dependencies in this scenario.

Imagining Status Quo

People differ in their view of where the limits should be for asserting your individual strengths versus the interests of the community. The COVID-19 pandemic brings this conflict to light. There will be enormous opportunities but also matching challenges.

What feelings do you get around Status Quo? Is it appealing?

Each scenario has fault lines (e.g., where people and interests clash).
Name a few such aspects of Status Quo.

Who do you think gains the most if aspects of this scenario play out?

CHAPTER 9:
CHARTING THE UNCHARTABLE

The following chapter is not fiction. Rather, it attempts compare and contrast each of the five scenarios with the aim of understanding our options and fallout in the post-COVID-19 society. I chart the implications for nation-states, businesses, and individuals. You would want to read this *after* you read each scenario, and ideally have begun a scenario process either in your organization, or at least in your mind, before you do so.

If I were to attempt to summarize what currently can be known about the coronavirus pandemic and the forces of disruption that are playing out, I would have to say this: we are in unchartered territory. Not completely unknown territory. Not doomsday territory. We are not facing an extinction event. We are not even close. Yet, the crisis has turned out to be so much more serious than almost anybody imagined. No amount of scenarios or disaster planning could have prepared us 100% for what is unfolding before our eyes.

Yet—and this must be stressed. Nothing that has come out on the biological severity of coronavirus and the COVID-19 disease it causes would have made it enter the radar as an outbreak-like scenario like the ones we have seen in movies such as *Outbreak*, based on a disease like Ebola. But as we also know, most of those movies end with the heroes successfully combatting and containing the disease before it reaches worldwide spread. Otherwise, it would be no fun to watch. After all, nobody wants to watch human extinction.

The importance of controlling the narrative around coronavirus is a thread running throughout my book. Not just in the sense of powerful networks trying to get their interpretations to prevail but also in a more fundamental sense: the world needs to get a common narrative before we can understand what is happening and what to do about it. One of the early challenges was that many observers, including the near entire public health establishment initially framed coronavirus in terms of influenza. That had two direct consequences, one, many underestimated it because even though the influenza pandemic of 1918 was immensely deadly, influenza epidemics occur annually and because of a tremendous investment in a vaccine there is typically a readily available vaccine (which most of us don't think about).

Second, the public health establishment and the political authorities (generally) also had only prepared for the scenario of a new influenza, although they had generally understood it to be a more serious threat. However, as a result, most of the stockpiling, many of the readiness discussions and the infrastructures put in place, were solely built with a future, and more severe, influenza epidemic in mind. This is readily visible through the plethora of articles surrounding the words "influenza" and "pandemic." The planning around any other scenario simply wasn't as thorough.

Because coronavirus was mishandled by a few key governments early on, and because of extensive pre-symptomatic and asymptomatic transmission, the disease got out of hand and into full-fledged, global community spread. We are now living with the consequences of that community spread, and the knowledge that flows from it, possibly that we will have another annual infectious disease, in addition to the flu, to contend with every year. The fact that *if* this had been an Ebola-like disease (but with a longer incubation period), the world would indeed have faced an extinction event, is hard to bear. Moreover, what does it mean for our future? Should we accept that we, with some probability, cannot withstand another pandemic that is significantly more severe? Should we attempt to do something about it? Can we?

The hard lessons from the scenarios

First off, in a typical scenario exercise, the discussion of the scenario is typically left to the client. Those who create the scenarios deliberately either just present the scenarios or they discuss them with a third party without inserting too many of their own opinions.

In this chapter, I will break with tradition, not to foreclose the discussion but to attempt to open it in new ways. You *can* choose not to read this chapter in order to preserve your own full interpretation of each of them. I would certainly suggest *not* reading this chapter before reading the scenarios. If you do so, you forego an important part of the reflection process. Scenarios are meant to be taken in deeply, experienced for what they are: imagined futures that the creators of the vision ask you to take as "deep fiction."

Scenarios are intense. They deliberately exaggerate. What they are is extrapolation of existing embryonic trends. At the same time, there is a certain logic to it. There are path dependencies within each of them and they are meant to be logically consistent.

Each of the five scenarios likely have pieces of truth in them. Even if one scenario is clearly intended as dystopian (Hobbesian Chaos) and one is utopian (Borderless World), the other three scenarios fall somewhere in the middle (Status Quo, Nation-State Renewal, and Two Worlds Apart), and each of the five reflect both positive and negative developments simultaneously. I wanted to reflect the reality of our world. No matter what we choose, no matter what happens despite what we try to choose or who or what chooses for us, we are always going to be faced with a hybrid world where some things go our way, and some don't.

In fact, if you take a closer look, the dystopian scenario has its advantages (regularly shifting fiefdoms means huge freedom of operation and few attempts to control social dynamics) and the utopian scenario its disadvantages (elite exceptionalism can become toxic and one dimensional), some would even say the scenario exposes a tragic flaw. What this should tell us, I will largely leave to the policy makers, executives, entrepreneurs, and regular citizens, like yourself, who pick up this book. What I wanted to do is to clearly lay out what the options are for the way forward. Not as a simple set of choices, more as a complex web of interrelated issues.

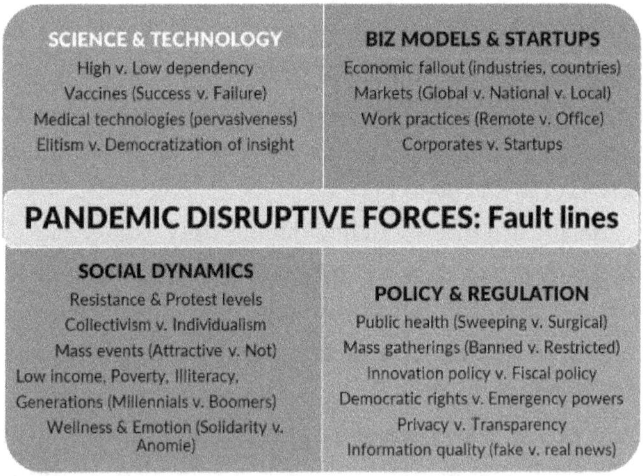
SCIENCE & TECHNOLOGY
High v. Low dependency
Vaccines (Success v. Failure)
Medical technologies (pervasiveness)
Elitism v. Democratization of insight
BIZ MODELS & STARTUPS
Economic fallout (industries, countries)
Markets (Global v. National v. Local)
Work practices (Remote v. Office)
Corporates v. Startups
PANDEMIC DISRUPTIVE FORCES: Fault lines
SOCIAL DYNAMICS
Resistance & Protest levels
Collectivism v. Individualism
Mass events (Attractive v. Not)
Low income, Poverty, Illiteracy,
Generations (Millennials v. Boomers)
Wellness & Emotion (Solidarity v. Anomie)
POLICY & REGULATION
Public health (Sweeping v. Surgical)
Mass gatherings (Banned v. Restricted)
Innovation policy v. Fiscal policy
Democratic rights v. Emergency powers
Privacy v. Transparency
Information quality (fake v. real news)

Figure 9.1 Pandemic Disruptive Forces—fault lines

The major fault lines in any scenario have to do with broad political and cultural disagreements that go back to the beginning of human society. This is why it has been somewhat surprising to watch the first 6 months of the coronavirus pandemic be mostly a discussion about either public health or the economy. Those two issues, while important, actually mask many of the other issues that will play out.

For example, as important as it is with a ventilator crisis, the true ethical issue of whether it makes sense to put all efforts in to make more of a product that only saves a median of 50% of the people who end up using it, and likely lead to major health risks and deteriorated health throughout that person's life, is more important and will become more significant in the aftermath (Hamilton, 2020). I'm not stating what the answer is, but it cannot simply be "let's never run out of ventilators." It has to do with a deep discussion of what a human life is and what quality of life is.

Pandemics seem to become an arena mostly for experts, at least in its initial phases. In fact, most of the scenarios that were run before this current crisis was *mostly* run by and for public sector *experts*. Yet, a pandemic is a mass phenomenon, and, as such, it is an area where common sense, popular opinion, grassroot action, and anthropological and sociological understanding of what the people's true sentiment is will become more important as time goes on.

We have commented on the varying degree of faith in science, technology, and innovation to "propel" us out of a pandemic. In truth, these endeavors take time and are fraught with pitfalls. As any survivalist knows, from British adventurer Bear Grylls and down, is that we should plan a crisis based on what's available there and then, not what we hope or ideally would have available.

On the regulatory side, the tension between privacy and freedom will seldom be put in more stark contrast than during a pandemic. Liberties are being sacrificed in the name of government oversight. Note that even Scandinavian governments that have a somewhat trusty population are getting into trouble for proposing digital tracking of its citizens "in the name of corona." Other countries, such as Hungary, have no such qualms, but their people do. On the other hand, what does it mean to have freedom, if our way of exercising that freedom takes away scores and scores of other people's lives? This is a classic liberal dilemma, but it cannot be solved by technology. It must be solved by discussion.

Lastly, I wanted to bring up the issue of economic rescue packages to large companies. These are controversial even in regular times but become even more so during a pandemic. Who does it serve to rescue an airline instead of paying out unemployment benefits to millions of individuals? If we need to prioritize, how do we do so? Can pure economic calculation be the only way to do it?

If we only take two opposing forces, communitarianism versus individualism, these are common counterpoints in any country's political culture, family structure, governance principles, and beyond. If you add survivalism into the mix as well, you get what's at stake during a pandemic. That third factor adds a potentially toxic powder to the mix, which might enflame the two others, which is what I'm trying to illustrate in the five scenarios we're now going through.

They are also not clear cut. Individuals may have aspects of each go into their decision making and how they apply this logic may vary depending on the context.

If we attempt to model what would happen in a given situation and we don't know what type of rationality citizens, states, or organizational actors will operate under, the probabilities we assign to our models won't make much sense.

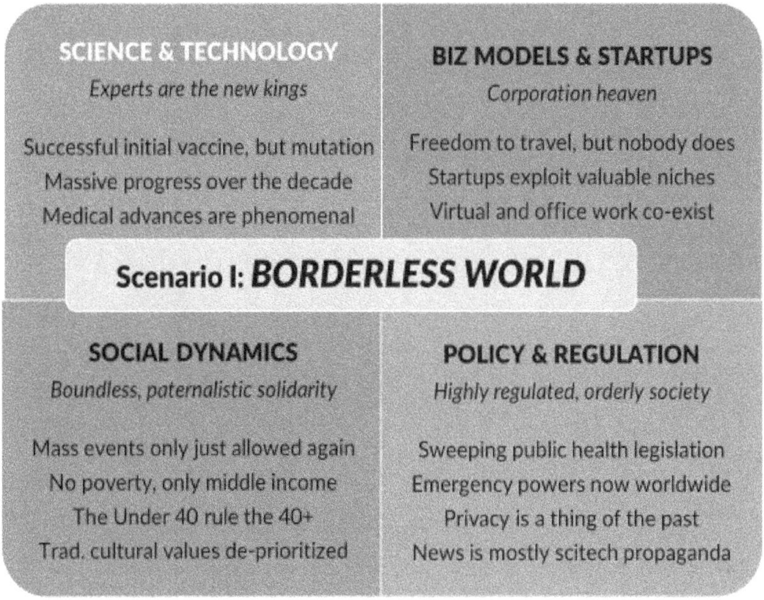

SCIENCE & TECHNOLOGY
Experts are the new kings
Successful initial vaccine, but mutation
Massive progress over the decade
Medical advances are phenomenal
BIZ MODELS & STARTUPS
Corporation heaven
Freedom to travel, but nobody does
Startups exploit valuable niches
Virtual and office work co-exist
Scenario I: BORDERLESS WORLD
SOCIAL DYNAMICS
Boundless, paternalistic solidarity
Mass events only just allowed again
No poverty, only middle income
The Under 40 rule the 40+
Trad. cultural values de-prioritized
POLICY & REGULATION
Highly regulated, orderly society
Sweeping public health legislation
Emergency powers now worldwide
Privacy is a thing of the past
News is mostly scitech propaganda

Figure 9.2 Scenario I: Borderless World

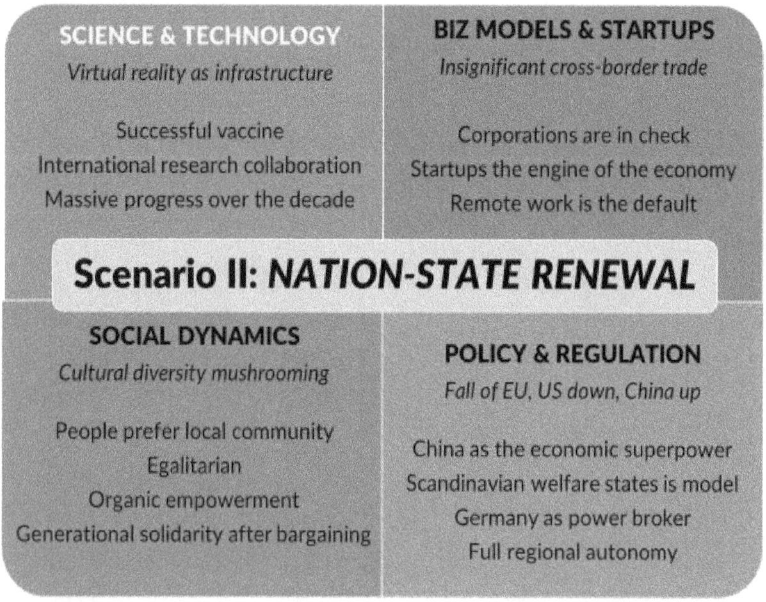
SCIENCE & TECHNOLOGY
Virtual reality as infrastructure
Successful vaccine
International research collaboration
Massive progress over the decade
BIZ MODELS & STARTUPS
Insignificant cross-border trade
Corporations are in check
Startups the engine of the economy
Remote work is the default
Scenario II: NATION-STATE RENEWAL
SOCIAL DYNAMICS
Cultural diversity mushrooming
People prefer local community
Egalitarian
Organic empowerment
Generational solidarity after bargaining
POLICY & REGULATION
Fall of EU, US down, China up
China as the economic superpower
Scandinavian welfare states is model
Germany as power broker
Full regional autonomy

Figure 9.3 Scenario II: Nation-State Renewal

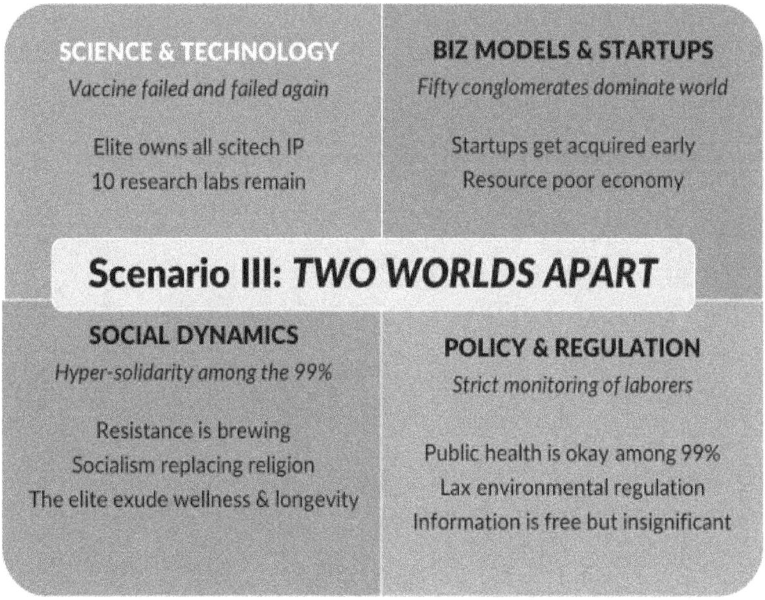
SCIENCE & TECHNOLOGY
Vaccine failed and failed again
Elite owns all scitech IP
10 research labs remain
BIZ MODELS & STARTUPS
Fifty conglomerates dominate world
Startups get acquired early
Resource poor economy
Scenario III: TWO WORLDS APART
SOCIAL DYNAMICS
Hyper-solidarity among the 99%
Resistance is brewing
Socialism replacing religion
The elite exude wellness & longevity
POLICY & REGULATION
Strict monitoring of laborers
Public health is okay among 99%
Lax environmental regulation
Information is free but insignificant

Figure 9.4 Scenario III: Two Worlds Apart

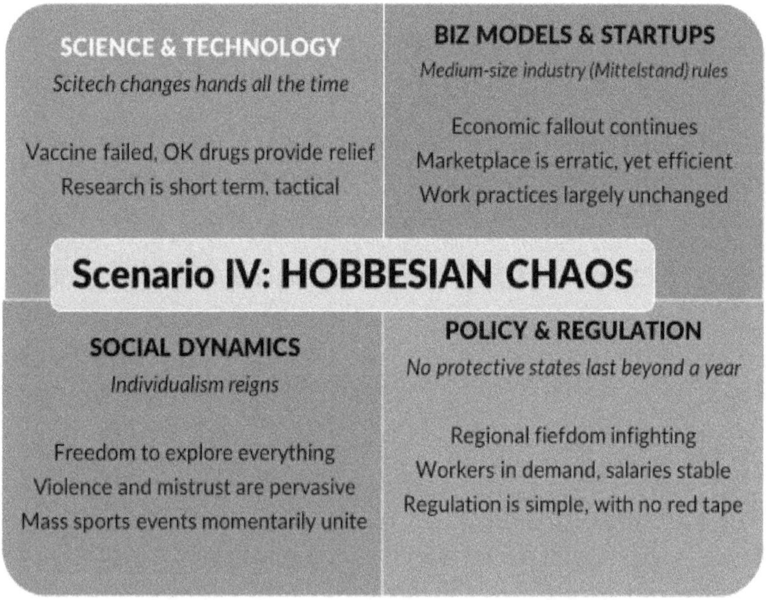
SCIENCE & TECHNOLOGY
Scitech changes hands all the time
Vaccine failed, OK drugs provide relief
Research is short term, tactical
BIZ MODELS & STARTUPS
Medium-size industry (Mittelstand) rules
Economic fallout continues
Marketplace is erratic, yet efficient
Work practices largely unchanged
Scenario IV: HOBBESIAN CHAOS
SOCIAL DYNAMICS
Individualism reigns
Freedom to explore everything
Violence and mistrust are pervasive
Mass sports events momentarily unite
POLICY & REGULATION
No protective states last beyond a year
Regional fiefdom infighting
Workers in demand, salaries stable
Regulation is simple, with no red tape

Figure 9.5 Scenario IV: Hobbesian Chaos

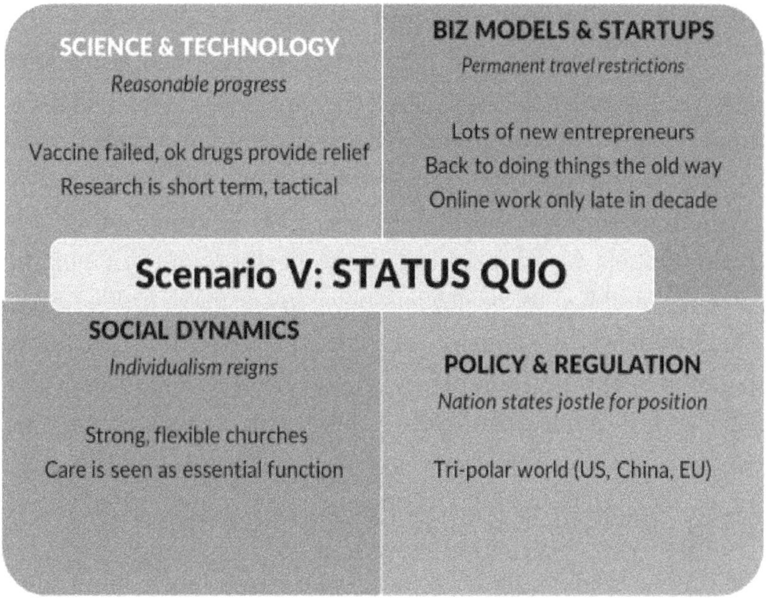

Figure 9.6. Status Quo

Beyond scenarios—lessons for the post-corona society

At the time of writing, the statistics are still emerging, so there is no point offering a final tally of the fallout. What's clear is this: a significant proportion of people across the world will have lost working hours or jobs when this is over, some will never again join the workforce due to psychological trauma, lack of skills, despair, or even death.

At the start of the outbreak, COVID-19 was dubbed "the rich people's disease" because contagion spread at ski resorts, cruise ships, country clubs, and the like.

At the end of it, the proportion of poor people to rich people who will have contracted the disease and who will have died from it will undoubtedly be overwhelmingly poor.

As pointed out by Health Poverty Action, the international NGO that was established in 1984 by a group of health professionals to address the social determinants of health, poverty, and health, *health and poverty are inextricably linked* (healthpovertyaction.org). In fact, the adverse correlation between poverty and quality of the health system one has access to is quite definitive on this point. In downturns, net worth of the wealthiest 10% generally increases, but the good news is that promoting economic equity may have broad health effects (Khullar & Chokshi, 2018).

Virus transmission is near optimized in a slum, for instance. Africa as a continent is also likely to get severely and disproportionately affected, just as it is with any other infectious disease. South America will also not be spared. The timelines of the spread and the intensity of the spread will differ across the world. We will not all be on one contagion cycle.

Normal but more intensely so

There are reasons to believe that a similar effect will come in the aftermath of a coronavirus-induced remote-work spree. Once the restrictive measures are relaxed, the great majority would want to go straight back to what they are used to. They might even become more extreme at doing things "the old way" and may become increasingly passionate, as well. Change is hard. Regression to the mean is far more probable. Habits are hard to break.

What that might look like is hard to say exactly, but it's not inconceivable that travel would spike in the first months after the major "back to normal" orders have been put in place. The consequences of unleashing a world population to do what they please, having been curtailed for months or in some cases perhaps a year or more, is anybody's guess but they won't be pretty. We could be looking at spikes or even massive outbreaks that make the first outbreak dwindle in its consequences.

Also, at the end of the day, the quality of the interaction matters. If we still, as a company or as an individual worker, discover that we can better accomplish our job by commuting, we might still want to do so, regardless of the opportunity to work from home. If we discover our ideas are ignored if presented in an online call but accepted if we walk into somebody's office and present the same (which is often the case), we will of course make sure we present important ideas face-to-face (Undheim, 2008).

The impact of this type of regression to the mean might be that a lot of the change we expect to happen around future of work changes will be reverted quite quickly. On the other hand, there is something to be said about seminal crisis events that are sustained over time. It may depend on how long these special restrictions are in place. It will also depend on how successful we are as companies, communities, groups, and individuals under these new conditions. Those who thrive under them might be more likely to sustain the activity even when given the choice to go back to the way it was done before. It will all play out in interesting ways, and there is no way of fully predicting which way a particular social group will go.

Postlude: Accepting the post-touch society or charting a new path?

We started this book by making a major leap—comparing the potential aftermath of COVID-19 to the impact of the Black Death. That plague had large scale social and economic effects. Some of these effects were seen in the first decade, others were only seen hundreds of years later. Arguably, it contributed to the Reformation: it broke up the Catholic Church and created massive, lasting persecution for the Jewish people around the world, but it also brought about, directly and indirectly, significant inventions, changed agriculture and the shape of towns and cities, including the emergence of the Italian city-state.

However, it is also important to remember that the demographic evolution, build-up of proper city structures and higher emphasis on learning gives rise to the Renaissance. That was a period that is striking in terms of artistic expression, built around patronage which became so important in the history of art through the support that kings, popes, and the wealthy provided to artists such as musicians, painters, and sculptors.

Long-term and short-term changes to the sense of touch

Could the same thing happen today? How deep are the changes that are coming, short and long term? To what extent will current or future epidemics be associated with these positive changes that may also occur? Who would the future recipients of patronage be? I know quite a few of us would hope that social entrepreneurs would receive this kind of support on a much wider basis and based on more transparent criteria, ideally.

The Renaissance was particularly known for its expansion of the human sense of vision. In contrast, the current progress in artificial sensors gives some hope that the future of artificial touch sensation might approximate—at a distance if necessary—some of the immense pleasure, experience, and humanity that is created by human touch. In virtual reality as well as robot teleoperation scenarios, this sense of touch must be artificially recreated by stimulating the human body (typically the hands, but also other body parts). The part our technological sensors are struggling the most with at present is how to register and interpret touch feedback—which unfortunately is the whole point of touch besides the physical manipulation itself, which of course is useful in a manufacturing facility and factory. Pandemics may bring forth a renewed emphasis on remedying the near impossibility (at the present time) of reproducing the *experience* of touch, the psychological perception itself.

The most urgent thing to regain in this post-pandemic discussion, which I feel is extremely important to commence on a global scale right now, in the middle of the pandemic, rather than afterward, when I feel it will be too late, is *the sense of touch*. If we as humans lose the incentive to touch each other, at least before we have learned to recreate it through technology, then much is lost. We might then need a social movement to emerge in order to regain the incentive, desire, and ability to touch one another. I'm not sure how that can play out, given the public health concerns short and medium term, but I know it must happen. Over time, and I don't mean necessarily in the next decade, but perhaps in some decade to come, we might be in a prime position to master the human psyche through some technological means.

Toward a Renaissance 2.0
Key milestones on the path to a Renaissance

Middle Ages (500–1500 AD)
Illiteracy among a vast majority of the world population

Renaissance 1.0 (1300–1600 AD)
In 1440, Gutenberg invents the printing press (mechanical movable type)
In 1503, Leonardo da Vinci paints the Mona Lisa
In 1508, Michelangelo begins his painting on the ceiling of the Sistine Chapel

Explosion of intellectual expression, starting in Europe and spreading throughout the world. Explosion of visual acuity (ability to encode visual impressions using art)—as our human world's material creations comes into focus for the first time.

Post-war era (1950–2020)
Tech illiteracy among a vast majority of the world population

Renaissance 2.0 (2030–2100)
In 1984, Charles Hull invents the 3D printer
In 1987, Jaron Lanier coins the term *virtual reality*
In 1992, Armstrong Labs invents *mixed reality*; throughout the 1990s, *augmented reality* gets commercialized through games and entertainment
In 1997, Deep Blue defeats world chess champion Garry Kasparov
In 1999, Kevin Ashton invents the Internet of Things (system connected by sensors)
In 2012, Crowdfunding creates the first Oculus VR headsets
In 2016, AlphaGo by Deep Mind defeats world Go champion Lee Sedol

Sometime between 2020 and 2050, distributed innovation platforms (e.g., digitalization, synthetic biology, 3D manufacturing, sensing) become simple enough and inexpensive enough for every human being to use without training and become widely available.

Explosion of intellectual expression on a global level for the second time in history. Explosion of haptic acuity (ability to encode the sense of touch using augmented and/or virtual reality)—likely as a result of our virtual creations starting to dominate and the natural world fading away (either because it is deteriorating, becoming diseased and dangerous to interact with or otherwise less desirable by comparison).

In my next book, I'll discuss in much more detail how the future of technology also is shaped by those larger forces, but I will emphasize how to truly understand the interplay of innovation and demand. The true nature of demand is not in the hands of a pollster or even of a marketer. Innovation corresponds to a deeper psychological need.

What I do know is that if I'm somebody who is innovating in the field human-computer interfaces (AR, MR, VR, sensors, neural links), human–human mediated interfaces (using both digital and neural stimulation) or interface design, including designing for a future with attentive interfaces that don't require users to do work (and don't require co-presence) in order to connect and feel things deeply and intensely, I would feel particularly excited about the future, given what we see unfolding right now.

What coronavirus indicates is that clear demand can channel specific evolutionary paths and pave the way for innovations that would have taken much longer to see the light of day otherwise. Equally, no matter how much you wish for something to be developed scientifically (say, a vaccine), no amount of money will get you there in an instant.

Achieving a fuller understanding of how our society works is a tremendous task in the contemporary climate. It is, nevertheless, an essential one. Moreover, many more people have realized that we cannot leave our most important choices only to our experts, whatever that means anymore, nor can we leave it to our political guardians.

As citizens, we are the arbiters. It's not that we are all experts, but we should all learn to have a healthy skepticism as well as a healthy dose of respect for people whose lives are dedicated to values many of us cannot afford to think about on a daily basis: truth, accuracy, and science.

If the post-touch society is fully implemented, the way our public health overlords would currently have it, it would be a qualitatively lower quality existence on many important levels: psychology, culture, economy, you name it. Even temporary restrictions on our ability to be in proximity to those we desire to be with, interact with, or trade with will have far-reaching consequences. No matter what technology we put in place, this is likely to produce a deficit of sorts, which will have to be compensated somehow.

We started this book with a look at the run-up to the first COVID-19 outbreak. We focused a lot of the lack of preparation, the public health debates and mandates, the early political response, and the shortages. What strikes me now, at the end of this discussion, is that even though there are clear and important path dependencies based on actions a government took or not (such as which country had the largest initial death toll), the ultimate results might not send up being so drastically impacted by the differing responses. Time will tell. The reason is, I think, that once a crisis is unleashed, you have what you have.

What we all could improve, in the end, is our response to adversity, both how we handle it logistically, the medical response, and our attitude, which is influenced by psychological factors that played out differently in each country. Furthermore, it is clear from past experience that any crisis exacerbates existing inequalities. We don't need another crisis to tell us that.

Importantly, I do not think, nor does any other scenario theorist, that any given scenario will work out the way the scenario is written. These are thought constructs. Imagined futures. However, some of this will happen, and it won't all be pleasant. But I take some comfort in having imagined a host of positive consequences as part of the fallout. There is a silver lining to everything, even COVID-19.

Path dependencies that matter

The ultimate path dependencies, the ones that mattered the most, seems to be a small set of things: (1) the economic situation of each country (*wealthy countries fared better*), (2) the public health readiness (*those scoring higher on health security fared better*), (3) cultural response (*those who managed to pull together fared better*), (4) trust in local governance (*those trusting state, region, city, and town government, with good reason, did well*), (5) relative differences in pandemic health and hygiene in nursing homes (*countries with stricter standards, more educated or better trained staff fared better*), (6) the average density during mass events (sports, culture, religion) and in big cities (subways, commuter trains, buses) matters (*crowding kills if there are even just a few superspreaders present*), (7) the power of (changing) habits, including learning the importance of social (physical) distancing (*those countries, cities and towns that can sustain their novel hygiene habits over long periods of time do better*), and (8) digitalization (*those becoming comfortable with online learning and videoconferences had better results and lasted longer doing distancing*). Short of any other more definitive data, I'm going to declare that those were the eight predictors of outcome in the first 4 months of the pandemic. What can we learn from that?

We can learn that a rising tide floats all boats. Until every health system has an acceptable minimum standard and/or we have a response system that can bring resources to the weakest points in greatest need at a sufficient speed, we cannot contain an event like this even in the future.

Furthermore, we can choose to isolate ourselves (as elites, as countries, as deniers that a crisis even exists), but the consequence will be that we all suffer even more. Conversely, congregating even closer together in cities does also not seem like the greatest idea. We need to find a happy medium that can sustain our life in a different way.

We can argue about global or national politics all we want, but local governance, time and again, proves itself vital to our well-being, regardless how insignificant it may seem in the big picture. Experts often have a blind spot in this respect; it is hard for them (and for us) to realize and even harder to accept, that to most people, the big picture is not what counts the most. What really matters is our proximate reality: our family, our long-term friends, our house, our town, and the emotional relationships we have built there (which may have since dispersed or we may have moved).

Lastly, we could legislate, regulate, force, nudge, or stimulate people to change their behavior all we want, but unless the new things that we now do (and you may think of 6-ft. social distancing in public, wearing a mask, not shaking hands, no hugging in public, the 20-seconds surgical scrub handwash, or more drastic changes such as traveling less, flying only as a last resort, not going to the movies, shunning cruise ships, consuming less, eating in) becomes new, ingrained habits, we will instantly revert once we get the chance.

There aren't that many habits we indeed can change overnight and not all public officials' dreams about perfect hygienic behavior will come true—certainly not across cultures. The question we need to ask is: *Which habits are worth changing and at what price?*

Learning compassion

Perhaps it's time anthropologists, sociologists, historians, and a host of other types of people (far beyond public health experts and economists) start voicing their opinions about what COVID-19 can and should mean for our life on this planet. I'd be interested in what emerging polls, ethnographies, and journalistic reporting uncovers about people's experiences with this period in human history.

Despite the initial myopic focus on health epidemiology, and the equally myopic focus on "opening up the economy" that followed in months three and four, even with a vaccine, the ultimate virus fallout is likely to be decided by non-medical factors such as emerging social movements, the tolerance of inequality in impact (the elderly, the poor, the immunocompromised, the severely obese, smokers, the immigrant population, and minorities seem disproportionally affected), mass psychology, and whether people's newly won "corona habits" regress to the mean or become lasting changes.

Having gone through a high number of pandemic scenarios, I find that the voice of (a) *the weakest links* (representing the elderly, nursing homes, minorities, the immune-compromised), (b) *representatives from sports and cultural events organizers of mass events* (sports associations, leagues, etc.), as well as (c) *religious congregations* (religious leaders), are each often missing in pandemic scenario planning. How on earth are we going to get a realistic picture of pandemics without those that either are most affected or those who can affect the outcome the most?

Similarly, most pandemic scenarios obsess with death toll and contagion and forget the emergent social dynamics, including about *how the perception of what's happening changes what's happening*. I'll state it a different way: don't lose sight of the *meaning* of what's happening while searching for and attempting to communicate the facts. Moreover, the facts don't exist in a vacuum, and are not always stable. Facts get created and re-created all the time. This is not peculiar and not worrisome, unless the process is opaque.

I find that it is often the simplest things that are the hardest to do or think about. It took me writing 400 pages on COVID-19 over several months to realize, that even more importantly than seeking deeper insight on the disease, in order to successfully move to the next chapter in the history of the earth, we need to learn and practice compassion.

We need to be thankful to those that bear the biggest burden. Speaking of the US reality which is the one I'm personally living right now; we need to appreciate the sacrifices made every day this pandemic goes on by African Americans, the elderly, the urban poor, the working class, and the new category of pandemic heroes: service workers in groceries and all those along the supply chain, including health workers. Extending it globally, we need to think of the two billion workers in the informal economy and we need to particularly remember refugees. Taking it inward, we need to be thankful to our kids, who had no part in creating this troubled world, yet are forced to live in it for years to come.

We need to be patient with those who, having lost all sense of safety due to loss of a job and being physically distant from everything they know, turn to anger. We need to understand that even if COVID-19 may not directly affect us, it has a negative impact on so many people that it cannot be ignored. We need to be concerned with how we can help others, in our community and abroad, in any way we can. We need to develop calm and find strength within to sustain physical distancing for long periods of time. Finally, we need to appreciate what we have, in the moment we have it, not just afterwards.

We need to come to terms with what the narrative should be around COVID-19. What *is it*, really? I tried to make clear that just like a brand, the disease must have a name, an identity, a trajectory that we both understand and can communicate in very simple terms. Otherwise, it is going to be foreign to us, it will be frightening, and it will be alienating in the same way that Durkheim in his classical studies of the *Division of Labor* (1893) and *Suicide* (1897) described the fragmentation of social identity would, at times, occur as a result of the rapid industrialization when it doesn't produce solidarity. Facing a lack of integrative restraint, or too much of it, can both lead astray. When our ambitions and coping mechanisms are overwhelmed by situational ambiguity, is when *anomie* looms. We should not withdraw from each other and from society permanently as a result of social distancing over a long period of time. We should rather find a new way of connecting.

For such a complicated crisis, it surprises me that the answers on how to prevent such a thing in the future is relatively easy to comprehend: slow globalization, build health security, deploy technology to monitor contagion (in a way that protects privacy), innovate for change (but through distributed platforms where all can part-take), develop a sophisticated strategy for long periods of intermittency (know how to quickly lock down *and* open up countries, regions, cities, and neighborhoods), start mapping risk in terms of its probabilities and consequences, not just as theoretical constructs. But implementing changes that could truly remedy this situation will take us decades. That's a hard lesson, too.

The German sociologist Ulrich Beck (1992:21) defines *risk society* as an entity that has a systematic way of dealing with hazards and insecurities. It strikes me that, despite the fact that the world has been under conditions of heightened risks due to a plethora of conditions associated with modernization and subsequently globalization for decades now, we haven't yet approached the situation as a true risk society would. In those instances, there is a system to lean on, it is frail, and needs a fix. Most of the time, there will be no system. Not yet. Perhaps not for years to come.

We have, in any case, significantly exaggerated our own ability to control the world. It is as if our own faith in the combined merits of the expanding global markets (neoliberalism), the increasing sophistication of science and technology (leading to the notion that humanity is making enormous progress), and the intense (and often exciting) proximity-induced cultural heterogeneity seen in megacities, have all *conspired against us*. In those few instances where we do have systems in place, they are set up by and favor elites. The downsides have now become painstakingly apparent. As I've tried to show in the scenarios, it is also not evident that the world order set in motion by elites has the ultimate staying power. Although the walls may (temporarily) be breaking down now, so to speak, new and more sophisticated walls may subsequently be raised.

As of 2020, international global organizations have convening power, but surprisingly little coordinating power, and little, if no traditional authority to act on their own. Nation-states do have systems in place, but those systems are woefully inadequate for the task at hand. Local governance is somewhat better placed but towns don't have a sufficient set of resources.

I'll leave the ultimate discussion of what to do and how to act to those who pick up this book. Discuss. Tear the book apart. Disagree. But please make up your mind on what coronavirus—whether it be COVID-19, a future genetically engineered bioweapon, or the next zoonotic virus—means for how we want to shape our next decade and beyond. Let's live through the crisis in a dignified and meaningful way. And let's start now, because as we all just discovered, whether we are experts or neophytes in either public health, politics, technology or compassion, tomorrow it may be too late.

The post-touch society

Let's imagine the next 10 years will have less physical contact between people than ever before. Let's also assume proximity-enhancing technologies will improve drastically (feel free to disagree).

What is the most likely balance to be had between safety from outbreak risks v. the two important imperatives of freedom and economic growth on the other hand?

We are all wondering about what the "new normal" will be. What's your take?

If you think about the four forces as areas that will change after COVID-19, which of them do you care the most about and why? (science & technology, policy & regulation, business models & startups, social & cultural dynamics)

Learning from history

Thinking about the two precedents to COVID-19: The Black Death and the Influenza of 1918, what are some parallels and what are some major differences?

Parallels: ______________________________

Differences: ______________________________

Charting the unchartable

After the introduction, I asked you about your first thoughts about each of the five scenarios. Having read through all of them and reflected on what they entail, what is your view now?

Which aspects do you like or dislike about them? If you could combine *two* scenarios, which ones would you choose and why? To what extent can you, with your role in society, influence which course the world moves in? Do you prefer any of them? Is your organization currently preparing for any of these or combinations of them, if so, how?

1. Borderless World________________________

2. Nation-State Renewal________________________

3. Two Worlds Apart________________________

4. Hobbesian Chaos________________________

5. Status Quo________________________

Are you currently ignoring or discounting any of these scenarios? Should you?

____

Tipping points for path dependency

Each of the five scenarios cover a decade's evolution. Pivotal events might create paths that are difficult to reverse, either fostering negative or positive change. Such events are typically related to the major forces of disruption (science and technology, politics and regulation, business models, startups and economics, sociocultural dynamics).

What do you see as the tipping points in each of them?

Remember that there can be several ways to argue this point. Ideally, you would have a group discussion or at least a talk with somebody else who has read this scenario to discuss.

1. Borderless World________________________

2. Nation-State Renewal________________________

3. Two Worlds Apart________________________

4. Hobbesian Chaos________________________

5. Status Quo________________________

Finally, what might your organization (and you personally) have to do differently, in order to benefit from each of these scenarios? What capabilities would you need?

____

Tabletop exercise—scenarios for the next decade

Scenarios are designed to be discussed and played out in a live setting, ideally over a few days. Half a day is the minimum amount of time advisable.

All scenarios, or simply one of them, could be chosen for an exercise. Each is independent from the other, even though they are most exciting when viewed together.

You could run a scenario exercise with your organization, government or with your workshop attendees, whether your challenges are to run a business, to run a government agency, to operate an NGO, or to innovate during uncertainty. In fact, these scenarios could be used for any challenge where readiness for change is important.

Preparing these scenarios for a large-scale tabletop exercise or workshop would take a little bit of work. Should you be interested in a live, guided scenario, which could also be executed online (if coronavirus dictates so), or a speech on the *Future of Public Health*, the *Future of Global Society*, the *Future of Infectious Diseases*, *Disruptive Innovation*, or on *Scenario Planning*, please contact the author at info@yegii.com or through the book's website: pandemic-aftermath.com.

Mini-scenario exercise (tabletop or online)
As a shortcut, here's a little exercise you could run in a small group:

Delegate some key roles: President, Head of a national CDC, Sec-Gen of WHO, Cabinet secretaries (Finance, Business, Health, Sports), Business (CEO of airline, supermarket chain, large e-retailer), Civil Society (Owner of a sports team, Organizer of mass events, Head of a chain of nursery homes), State or Local official.

Play out three discussions: (1) At first news of outbreak, (2) Mid-way, after X, Y, and Z happened (pick one of the scenarios), and (3) At the end of the outbreak (summarize the experience and make recommendations for the future).

BIBLIOGRAPHY

Abaday, A (2020) Germany's 2012 Covid scenario became real in 2020. Foreigner.fi, 25 March. Available from: https://www.foreigner.fi/articulo/Coronavirus/germany-s-2012-covid-scenario-became-real/20200325014404004958.html [Last accessed 15 April 2020]

Abbot (2020) Detect COVID-19 in as little as 5 minutes. 27 March. Available from: https://www.abbott.com/corpnewsroom/product-and-innovation/detect-COVID-19-in-as-little-as-5-minutes.html [Last accessed 16 April 2020]

AFP (2020) Israeli scientists have not developed a COVID-19 vaccine– they were still working to develop one in February 2020. AFP Sri Lanka, 5 March. Available from: https://factcheck.afp.com/israeli-scientists-have-not-developed-COVID-19-vaccine-they-were-still-working-develop-one-february [Last accessed 16 April 2020]

Ahmed, AS (2020) Sweden's unique response to coronavirus is hurting its minority communities. Huffington Post, 8 April. Available from https://www.huffpost.com/entry/sweden-Coronavirus-minorities_n_5e8dfba3c5b670b4330a3977 [Last accessed 17 April 2020]

Akst, J (2020) COVID-19 Vaccine frontrunners. The Scientist, Available from: https://www.the-scientist.com/news-opinion/COVID-19-vaccine-frontrunners-67382 [Last accessed 15 April 2020]

Aldridge, B (2020) 'Super spreaders' of coronavirus may be among us, experts say. What does that mean? The News & Observer, 3 March. Available from: https://www.newsobserver.com/news/nation-world/national/article241209786.html [Last accessed 24 March 2020]

Alexander, H (2019) Disease X dummy run: World health experts prepare for a deadly pandemic and its fallout. The Telegraph, 21 October. Available from: https://www.telegraph.co.uk/global-health/science-and-disease/disease-x-dummy-run-world-health-experts-prepare-deadly-pandemic/ [Last accessed 16 April 2020]

Al Jazeera (2020) China approves two coronavirus vaccines for human trials. Al Jazeera, 14 April. Available from: https://www.aljazeera.com/news/2020/04/china-approves-Coronavirus-vaccines-human-trials-200414083310079.html [Last accessed 15 April 2020]

Allen, K (2016) How a Toronto company used big data to predict the spread of Zika. The Toronto Star, 22 February. Available from: https://www.thestar.com/news/insight/2016/02/22/how-a-toronto-company-used-big-data-to-predict-the-spread-of-zika.html [Last accessed 17 April 2020]

Andersen, KG et al. (2020) The proximal origin of SARS-CoV-2. Nature Medicine 26, 450–452 (2020). Available from: https://doi.org/10.1038/s41591-020-0820-9 [Last accessed 20 April 2020]

Ankel, S (2020) How Singapore went from being applauded for its coronavirus response to facing an alarming second wave with thousands of new cases, Business Insider, 22 April.

Available from:
https://www.businessinsider.com/coronavirus-singapore-lost-control-second-wave-2020-4 [Last accessed 20 April 2020]

Arendt, H (1951) The Origins of Totalitarianism. Schocken Books.

Army Mobility Command (2020) Transport Isolation System (TIS). 1 April. Available from: https://www.amc.af.mil/About-Us/Fact-Sheets/Display/Article/2132917/transport-isolation-system-tis/ [Last accessed 15 April 2020]

Army Technology (2020) EpiGuard: Medical isolation and transportation units for the defence industry. Company profile. Available from:
https://www.army-technology.com/contractors/field_hospitals/epiguard/#company-details [Last accessed 15 April 2020]

ASEF–ASAP Scenarios (2011) ASEF–ASAP scenarios: Accurate scenarios, active preparedness. Asia-Europe Foundation. Available from:
https://asef.org/ebooks/public-health/scenarios/pdf/report.pdf [Last accessed 7 April 2020]

Asia Pacific Strategy for Emerging Diseases (APSED 2011) Available from:
https://www.ncbi.nlm.nih.gov/pmc/articles/PMC3729053/ [Last accessed 7 April 2020]

Atlantic Storm (2005) Tabletop exercise. University of Pittsburgh Medical Center. Available from:
https://www.centerforhealthsecurity.org/our-work/events-archive/2005_atlantic_storm/ [Last accessed 20 April 2020]

Baier, B and Re, G (2020) Sources believe coronavirus outbreak originated in Wuhan lab as part of China's efforts to compete with US, Fox News, 15 April. Available from: https://www.foxnews.com/politics/coronavirus-wuhan-lab-china-compete-us-sources [Last accessed 2 May 2020]

Barry, E (2020) An army of contact tracers take shape in Massachusetts. New York Times, Available from: https://www.nytimes.com/2020/04/16/us/Coronavirus-massachusetts-contact-tracing.html [Last accessed 16 April 2020]

Basu, O (2020) In numbers: corona, people dominate PM Modi's lockdown speech. India Today, 24 March. Available from: https://www.indiatoday.in/india/story/in-numbers-corona-people-dominate-pm-modi-lockdown-speech-1659301-2020-03-24 [Last accessed 24 March 2020]

BBC News (2020) Coronavirus: India 'super spreader' quarantines 40,000 people. BBC News, 27 March. Available from: https://www.bbc.com/news/world-asia-india-52061915 [Last accessed 16 April 2020]

Beaumont, P (2020) Wuhan eases quarantine as coronavirus cases in US pass 100,000. The Guardian, 28 March. Available from: https://www.theguardian.com/world/2020/mar/28/quarantine-eased-in-wuhan-as-Coronavirus-cases-in-us-pass-100000 [Last accessed 28 March 2020]

Beck, U (1992). Risk society: Towards a new modernity. London: Sage Publications.

Bilodeau, A and Potvin, L (2018) Unpacking complexity in public health interventions with the Actor–Network Theory. Health Promotion International, Volume 33, Issue 1, February 2018, Pages 173–181. Available from: https://doi.org/10.1093/heapro/daw062 [Last accessed 19 April 2020]

Boselely, S. and Belam, M (2020) Super-spreaders: What are they and how are they transmitting coronavirus? The Guardian, 27 February. https://www.theguardian.com/world/2020/feb/27/what-are-super-spreaders-and-how-are-they-transmitting-Coronavirus [Last accessed 28 March 2020]

Boulos, MN and Geraghty, EM (2020) Geographical tracking and mapping of coronavirus disease COVID-19/severe acute respiratory syndrome coronavirus 2 (SARS-CoV-2) epidemic and associated events around the world: How 21st century GIS technologies are supporting the global fight against outbreaks and epidemics. International Journal of Health Geographics, 19, Article number: 8 (2020). Available from: https://www.theguardian.com/world/2020/feb/27/what-are-super-spreaders-and-how-are-they-transmitting-Coronavirus [Last accessed 24 March 2020]

Boyd, C and Matthews, S (2020) How Italian doctors failed to stop coronavirus super-spreader: Marathon runner at outbreak epicentre infected 13 people including his pregnant wife, two doctors, three bar-goers and a 77-year-old woman who died. Daily Mail, 27 February. Available from: https://www.dailymail.co.uk/health/article-8050705/Trail-Italian-Coronavirus-super-spreader-Marathon-runner-38-heart-crisis-Europe.html [Last accessed 24 March 2020]

Brand, R (2020) How to make an N95 mask out of a bra: DIY

respirator mask. In My Opinion, YouTube, 9 March. Available from:
https://www.youtube.com/watch?v=Dy590QArwXI&app=desktop [Last accessed 23 March 2020]

Brannen, SB and Hicks, K (2020) We predicted a coronavirus pandemic: Here's what policymakers could have seen coming. Politico, 7 March. Available from:
https://www.politico.com/news/magazine/2020/03/07/Coronavirus-epidemic-prediction-policy-advice-121172
[Last accessed 7 April 2020]

Brennan, D (2020) Iran official says Trump sanctions are 'medical terrorism' during coronavirus pandemic. Newsweek, 1 April. Available from: https://www.newsweek.com/iran-official-says-donald-trump-sanctions-medical-terrorism-during-coronavirus-pandemic-1495415 [Last accessed 15 April 2020]

Brownlie, J et al. (2006) Infectious diseases: Preparing for the future. Future Threats. Office of Science and Innovation, London. Available from:
https://assets.publishing.service.gov.uk/government/uploads/system/uploads/attachment_data/file/294762/06-761-infectious-diseases-futures.pdf [Last accessed 9 April 2020]

Bruchner, T (2020) All COVID-19 clinical trials at a glance. TranspariMed, 9 Apr 2020. Available from:
https://www.transparimed.org/single-post/2020/03/27/COVID-19-clinical-trials-information-sources [Last accessed 15 April 2020]

Brunson, EK et al. (2020) The SPARS pandemic 2025–2028: A futuristic scenario to facilitate medical countermeasure communication. Journal of International Crisis and Risk, Communication Research, 2020, Volume 3, Issue 1, Pages 71–102. Available from: https://doi.org/10.30658/jicrcr.3.1.4 [Last accessed 15 April 2020]

Campbell, J et al. (2020) US explores possibility that coronavirus spread started in Chinese lab, not a market. CNN, 16 April. Available from: https://www.cnn.com/2020/04/15/politics/us-intelligence-virus-started-chinese-lab/index.html [Last accessed 17 April 2020]

Campbell, J (2020) Principal Nigerian religious leaders largely in lockstep with government on lockdowns. Council on Foreign Relations, 14 April. Available from: https://www.cfr.org/blog/principal-nigerian-religious-leaders-largely-lockstep-government-lockdowns [Last accessed 9 April 2020]

Caprioli, M and Boyer, MA (2001) Gender, Violence, and International Crisis, Journal of Conflict Resolution, 45(4), pp. 503–518. Available from: doi: 10.1177/0022002701045004005 [Last accessed 3 May 2020]

Carrol, T (2020) Pandemics: An essential reading list. Vulture, 10 March. Available from: https://www.vulture.com/article/best-pandemic-books.html [Last accessed 8 April 2020]

CEPI (2020) The Coalition for Epidemic Preparedness Innovations (CEPI). Available from: https://cepi.net/ [Last accessed 16 April 2020]

Chandra S, Kassens-Noor E, Kuljanin G, Vertalka J (2013) A geographic analysis of population density thresholds in the influenza pandemic of 1918-19. International Journal of Health Geography 2013;12:9. Published 2013 Feb 20. Available from: doi:10.1186/1476-072X-12-9 [Last accessed 2 May 2020]

Cheung, G, Wong, N, and Lum, A (2020) Coronavirus: Hong Kong will close borders to visitors and plans to ban sale of alcohol at bars in bid to stop spread of infections. South China Morning Post, 23 March. Available from: https://www.indiatoday.in/india/story/in-numbers-corona-people-dominate-pm-modi-lockdown-speech-1659301-2020-03-24 [Last accessed 24 March 2020]

Chiu, A and Armus, T (2020) Autopsies find first U.S. coronavirus death occurred in early February, weeks earlier than previously thought, Washington Post, 22 April. Available from: https://www.washingtonpost.com/nation/2020/04/22/death-coronavirus-first-california/ [Last accessed 2 May 2020]

Christakis, NA and Fowler, JH (2011) Connected: The surprising power of our social networks and how they shape our lives. Little, Brown Spark, New York. Available from: https://www.amazon.com/Connected-Surprising-Networks-Friends-Everything/dp/0316036137 [Last accessed 26 March 2020]

CIDRAP (2020) COVID-19: The CIDRAP Viewpoint, The Center for Infectious Disease Research and Policy (CIDRAP), 30 April. Available from: https://www.cidrap.umn.edu/sites/default/files/public/downloads/cidrap-covid19-viewpoint-part1_0.pdf [Last accessed 2 May 2020]

Clade X (2018) Clade X exercise. The Johns Hopkins Center for Health Security, 15 May. Accessible from:

https://www.centerforhealthsecurity.org/our-work/events/2018_clade_x_exercise/ [Last accessed 17 April 2020]

Cohen, E (2020) Infected people without symptoms might be driving the spread of coronavirus more than we realized. 19 March. Available from: https://www.cnn.com/2020/03/14/health/Coronavirus-asymptomatic-spread/index.html [Last accessed 24 March 2020]

Cohen, J (2020) Not wearing masks to protect against coronavirus is a 'big mistake,' top Chinese scientist says. Science, 27 March. https://www.sciencemag.org/news/2020/03/not-wearing-masks-protect-against-coronavirus-big-mistake-top-chinese-scientist-says# [Last accessed 20 April 2020]

Cookson, C (2020) Coronavirus may have infected half of UK population – Oxford study, Financial Times, 24 March. Available from: https://www.ft.com/content/5ff6469a-6dd8-11ea-89df-41bea055720b [Last accessed 2 May 2020]

Cordis (2020) Taking to market a novel filtration system for air purification. CORDIS. Available from: https://cordis.europa.eu/project/id/811822 [Last accessed 20 April 2020]

Council on Foreign Relations, With Michelle D. Gavin (2020) The coronavirus's impact throughout Africa. 14 April. Available from: https://www.cfr.org/podcasts/Coronaviruss-impact-throughout-africa-michelle-d-gavin [Last accessed 15 April 2020]

Council on Foreign Relations (2020) Latin America's Response

to COVID-19. 14 April. Available from:
https://www.cfr.org/conference-calls/latin-americas-response-COVID-19 [Last accessed 15 April 2020]

COVID-19 Dashboard (2020) COVID-19 Dashboard by the Center for Systems Science and Engineering (CSSE) at Johns Hopkins University (JHU). Available from:
https://Coronavirus.jhu.edu/map.html [Last accessed 16 April 2020]

Crimson Contagion (2019) Crimson Contagion Functional Exercise Draft Findings. HHS, October. Available from:
https://int.nyt.com/data/documenthelper/6824-2019-10-key-findings-and-after/05bd797500ea55be0724/optimized/full.pdf [Last accessed 20 April 2020]

Crowcroft, O (2020) Is Sweden's COVID-19 strategy working?, Euronews, 13 April. Available from:
https://www.euronews.com/2020/04/12/is-sweden-s-COVID-19-strategy-working [Last accessed 17 April 2020]

CSIS (2019) Ending the cycle of crisis and complacency in U.S. global health security. CSIS Commission on Strengthening America's Health Security, 18 November. Available from:
https://healthsecurity.csis.org/final-report/ [Last accessed 17 April 2020]

Curtis, N et al. (2020) Considering BCG vaccination to reduce the impact of COVID-19, Lancet, 30 April. Available from:
https://doi.org/10.1016/S0140-6736(20)31025-4 [Last accessed 2 May 2020]

Dandan, N (2020) How Wenzhou, 900 km from Wuhan, went into total lockdown. Sixth Tone, 14 February. Available from:

https://www.sixthtone.com/news/1005197/how-wenzhou%2C-900-km-from-wuhan%2C-went-into-total-lockdown [Last accessed 28 March 2020]

Delivorias, A and Scholz, N (2020) Economic impact of epidemics and pandemics. European Parliament Think Tank. 27 February. Available from: https://www.europarl.europa.eu/thinktank/en/document.html?reference=EPRS_BRI(2020)646195 [Last accessed 8 April 2020]

Deloitte (2020) The world remade by COVID-19. Recover: Planning scenarios for resilient leaders. Available from: https://www2.deloitte.com/global/en/pages/about-deloitte/articles/covid-19/covid-19-scenarios-and-impacts-for-business-and-society-world-remade.html [Last accessed 2 May 2020]

Deluca, D (2004) Networks of the Chinese community in Milan. Revue Européenne des Migrations Internationales, Vulume 20, Issue 3. Available from: https://journals.openedition.org/remi/2016?lang=en [Last accessed 13 April 2020]

Deutscher Bundestag (2013) Bericht zur risikoanalyse im bevölkerungsschutz 2012, Drucksache 17/12051, 3 January. Available from: https://www.bbk.bund.de/SharedDocs/Downloads/BBK/DE/Downloads/Krisenmanagement/BT-Bericht_Risikoanalyse_im_BevSch_2012.pdf?__blob=publicationFile [Last accessed 15 April 2020]

Devlin, H (2020) Do not relax COVID-19 measures in Wuhan too soon, scientists warn. The Guardian, 26 March. Available from:

https://www.theguardian.com/world/2020/mar/26/do-not-relax-COVID-19-measures-in-wuhan-too-soon-scientists-warn [Last accessed 28 March 2020]

Disley, J (2016) FLU WARNING: NHS would be 'unable to cope' in face of major pandemic, says medical officer. The Express, 27 December. Available from: https://www.express.co.uk/news/uk/747672/flu-pandemic-nhs-warning-world-innovation-summit-for-health [Last accessed: 4/29/2020]

Doward, J (2020) If ministers fail to reveal 2016 flu study, they 'will face court.' The Observer, 26 April. Available from: https://www.theguardian.com/uk-news/2020/apr/26/doctor-sue-results-operation-cygnus [Last accessed: 4/29/2020]

Dunleavey, J (2020) Pentagon denies existence of November coronavirus intelligence report warning of 'cataclysmic event.' 9 April. Available from: https://www.washingtonexaminer.com/news/pentagon-denies-existence-of-november-Coronavirus-intelligence-report-warning-of-cataclysmic-event [Last accessed 8 April 2020]

Durkheim, E (1997) The Division of Labour in Society. Trans. W. D. Halls, intro. Lewis A. Coser. New York: Free Press, 1893.

Durkheim, E (1951) Suicide: A study in sociology. Trans. by JA Spaulding and George Simpson. New York: The Free Press, 1897.

DW (2020) What do futurists imagine for the post-coronavirus-pandemic world? 10 March. Available from: https://www.dw.com/en/what-do-futurists-imagine-for-the-post-Coronavirus-pandemic-world/a-52993740 [Last accessed 8 April 2020]

ECDC (2016) Assessing communicable disease control and prevention in EU enlargement countries: Disease surveillance, preparedness and response, health governance and public health capacity development. (Technical Document.) Available from: https://www.ecdc.europa.eu/sites/default/files/media/en/publications/Publications/communicable-disease-control-assessment-EU-enlargement-countries.pdf [Last accessed 8 April 2020]

Edelman, S (2020) Gov. Cuomo urged to shut down NYC subways to stop coronavirus spread. New York Post, 18 April. Available from: https://nypost.com/2020/04/18/gov-cuomo-urged-to-shut-down-nyc-subways-to-stop-coronavirus-spread/ [Last accessed 8 April 2020]

Eletreby, R et al. (2020) The effects of evolutionary adaptations on spreading processes in complex networks. PNAS March 17, 2020 117 (11) 5664-5670. Available from: https://www.pnas.org/content/117/11/5664 [Last accessed 2 May 2020]

Emanuel, EJ, Ellenberg, S and Levy, M (2020) The coronavirus is here to stay, so what happens Next? New York Times, 17 March. Available from: https://www.nytimes.com/2020/03/17/opinion/Coronavirus-social-distancing-effect.html [Last accessed 23 March 2020]

Erichsen, VM (2020) Epiguard kastet seg rundt for å levere smittevern-kuvøser til norske redningshelikoptre. Shifter, 23 Mars. Available from: https://shifter.no/nyheter/epiguard-kastet-seg-rundt-for-a-levere-smittevern-kuvoser-til-norske-redningshelikoptre/121391 [Last accessed 8 April 2020]

Event 201 (2019) Event 201. The Johns Hopkins Center for Health Security, 18 October. Available from: https://www.centerforhealthsecurity.org/event201/ [Last accessed 15 April 2020]

Fallon, K (2020) Greece: 148 refugees test positive for COVID-19, all asymptomatic, Al Jazeera, 21 April. Available from: https://www.aljazeera.com/news/2020/04/greece-148-refugees-test-positive-covid-19-asymptomatic-200421134039733.html [Last accessed 15 April 2020]

Feng, E and Cheng A (2020) Mystery in Wuhan: Recovered coronavirus patients test negative...then positive. NPR, 27 March. Available from: https://www.npr.org/sections/goatsandsoda/2020/03/27/822407626/mystery-in-wuhan-recovered-Coronavirus-patients-test-negative-then-positive [Last accessed 28 March 2020]

Ferguson, N et al. (2020) Report 9: Impact of non-pharmaceutical interventions (NPIs) to reduce COVID-19 mortality and healthcare demand, Imperial College, 16 March. Available from: https://doi.org/10.25561/77482 [Last accessed 2 May 2020]

Feuerstein, A and Herper, M (2020) Early peek at data on Gilead coronavirus drug suggests patients are responding to treatment. Statnews, 16 April. Available from: https://www.statnews.com/2020/04/16/early-peek-at-data-on-gilead-Coronavirus-drug-suggests-patients-are-responding-to-treatment/ [Last accessed 16 April 2020]

Finley, K (2020) Data sharing and open source software help

combat COVID-19. Wired, 13 March. Avaiable from: https://www.wired.com/story/data-sharing-open-source-software-combat-COVID-19/ [Last accessed 16 April 2020]

Foreigner.fi (2020) Finland responds to Trump's announcement with increased funding to WHO. Foreigner.fi, 15 April. Available from:
https://www.foreigner.fi/articulo/news/finnish-government-agrees-to-increase-funding-for-who/20200415175435005324.html [Last accessed 15 April 2020]

Fox, EA (2020) CEOs lead the coronavirus response with unparalleled innovation. Forbes, 20 March. Available from: https://www.forbes.com/sites/ericaarielfox/2020/03/20/ceos-lead-the-Coronavirus-response-with-unparalleled-innovation/#6a0115085355 [Last accessed 17 April 2020]

Frieden, TR and Lee, CT (2020) Identifying and interrupting superspreading events—Implications for control of Severe Acute Respiratory Syndrome Coronavirus 2. Emerging Infectious Diseases. Volume 26, Issue 6—June 2020. Available from:
https://wwwnc.cdc.gov/eid/article/26/6/20-0495_article [Last accessed 24 March 2020]

Friedman, U (2020) We were warned. The Atlantic, 18 March. Available from:
https://www.theatlantic.com/politics/archive/2020/03/pandemic-Coronavirus-united-states-trump-cdc/608215/ [Last accessed 8 April 2020]

Fu, F, Christakis, NA and Fowler, JH (2017) Dueling biological and social contagions. Scientific Reports. Volume 7, Article number: 43634 (2017). 2 March. Available from:

https://www.nature.com/articles/srep43634 [Last accessed 24 March 2020]

FullFact (2019) How long does the average government last?, FullFact, 11 October. Available from: https://fullfact.org/news/how-long-does-average-government-last/ [Last accessed 2 May 2020]

Gan, N (2020) China lifts 76-day lockdown on Wuhan as city reemerges from coronavirus crisis. CNN, 8 April. Available from: https://www.cnn.com/2020/04/07/asia/Coronavirus-wuhan-lockdown-lifted-intl-hnk/index.html [Last accessed 8 April 2020]

Gates, B. (2015) The next outbreak: We're not ready. TED Talk, March 2015. Available from: https://www.ted.com/talks/bill_gates_the_next_outbreak_we_re_not_ready?language=dz [Last accessed 28 March 2020]

Georgia Department of Public Health (2020) Georgia Department of Public Health Daily Status Report. Available from: https://dph.georgia.gov/covid-19-daily-status-report [Last accessed 2 May 2020]

Gorvett, Z (2020) The tricky politics of naming the new coronavirus. BBC, 16 February. Available from: https://www.bbc.com/future/article/20200214-Coronavirus-swine-flu-and-sars-how-viruses-get-their-names [Last accessed 8 April 2020]

Ghosh, I (2019) 70 years of urban growth in 1 infographic. World Economic Forum, 3 September. Available from: https://www.weforum.org/agenda/2019/09/mapped-the-dramatic-global-rise-of-urbanization-1950-2020/ [Last accessed 8 April 2020]

Gibbs, WW and Soares, C (2005) Preparing for a pandemic. Scientific American. Available from: https://www.scientificamerican.com/article/preparing-for-a-pandemic-2005-11/ [Last accessed 8 April 2020]

Giddens, A. (1991) Modernity and Self-Identity. Stanford: Stanford University Press.

Global Preparedness Monitoring Board (2019) World at risk from deadly pandemics. (Press Release.) 17 September. Available from: https://apps.who.int/gpmb/assets/annual_report/GPMB%20Press%20Release%2017%20Sep.pdf [Last accessed 28 March 2020]

Global Times (2020) Some Chinese medics may be injected with newly developed COVID-19 vaccine by end of 2020: Head of Chinese CDC. Global Times, 20 April. Available from: https://www.globaltimes.cn/content/1186197.shtml [Last accessed 20 April 2020]

Goñi, U (2020) Half of Uruguay's coronavirus cases traced to a single guest at a society party. The Guardian, 19 March. Available from: https://www.theguardian.com/world/2020/mar/19/uruguay-Coronavirus-party-guest-argentina [Last accessed 24 March 2020]

Graff, GM (2020) An oral history of the pandemic warnings Trump ignored. Wired, 17 April. Available from: https://www.wired.com/story/an-oral-history-of-the-pandemic-warnings-trump-ignored/ [Last accessed 15 April 2020]

Green, MJ (2020) Geopolitical scenarios for Asia after COVID-19. CSIS, 31 March. Available from: https://www.csis.org/analysis/geopolitical-scenarios-asia-after-COVID-19 [Last accessed 20 April 2020]

Green, M and Medeiros, ES (2020) The pandemic won't make China the world's leader. Foreign Affairs, 15 April. Available from: https://www.foreignaffairs.com/articles/united-states/2020-04-15/pandemic-wont-make-china-worlds-leader [Last accessed 15 April 2020]

Greer, B (2020) The female world leaders defeating coronavirus, The New European, 24 April. Available from: https://www.theneweuropean.co.uk/top-stories/women-world-leaders-taking-control-during-coronavirus-1-6620730 [Last accessed 3 May 2020]

Grein et al (2020) Compassionate use of Remdesivir for patients with severe COVID-19. New England Journal of Medicine, 10 April. Available from: DOI: 10.1056/NEJMoa2007016 [Last accessed 15 April 2020]

Grubaugh, M et al. (2019) Tracking virus outbreaks in the twenty-first century. Nature Microbiology, Volume 4, Pages 10–19. Available from: https://doi.org/10.1038/s41564-018-0296-2 [Last accessed 15 April 2020]

Grüll, P (2020) How an Austrian ski paradise became a COVID-19 hotspot. Euractiv, 20 March. Available from: https://www.euractiv.com/section/Coronavirus/news/ischgl-oesterreichisches-skiparadies-als-corona-hotspot/ [Last accessed 19 March 2020]

Guo, R (2020) China's economic powerhouse Guangdong

lowers coronavirus threat level amid drive to get economy going again. South China Morning Post, 24 February. Available from:
https://www.scmp.com/news/china/politics/article/3052157/chinas-economic-powerhouse-guangdong-lowers-Coronavirus-threat [Last accessed 28 March 2020]

Haas, R (2020) The pandemic will accelerate history rather than reshape it. Foreign Affairs, May/June, 8 April. Available from:
https://www.foreignaffairs.com/articles/united-states/2020-04-07/pandemic-will-accelerate-history-rather-reshape-i [Last accessed 7 April 2020]

Hadfield, J et al. (2018) Nextstrain: Real-time tracking of pathogen evolution. Bioinformatics, Volume 34, Issue 23, 1 December, Pages 4121–4123. Available from:
https://doi.org/10.1093/bioinformatics/bty407
[Last accessed 16 April 2020]

Hamilton, J (2020) Ventilators can save lives of some COVID-19 patients, but they're no panacea, all things considered. NPR, 1 April. Available from:
https://www.npr.org/2020/04/01/825499422/ventilators-can-save-lives-of-some-COVID-19-patients-but-theyre-no-panacea [Last accessed 16 April 2020]

Health Europa (2020) EpiGuard: Providing solutions for medical isolation and transportation. Health Europa, 15 April. Available from:
https://www.healtheuropa.eu/epiguard-providing-solutions-for-medical-isolation-and-transportation/99358/
[Last accessed 16 April 2020]

Helm, T et al. (2020) How did Britain get its coronavirus

response so wrong? The Guardian, 19 April. Available from: https://www.theguardian.com/world/2020/apr/18/how-did-britain-get-its-response-to-coronavirus-so-wrong [Last accessed 21 April 2020]

History-computer.com (2020) History of Skype. Available from: https://history-computer.com/Internet/Conquering/Skype.html [Last accessed 16 April 2020]

Hoare, C (2020) How shop assistant 'super-spreader' infected eight people in BBC UK town pandemic study. Express, 21 March. Available from: https://www.express.co.uk/news/uk/1258415/Coronavirus-shop-superspreader-covid19-bbc-pandemic-haslemere-boris-johnson-spt [Last accessed 24 March 2020]

Huang, Y (2008) Capitalism with Chinese Characteristics: Entrepreneurship and the State. Cambridge, UK: Cambridge University Press.

Humphries, J (2014) No, the Black Death did not create more jobs for women. 8 April. Available from: http://theconversation.com/no-the-black-death-did-not-create-more-jobs-for-women-25298 [Last accessed 9 April 2020]

ICNARC (2020) ICNARC report on COVID-19 in critical care, 27 March. Available from: https://www.icnarc.org/DataServices/Attachments/Download/b5f59585-5870-ea11-9124-00505601089b [Last accessed 16 April 2020]

Imperial College COVID-19 (2020) Available from:

http://www.imperial.ac.uk/mrc-global-infectious-disease-analysis/COVID-19/ [Last accessed 20 April 2020]

Ip, G (2020) Shoes to masks: Corporate innovation flourishes in coronavirus fight. Wall Street Journal, 16 April. Available from: https://www.wsj.com/articles/american-companies-innovate-to-fight-the-Coronavirus-in-echo-of-world-war-ii-11587045652 [Last accessed 16 April 2020]

IHME (2020) COVID-19 Projections. Institute for Health Metrics and Evaluation, University of Washington. Available from:
https://covid19.healthdata.org/united-states-of-america
[Last accessed 2 May 2020]

ILO (2020) ILO: As job losses escalate, nearly half of global workforce at risk of losing livelihoods, ILO, 29 April. Available from:
https://www.ilo.org/global/about-the-ilo/newsroom/news/WCMS_743036/lang--en/index.htm
[Last accessed 2 May 2020]

Institute of Medicine (1992) Emerging infections: Microbial threats to health in the United States. Institute of Medicine (US) Committee on Emerging Microbial Threats to Health; Lederberg J, Shope RE, Oaks SC Jr, eds. Washington, DC: National Academies Press. Available from:
https://www.ncbi.nlm.nih.gov/pubmed/25121245
[Last accessed 20 April 2020]

IRC (2020) IRC: World risks up to 1 billion cases and 3.2 million deaths from COVID-19 across fragile countries, IRC, 29 April. Available from:
https://www.rescue.org/press-release/irc-world-risks-1-billion-cases-and-32-million-deaths-covid-19-across-fragile

[Last accessed 2 May 2020]

Jacobsen, K (2020) Will COVID-19 generate global preparedness? Lancet, 18 March. Available from: https://www.thelancet.com/journals/lancet/article/PIIS0140-6736(20)30559-6/fulltext [Last accessed 23 March 2020]

Jones, K et al. (2008) Global trends in emerging infectious diseases. Nature, Volume 451, Issue 7181, Pages 990–993. Available from: https://dx.doi.org/10.1038%2Fnature06536 [Last accessed 8 April 2020]

Kalehsar, O (2019) Iran's interests in China's one belt one road policy. United World International, 3 August. Available from: https://uwidata.com/4707-irans-interests-in-chinas-one-belt-one-road-policy/ [Last 13 April 2020]

Kasulis, K (2020) 'Patient 31' and South Korea's sudden spike in coronavirus cases. Al Jazeera, 3 March. Available from: https://www.aljazeera.com/news/2020/03/31-south-korea-sudden-spike-Coronavirus-cases-200303065953841.html [Last accessed 24 March 2020]

Kent, C (2020) UK businesses launch VentilatorChallengeUK consortium. Verdict Medical Devices, 30 March. Available from: https://www.medicaldevice-network.com/news/ventilatorchallengeuk/ [Last accessed 16 April 2020]

KFF (2020) The US Government and the World Health Organization. Kaiser Family Foundation, 16 April. Available from: https://www.kff.org/global-health-policy/fact-sheet/the-u-s-government-and-the-world-health-organization/

[Last accessed 16 April 2020]

Khullar, D and Chokshi, DA (2018) Health, income & poverty: Where we are & what could help. Health Affairs, 4 October. Available from: https://www.healthaffairs.org/do/10.1377/hpb20180817.901935/full/ [Last accessed 17 April 2020]

Kirkwood, I (2016) Bluedot announces second series a round, this time worth $9.2 million CAD. Betakit, 7 August. Available from: https://betakit.com/bluedot-announces-second-series-a-round-this-time-worth-9-2-million-cad/ [Last accessed 16 April 2020]

Kissler, SM et al. (2020) Social distancing strategies for curbing the COVID-19 epidemic, Medrxiv, 24 March. Available from: https://doi.org/10.1101/2020.03.22.20041079 [Last accessed 2 May 2020]

Klass, P (2018) A centennial of death: The great influenza pandemic of 1918. New York Times, 22 October. Available from: https://www.nytimes.com/2018/10/22/well/family/a-centennial-of-death-the-great-influenza-pandemic-of-1918.html [Last accessed 28 March 2020]

Klein, A (2020) After coronavirus outbreak at Biogen meeting, company foundation commits $10M for relief. NBC Boston, 16 March. Available from: https://www.nbcboston.com/news/Coronavirus/after-Coronavirus-outbreak-at-biogen-meeting-company-foundation-commits-10m-for-relief/2092143/
[Last accessed 24 March 2020]

Krieg, G (2020) Maryland Gov. Larry Hogan defies Trump with aggressive coronavirus response. CNN, 24 March.

Available from:
https://www.cnn.com/2020/03/24/politics/Coronavirus-larry-hogan-maryland-governor/index.html [Last accessed 24 March 2020]

Kupferschmidt, K and Cohen, J (2020) China's aggressive measures have slowed the coronavirus: They may not work in other countries. Science Magazine, 2 March. Accessible from: https://www.sciencemag.org/news/2020/03/china-s-aggressive-measures-have-slowed-Coronavirus-they-may-not-work-other-countries [Last accessed 28 March 2020]

Kurilla, MG and Zhang, R (2020) Harvard announces salary and hiring freezes, discretionary spending reductions, potential deferral of capital projects, and leadership salary cuts. The Harvard Crimson, 14 April. Accessible from: https://www.thecrimson.com/article/2020/4/14/harvard-Coronavirus-hiring-salary-freeze/ [Last accessed 28 March 2020]

Kwok et al. (2020) Community responses during early phase of COVID-19 epidemic. Hong Kong, Emerging Infectious Diseases, Volume 26, Issue 7, July 2020. Accessible from: https://wwwnc.cdc.gov/eid/article/26/7/20-0500_article [Last accessed 9 April 2020]

Lakoff, A (2017) Unprepared: Global health in a time of emergency. University of California Press. Available from: https://www.ucpress.edu/book/9780520295766/unprepared [Last accessed 9 April 2020]

Lanese, N (2020) What is a coronavirus?, LiveScience, 7 February. Available from:
https://www.livescience.com/what-are-coronaviruses.html [Last accessed 2 May 2020]

Langenhove, LF (2012) Foresight is 20/20: Scenario building for policy analysis and strategy development. Available from: https://www.researchgate.net/publication/237079050_Foresight_is_2020_Scenario_Building_for_Policy_Analysis_and_Strategy_Development [Last accessed 9 April 2020]

Latour, B (1983) Give me a laboratory and I will raise the world. In Knorr-Cetina, K and Mulkay, M, Science Observed. London: Sage Publications. Available from: http://www.bruno-latour.fr/sites/default/files/12-GIVE-ME-A-LAB-GB.pdf [Last accessed 19 April 2020]

Laughland , O and Holpuch, A (2020) 'We're modern slaves': How meat plant workers became the new frontline in Covid-19 war, The Guardian, 2 May. Available from: https://www.theguardian.com/world/2020/may/02/meat-plant-workers-us-coronavirus-war [Last accessed 2 May 2020]

Laughlin, D (2020) Coronavirus reveals the downsides of urbanization. National Review, 19 March. Accessible from: https://www.nationalreview.com/2020/03/Coronavirus-reveals-the-downsides-of-urbanization/ [Last accessed 28 March 2020]

Leichmann, AK (2020) 30 Israeli medical innovations to fight coronavirus. Israel 21c, 30 March. Available from: https://www.israel21c.org/30-israeli-medical-tech-solutions-to-help-fight-Coronavirus/ [Last accessed 16 April 2020]

Li, D et al (2020) Estimating the scale of COVID-19 epidemic in the United States: Simulations based on air traffic directly from Wuhan, China. MedRxiv, 8 March. Available from: https://doi.org/10.1101/2020.03.06.20031880 [Last accessed

28 March 2020]

Lin, K (2016) Exploring China's former 'Capital of Sex.' Global Times, 13 May. Accessible from: http://www.globaltimes.cn/content/982835.shtml [Last accessed 28 March 2020]

Lipton, J (2020) What Ebola taught me about coronavirus: Panic will get us nowhere. The Guardian, 11 March. Available from: https://www.theguardian.com/commentisfree/2020/mar/11/what-ebola-taught-me-about-Coronavirus-panic-will-get-us-nowhere [Last accessed 23 March 2020]

Liu, A (2020) Biogen parts ways with employee who hid coronavirus symptoms and lied her way back to China. Fierce Pharma, 20 March. Available from: https://www.fiercepharma.com/pharma/biogen-parts-way-employee-who-hid-Coronavirus-symptoms-and-lied-her-way-back-to-china [Last accessed 24 March 2020]

Liu, Y, Li, J and Feng, Y (2020) Critical care response to a hospital outbreak of the 2019-nCoV infection in Shenzhen, China. Critical Care Volume 24, Issue 56, 19 February. Available from: https://doi.org/10.1186/s13054-020-2786-x [Last accessed 28 March 2020]

Lourenco, J el al. (2020) Fundamental principles of epidemic spread highlight the immediate need for large-scale serological surveys to assess the stage of the SARS-CoV-2 epidemic, Medrxiv, 26 March. Available from: https://doi.org/10.1101/2020.03.24.20042291 [Last accessed 2 May 2020]

Lowy, F (2018) Australia must recapture its sense of ambition,

The Sydney Morning Herald, 13 September. Available from: https://www.smh.com.au/politics/federal/australia-must-recapture-its-sense-of-ambition-20180913-p503kw.html [Last accessed 2 May 2020]

NEOM (2020) Top 10 largest megacities in the world 2020. NEOM, 20 January. Available from:
https://neomsaudicity.net/top-largest-megacities-2017/
[Last accessed 24 March 2020]

Loria, K. (2018) A leading medical institution created a simulation that shows how a new disease could kill 900 million people—and it reveals how unprepared we are. Business Insider, 29 July. Available from:
https://www.businessinsider.com/pandemic-virus-simulation-johns-hopkins-shows-vulnerability-2018-7 [Last accessed 15 April 2020]

Lou Corpuz-Bosshart, L (2020) The post-pandemic city: Expert on how the coronavirus will impact future cities, Phys.org, 24 March. Available from:
https://phys.org/news/2020-03-post-pandemic-city-expert-Coronavirus-impact.html [Last accessed 8 April 2020]

Lowy Institute (2020) The world after COVID-19 Available from:
https://www.lowyinstitute.org/publications/world-after-COVID-19 [Last accessed 15 April 2020]

Mahajan, AS (2020) Time to blame or learn: Punjab's 1st coronavirus death sparks 'super-spreader' fears with 40,000 under quarantine. India Today, 30 March. Available from:
https://www.indiatoday.in/india/story/time-to-blame-or-learn-punjab-s-1st-Coronavirus-death-sparks-super-spreader-fears-with-40-000-under-quarantine-1661337-

2020-03-30 [Last accessed 15 April 2020]

Mackenzie, D (2001) Did bubonic plague really cause the Black Death?, New Scientist, 24 November. Available from: https://www.newscientist.com/article/mg17223184-000-did-bubonic-plague-really-cause-the-black-death/ [Last accessed 2 May 2020]

Margolin, J and Meek, JG (2020) Intelligence report warned of coronavirus crisis as early as November, Sources. ABC News, 8 April. Available from: https://abcnews.go.com/Politics/intelligence-report-warned-Coronavirus-crisis-early-november-sources/story?id=7003127 [Last accessed 15 April 2020]

Marin, C and Moseley, D (2020) 'Crimson Contagion 2019' simulation warned of pandemic implications in US. NBC News Chicago, 24 March. Available from: https://www.nbcchicago.com/news/local/crimson-contagion-2019-simulation-warned-of-pandemic-implications-in-us/2243832/ [Last accessed 20 April 2020]

Maron, DF (2014) Weaponized Ebola: Is it really a bioterror threat? Scientific American, 25 September. Available from: https://www.scientificamerican.com/article/weaponized-ebola-is-it-really-a-bioterror-threat/ [Last accessed 13 April 2020]

Martin, B (2020) Texas anti-vaxxers fear mandatory COVID-19 vaccines more than the virus Itself. Texas Monthly, 18 March. Available from: https://www.texasmonthly.com/news/texas-anti-vaxxers-fear-mandatory-Coronavirus-vaccines/ [Last accessed 15 April 2020]

McFall-Johnsen, M and Bendix, A (2020) An average coronavirus patient infects at least 2 others. To end the pandemic, that crucial metric needs to drop below 1—here's how we get there. Business Insider, 18 April. Available from: https://www.businessinsider.com/Coronavirus-contagious-r-naught-average-patient-spread-2020-3 [Last accessed 15 April 2020]

McKinsey (2020) COVID-19: Implications for business, Executive Briefing. April. Available from: https://www.mckinsey.com/business-functions/risk/our-insights/COVID-19-implications-for-business [Last accessed 15 April 2020]

Med-Tech Innovation News (2020) Government orders 15,000 Penlon ventilators following MHRA approval. Med-Tech Innovation News, 16 April. Available from: https://www.med-technews.com/news/government-orders-15-000-penlon-ventilators-following-mhra-a/ [Last accessed 15 April 2020]

Metabiota (2020) Metabiota Risk Report No. 3: February 25, 2020. Available from: https://metabiota.com/sites/default/files/inline-files/Metabiota_Risk_Report_No.3-25Feb2020-COVID-2019_0.pdf [Last accessed 17 April 2020]

Miller, AM (2020) Imperial College scientist who predicted 500K coronavirus deaths in UK adjusts figure to 20K or fewer, Washington Examiner, 26 March. Available from: https://www.washingtonexaminer.com/news/imperial-college-scientist-who-predicted-500k-coronavirus-deaths-in-uk-revises-to-20k-or-less [Last accessed 17 April 2020]

Mitchell, SP (2020) Exploring the mysterious and beautiful island of Vis, International Living, 7 February. Croatia. Available from: https://internationalliving.com/exploring-the-mysterious-and-beautiful-island-of-vis-croatia-trl/ [Last accessed 13 April 2020]

MOHFW (2020) COVID-19 INDIA. Indian Ministry of Health and Family Welfare. Available from: https://www.mohfw.gov.in/ [Last accessed 2 May 2020]

Monaco, L (2020) Pandemic disease is a threat to national security. Foreign Affairs, 3 March. https://www.foreignaffairs.com/articles/2020-03-03/pandemic-disease-threat-national-security [Last accessed 9 April 2020]

Money et al. (2020) Backlash over closing California beaches grows in some coastal communities, Los Angeles Times, 30 April. Available from: https://www.latimes.com/california/story/2020-04-30/backlash-over-closing-calfornia-beaches-grows-in-some-coastal-communities [Last accessed 2 May 2020]

Morens, DM and Fauci, AS (2012) Emerging infectious diseases in 2012: 20 years after the Institute of Medicine report. mBio. November/December 2012, Volume 3, Issue 6, e00494-12. Available from: https://mbio.asm.org/content/mbio/3/6/e00494-12.full.pdf [Last accessed 21 April 2020]

Morris, C (2020) Social distancing creates $8 trillion in economic benefits, Fortune, 20 March. Available from: https://fortune.com/2020/03/30/social-distancing-economic-benefits-coronavirus/ [Last accessed 16 April 2020]

Morrison, JS and Carrol, A (2020) Which COVID-19 future will we choose? CSIS, 1 April. Available from: https://www.csis.org/analysis/which-COVID-19-future-will-we-choose [Last accessed 16 April 2020]

Moritsugu, K (2020) China, on virus PR offensive, sends masks and experts abroad. ABC News, Associated Press, 21 March. Available from: https://abcnews.go.com/Health/wireStory/china-virus-pr-offensive-sends-masks-experts-abroad-69723923 [Last accessed 23 March 2020]

Morrell, M (2020) Transcript: Lisa Monaco speaks with Michael Morell on "intelligence matters." Intelligence Matters, CBS News, 15 April. Available from: https://www.cbsnews.com/news/transcript-lisa-monaco-speaks-with-michael-morell-on-intelligence-matters/ [Last accessed 20 April 2020]

National Strategy for Pandemic Influenza Implementation Plan (2006) Available from: https://www.cdc.gov/flu/pandemic-resources/pdf/pandemic-influenza-implementation.pdf [Last accessed 16 April 2020]

Nationmaster (2020) Failed states: Statistical profile. Available from: https://www.nationmaster.com/country-info/groups/failed-states [Last accessed 13 April 2020]

NERVTAG (2016) The New and Emerging Respiratory Virus Threats Advisory Group (NERVTAG): 2nd Annual Report, January-December. Prepared by: Fran Parry-Ford. Available from: https://app.box.com/s/3lkcbxepqixkg4mv640dpvvg978ixjtf/

file/428772311641 [Last accessed: 4/29/2020]

Nextstrain (2020) Genomic epidemiology of novel coronavirus—Global subsampling. Available from: https://nextstrain.org/ncov/global [Last accessed 16 April 2020]

NHS England (2017) Emergency Preparedness, Resilience and Response (EPRR), Board Paper NHS England, No. 10, 30 March. Available from: https://www.england.nhs.uk/wp-content/uploads/2017/03/board-paper-300317-item-10.pdf [Last accessed: 4/29/2020]

Nuki, P (2020) Exercise Cygnus uncovered: The pandemic warnings buried by the government. The Telegraph, 28 March. Available from: https://www.telegraph.co.uk/news/2020/03/28/exercise-cygnus-uncovered-pandemic-warnings-buried-government/ [Last accessed: 4/29/2020]

Ogilvy, J and Schwartz, P (2004). Plotting your scenarios. Global Business Network. Available from: https://web.archive.org/web/20190803235747/http://www.meadowlark.co/plotting_your_scenarios.pdf [Last accessed 20 April 2020]

O'Toole, T, Mair, M, and Inglesby, TV (2002) Shining light on "dark winter." Clinical Infectious Diseases, Volume 34, Issue 7, 1 April, Pages 972–983. Available from: https://doi.org/10.1086/339909 [Last accessed 21 April 2020]

Oliveira, N (2020) Coronavirus 'super spreader' who unintentionally infected at least 11 people comes forward. New York Daily News, 11 February. Available from:

https://www.nydailynews.com/news/world/ny-Coronavirus-super-spreader-steve-walsh-speaks-up-20200211-ghn7wvvh6vb7nne5unqrawxy5u-story.html [Last accessed 24 March 2020]

Omondi, S (2018) What is a megacity? WorldAtlas, 28 June. Available from: https://www.worldatlas.com/articles/what-is-a-megacity.html [Last accessed 28 March 2020]

Oruko, I (2020) How church became coronavirus super-spreader. Daily Nation, 23 March. Available from: https://www.nation.co.ke/news/How-church-became-Coronavirus-super-spreader/1056-5500834-2i1qwe/index.html [Last accessed 24 March 2020]

O'Toole, S et al. (2002) Shining light on "dark winter." Clinical Infectious Diseases, Volume 34, Issue 7, 1 April, Pages 972–983. Available from: https://doi.org/10.1086/339909 [Last accessed 20 April 2020]

Owoseje, T (2020) Coronavirus is 'the great equalizer,' Madonna tells fans from her bathtub. CNN, 23 March. Available from: https://www.cnn.com/2020/03/23/entertainment/madonna-Coronavirus-video-intl-scli/index.html [Last accessed 23 March 2020]

Palmer, M (2020) How to prepare your business for a post-pandemic future. Sifted, 7 April. Available from: https://sifted.eu/articles/business-post-pandemic/ [Last accessed 15 April 2020]

Panovska-Griffiths J (2020). Can mathematical modelling solve the current Covid-19 crisis?. BMC public health, 20(1), 551. Available from: https://doi.org/10.1186/s12889-020-

08671-z [Last accessed 2 May 2020]

Patel, NV (2020) The best, and the worst, of the coronavirus dashboards. MIT Tech Review, 6 March. Available from: https://www.technologyreview.com/2020/03/06/905436/best-worst-Coronavirus-dashboards/ [Last accessed 20 April 2020]

Perry, M (2020) America's pandemic war games don't end well. Foreign Policy, 1 April. Available from: https://foreignpolicy.com/2020/04/01/Coronavirus-pandemic-war-games-simulation-dark-winter/ [Last accessed 20 April 2020]

Perry, TS (2020) Satellites and AI monitor Chinese economy's reaction to coronavirus. IEEE Spectrum, 10 March. Available from: https://spectrum.ieee.org/view-from-the-valley/artificial-intelligence/machine-learning/satellites-and-ai-monitor-chinese-economys-reaction-to-Coronavirus [Last accessed 17 April 2020]

Picheta, R. (2020) Coronavirus pandemic will cause global famines of 'biblical proportions,' UN warns, CNN, 22 April. Available from: https://www.cnn.com/2020/04/22/africa/coronavirus-famine-un-warning-intl/index.html [Last accessed 2 May 2020]

Porterfield, C (2020) Report: CDC director warns a second coronavirus wave would be 'even more difficult', Forbes, 21 April. Available from: https://www.forbes.com/sites/carlieporterfield/2020/04/21/report-cdc-director-warns-a-second-coronavirus-wave-would-be-even-more-difficult/#1946a94f43d0 [Last accessed

2 May 2020]

Prem, K et al. (2020) The effect of control strategies to reduce social mixing on outcomes of the COVID-19 epidemic in Wuhan, China: a modelling study, The Lancet Public Health. Available from:
https://doi.org/10.1016/S2468-2667(20)30073-6
[Last accessed 2 May 2020]

Pronker, ES et al (2013) Risk in vaccine research and development quantified. PLoS One, Volume 8, Issue 3, e57755. Available from:
https://www.ncbi.nlm.nih.gov/pmc/articles/PMC3603987/
[Last accessed 23 March 2020]

Prospex (2020) Preparing for the pandemics of the future http://www.prospex.com/client-success/preparing-for-the-pandemics-of-the-future/ [Last accessed 7 April 2020]

Qiu, J (2020) How China's "Bat Woman" hunted down viruses from SARS to the new coronavirus., Scientific American, 11 March. Available from:
https://www.scientificamerican.com/article/how-chinas-bat-woman-hunted-down-viruses-from-sars-to-the-new-Coronavirus1/ [Last accessed 5 April 2020]

Qureshi, M (2020) What are the Government hiding about their response to Covid-19? Available from:
https://www.crowdjustice.com/case/jrcovid19/
[Last accessed: 4/29/2020]

Radjou, N (2020) Corporate America must learn to innovate frugally to get through the coronavirus crisis. Fast Company, 27 March. Available from:
https://www.fastcompany.com/90482825/corporate-

america-must-learn-to-innovate-frugally-to-get-through-the-Coronavirus-crisis [Last accessed 17 April 2020]

Radu, S (2020) How AI tracks the coronavirus spread. US News and World Report, 11 March. Available from: https://www.usnews.com/news/best-countries/articles/2020-03-11/how-scientists-are-using-artificial-intelligence-to-track-the-Coronavirus [Last accessed 17 April 2020]

Rand Corporation (2012) Threats without threateners? Rand Corporation. Available from: https://www.rand.org/content/dam/rand/pubs/occasional_papers/2012/RAND_OP360.pdf [Last accessed 7 April 2020]

Rainey, J et al. (2020) A sunny California weekend of social distancing, neighborly love—and some overcrowding. LA Times, 21 March. Available from: https://www.latimes.com/california/story/2020-03-21/southern-california-settles-into-first-weekend-of-Coronavirus-shut-down [Last accessed 23 March 2020]

Rasheed, Z (2020) Our lives after the coronavirus pandemic. Al Jazeera, 26 March. Available from: https://www.aljazeera.com/news/2020/03/world-Coronavirus-pandemic-200326055223989.html [Last accessed 14 April 2020]

Raskin, R (2020) Are we ready for a do-not-touch World? Techonomy, 21 March. Available from: https://techonomy.com/2020/03/are-we-ready-for-a-do-not-touch-world/ [Last accessed 19 March 2020]

Rathi, A (2020) Nations with mandatory TB vaccines show fewer coronavirus deaths, Bloomberg, 2 April. Available from:

https://www.bloomberg.com/news/articles/2020-04-02/fewer-coronavirus-deaths-seen-in-countries-that-mandate-tb-vaccine [Last accessed 2 May 2020]

Reuters (2020) US health worker counter-protest. Available from:
https://www.theguardian.com/us-news/2020/apr/20/us-protests-lockdown-coronavirus-cases-surge-warning#img-3 [Last accessed 17 April 2020]

Reuters (2020) Coronavirus epidemic 'under control' in Norway: health minister, Reuters, 6 April. Available from: https://www.reuters.com/article/us-health-coronavirus-norway/coronavirus-epidemic-under-control-in-norway-health-minister-idUSKBN21O27H [Last accessed 2 May 2020]

Rincon, P (2020) Coronavirus: Is there any evidence for lab release theory? BBC, 16 April. Available from:
https://www.bbc.com/news/science-environment-52318539 [Last accessed 17 April 2020]

Roos, D (2020) Why the Second Wave of the 1918 Spanish Flu Was So Deadly, History.com, 3 March. Available from: https://www.history.com/news/spanish-flu-second-wave-resurgence Last accessed 3 May 2020]

Rosling, H (2018) Factfulness. New York: Flatiron Books.

Sadati, AK et al. (2020) Risk society, global vulnerability and fragile resilience: Sociological view on the coronavirus outbreak. Shiraz E-Medical Journal, Online ahead of Print, Volume 21, Issue 4, e102263. Available from: doi:10.5812/semj.102263 [Last accessed 20 April 2020]

Salathe, M and Case, N (2020) What Happens Next? COVID-

19 Futures, Explained With Playable Simulations. Free, open-source guide, May 2020. Available from: https://ncase.me/covid-19/ [Last accessed 2 May 2020]

Salo, J (2020) Sweden grapples with high death toll after controversially refusing to lock down. New York Post, 16 April. Available from: https://nypost.com/2020/04/16/sweden-grapples-with-high-death-toll-after-controversially-refusing-to-lockdown/ [Last accessed 16 April 2020]

Sanger, D et al. (2020) Before virus outbreak, a cascade of warnings went unheeded. New York Times 19 March. Available from: https://www.nytimes.com/2020/03/19/us/politics/trump-Coronavirus-outbreak.html [Last accessed 19 March 2020]

Schmidt, C (2020) The COVID-19 crisis and risk society in the second modernity. Japan Today, 24 March. Available from: https://japantoday.com/category/features/opinions/the-COVID-19-crisis-and-risk-society-in-the-second-modernity [Last accessed 20 April 2020]

Schnirring, L (2015) Study notes MERS, SARS virus shedding similarities. CIDRAP News, 13 November. Available from: http://www.cidrap.umn.edu/news-perspective/2015/11/study-notes-mers-sars-virus-shedding-similarities [Last accessed 24 March 2020]

Schwartz, P (2020) 4 Possible Pandemic Outcomes Every Company Needs to Consider, Salesforce Blog, 17 April. Available from: https://www.salesforce.com/blog/2020/04/four-possible-pandemic-outcomes.html [Last accessed 2 May 2020]

Schwartz, J and Yen, M (2016) Toward a collaborative model

of pandemic preparedness and response: Taiwan's changing approach to pandemics. Journal of Microbiology, Immunology and Infection, Volume 50, Issue 2, April 2017, Pages 125–132. Available from: https://doi.org/10.1016/j.jmii.2016.08.010 [Last accessed 15 April 2020]

Science Daily (2020) Researchers hope to improve future epidemic predictions, Science Daily, 6 April. Available from: https://www.sciencedaily.com/releases/2020/04/200406110719.htm [Last accessed 2 May 2020]

Scott, S and Duncan CJ (2001) Biology of Plagues: Evidence from Historical Populations. Cambridge, UK: Cambridge University Press.

Scutti, S (2017) How countries around the world try to encourage vaccination. CNN, 6 June. Available from: https://www.cnn.com/2017/06/06/health/vaccine-uptake-incentives/index.html [Last accessed 15 April 2020]

Segaard SB and Saglie J (2017) Education and Elderly Care in Denmark, Norway and Sweden: National Policies and Legal Frameworks for Private Providers. In: Sivesind K., Saglie J. (eds) Promoting Active Citizenship. Palgrave Macmillan, Cham. Available from: https://link.springer.com/chapter/10.1007/978-3-319-55381-8_3 [Last accessed 17 April 2020]

Sefton, T (2020) Norway and Sweden: Battling coronavirus in two different worlds. PRIO Blog, 30 March. Available from: https://blogs.prio.org/2020/03/norway-and-sweden-battling-Coronavirus-in-two-different-worlds/ [Last accessed 17 April 2020]

Shapiro, D (2020) Taiwan shows its mettle in coronavirus

crisis, while the WHO is MIA. (Blog.) Brookings Institution, 19 March. Available from: https://www.brookings.edu/blog/order-from-chaos/2020/03/19/taiwan-shows-its-mettle-in-Coronavirus-crisis-while-the-who-is-mia/ [Last accessed 15 April 2020]

Shapiro, W (2020) How America's newspapers covered up a pandemic., The New Republic, 31 March. Available from: https://newrepublic.com/article/157094/americas-newspapers-covered-pandemic [Last accessed 7 April 2020]

Siegel, Z (2018) Is the U.S. knee-deep in 'epidemics,' or is that just wishful thinking? New York Times, 8 August. Available from: https://www.nytimes.com/2018/08/14/magazine/epidemic-disaster-tragedy.html [Last accessed 15 April 2020]

Silverman H and Moon, S (2020) Crowds packed California beaches despite shelter in place order. CNN, 23 March. Available from: https://www.cnn.com/2020/03/23/us/california-stay-at-home-beach-goers/index.html [Last accessed 23 March 2020]

Soucheray, S (2020) Officials say most Americans not at risk of coronavirus. CIDRAP News, 28 January. Available from: https://www.cidrap.umn.edu/news-perspective/2020/01/officials-say-most-americans-not-risk-Coronavirus [Last accessed 15 April 2020]

SPARS Pandemic Scenario (2017) Available from: https://www.centerforhealthsecurity.org/our-work/Center-projects/completed-projects/spars-pandemic-scenario.html [Last accessed 20 April 2020]

Standish, R (2020) Will Putin be Russia's president for life?

Foreign Policy. Available from: https://foreignpolicy.com/2020/03/10/will-putin-be-russia-president-for-life-constitutional-changes/ [last accessed 7 April 2020]

Staresinic, C (2014) Lessons from a dark winter. PittMeD, U Pittsburgh. Available from: https://www.pittmed.health.pitt.edu/story/lessons-dark-winter [last accessed 20 April 2020]

Stein, RA (2011) Superspreaders in infectious diseases. International Journal of Infectious Diseases, Volume 15, e510–e513. Available from: https://www.sciencedirect.com/science/article/pii/S1201971211000245 [Last accessed 24 March 2020]

Stieg, C (2020) How this Canadian start-up spotted coronavirus before everyone else knew about it. CNBC Make It, 3 March. Available from: https://www.cnbc.com/2020/03/03/bluedot-used-artificial-intelligence-to-predict-Coronavirus-spread.html [Last accessed 24 March 2020]

Stracqualursi, V (2020) New York Times: HHS' pandemic simulation showed how US was ill prepared for coronavirus. CNN, 19 March. Available from: https://www.cnn.com/2020/03/19/politics/hhs-pandemic-simulation-crimson-contagion-report/index.html [Last accessed 20 April 2020]

Subbaraman, N (2020) Coronavirus tests: researchers chase new diagnostics to fight the pandemic. Nature, 23 March. Available from: https://www.nature.com/articles/d41586-020-00827-6 [Last accessed 16 April 2020]

Suk, JE et al. (2008) Mapping the future dynamics of disease transmission: Risk analysis in the United Kingdom Foresight Programme on the detection and identification of infectious diseases. Eurosurveillance, Volume 13, Issue 44, 30 October. Available from:
https://www.eurosurveillance.org/content/10.2807/ese.13.44.19021-en [Last accessed 7 April 2020]

Suk, JE and Semenza JC (2011) Future infectious disease threats to Europe. American Journal of Public Health, Volume 101, Issue 11, Pages 2068–2079, November. Available from: https://dx.doi.org/10.2105%2FAJPH.2011.300181
[Last accessed 7 April 2020]

Taleb, NN (2007) The Black Swan: The Impact of the Highly Improbable. New York: Random House.

Taleb, NN (2007) Fooled by Randomness: The Hidden Role of Chance in Life and in the Markets. New York: Random House.

Taylor, D (2020) The timeline of the coronavirus. New York Times, 19 March. Available from:
https://www.nytimes.com/article/Coronavirus-timeline.html [Last accessed 19 March 2020]

Taylor, P (2020) First study of Gilead's Remdesivir in COVID-19 reveals little. Pharmaphorum, 13 April. Available from: https://pharmaphorum.com/news/first-study-of-gileads-remdesivir-in-COVID-19-reveals-little/ [Last accessed 16 April 2020]

Taylor, M (2020) Exclusive: U.S. axed CDC expert job in China months before virus outbreak. Reuters, 22 March. Available from:
https://www.reuters.com/article/us-health-Coronavirus-

china-cdc-exclusiv/exclusive-u-s-axed-cdc-expert-job-in-china-months-before-virus-outbreak-idUSKBN21910S [Last accessed 8 April 2020]

Taylor DL and Kahawita TM and Cairncross S and Ensink JH (2015) The Impact of Water, Sanitation and Hygiene Interventions to Control Cholera: A Systematic Review. PLoS One. 2015;10(8):e0135676. Published 2015 Aug 18. Available from: 10.1371/journal.pone.0135676 [Last accessed 2 May 2020]

The Lancet (2018). Pandemic influenza: 100 years. Available from: https://info.thelancet.com/pandemic-flu-100 [Last accessed 5 April 2020]

Tercatin, R and Jean, C (2000) Coronavirus: Israeli researchers develop innovative diagnostic method. The Jerusalem Post, 1 April. Available from: https://www.jpost.com/health-science/israeli-researchers-develop-innovative-diagnostic-method-for-Coronavirus-621617 [Last accessed 16 April 2020]

Thai PBS (2020) Thailand facing coronavirus from Italy which may be more virulent than the Asian virus. Thai PBS World, 23 March. Available from: https://www.thaipbsworld.com/thailand-facing-Coronavirus-from-italy-which-may-be-more-virulent-than-the-asian-virus/ [Last accessed 24 March 2020]

Tisoncik JR, Korth MJ, Simmons CP, Farrar J, Martin TR, Katze MG (2012) Into the eye of the cytokine storm. Microbiol Mol Biol Rev. 2012;76(1):16-32. Available from: doi:10.1128/MMBR.05015-11 [Last accessed 3 May 2020]

Togoh, I (2020) Singapore, praised for its initial coronavirus response, closes schools and offices to prevent second wave of infections. Forbes, 3 April. Available from: https://www.forbes.com/sites/isabeltogoh/2020/04/03/singapore-praised-for-its-initial-Coronavirus-response-closes-schools-and-offices-to-prevent-second-wave-of-infections/#37a27dc473f0 [Last accessed 16 April 2020]

Tolan et al. (2020) Rural hospitals are facing financial ruin and furloughing staff during the coronavirus pandemic. CNN, 21 April. Available from: https://www.cnn.com/2020/04/21/us/coronavirus-rural-hospitals-invs/index.html [Last accessed 21 April 2020]

Undheim, TA (2020) Disruption Games. Texas: Atmosphere Press.

Undheim, TA (2008) Leadership From Below. Morrisville, North Carolina: Lulu Press.

University of Michigan Library Research Guides Community Health Special Topic: Novel Coronavirus (COVID-19). Available from: https://guides.lib.umich.edu/n456 [Last accessed 16 April 2020]

van Elsland, SL and O'Hare, R (2020) COVID-19: Imperial researchers model likely impact of public health measures. Imperial College London, 17 March. Available from: https://www.imperial.ac.uk/news/196234/COVID-19-imperial-researchers-model-likely-impact/ [Last accessed 23 March 2020]

Zalman, A (2020) Imagination: Powering post-COVID pandemic planning. 13 April. Available from: https://www.theglobalist.com/Coronavirus-pandemic-planning-risk-management-innovation-imagination-future-strategy/ [Last accessed 15 April 2020]

Vanderklippe, N (2020) Violence erupts in China as people try to leave coronavirus-stricken Hubei. The Globe and Mail, 27 March. Available from: https://www.theglobeandmail.com/world/article-violence-erupts-in-china-as-people-try-to-leave-Coronavirus-stricken/ [Last accessed 28 March 2020]

Van Buul, Laura W. et al. (2020) Antibiotic Stewardship in European Nursing Homes: Experiences From the Netherlands, Norway, Poland, and Sweden. Journal of the American Medical Directors Association, Volume 21, Issue 1, 34 - 40. Available from: https://doi.org/10.1016/j.jamda.2019.10.005 [Last accessed 2 May 2020]

Wee, RY (2019) The largest cities in China. WorldAtlas, 9 July. Available from: https://www.worldatlas.com/articles/20-biggest-cities-in-china.html [Last accessed 28 March 2020]

Wei, D et al (2020) China pushes factories to reopen, risking renewed virus spread. Bloomberg News, 23 February. Available from: https://www.bloomberg.com/news/articles/2020-02-23/china-is-pushing-factories-to-resume-even-as-death-toll-rises [Last accessed 28 March 2020]

WHO (2005) Pandemic influenza preparedness planning: Report on the second joint WHO/European Commission workshop, 24-26 October 2005. Available from: https://ec.europa.eu/health/ph_threats/com/Influenza/second_workshop.pdf [Last accessed 15 April 2020]

WHO (2020) Naming the coronavirus disease (COVID-19) and

the virus that causes it. Available from: https://www.who.int/emergencies/diseases/novel-Coronavirus-2019/technical-guidance/naming-the-Coronavirus-disease-(covid-2019)-and-the-virus-that-causes-it [Last accessed 19 April 2020]

WHO R&D blueprint (2020) Public statement for collaboration on COVID-19 vaccine development. 13 April. Available from: https://www.who.int/news-room/detail/13-04-2020-public-statement-for-collaboration-on-COVID-19-vaccine-development [Last accessed 15 April 2020]

WHO (2020) WHO Director-General's opening remarks at the media briefing on COVID-19. 3 March. Available from: https://www.who.int/dg/speeches/detail/who-director-general-s-opening-remarks-at-the-media-briefing-on-COVID-19---3-march-2020 [Last accessed 17 April 2020]

Wollan, M (2018) How to survive a flue pandemic. New York Times, 28 November. Available from: https://www.nytimes.com/2018/11/28/magazine/how-to-survive-a-flu-pandemic.html [Last accessed 15 April 2020]

World Justice Project (2020) World Justice Project Rule of Law Index 2020. Available from: https://worldjusticeproject.org/ [Last accessed 15 April 2020]

World Shipping Council (2020) Top 50 world container ports. Available from: http://www.worldshipping.org/about-the-industry/global-trade/top-50-world-container-ports [Last accessed 28 March 2020]

Williamson, E and Hussey K (2020) Party zero: How a soirée in Connecticut became a coronavirus ‘super spreader.’ Chicago Tribune, 23 March. Available from:

https://www.chicagotribune.com/Coronavirus/ct-nw-nyt-Coronavirus-connecticut-super-spreader-20200323-akznc44v4zhhzpajkmb7w6kftq-story.html [Last accessed 24 March 2020]

Wu, H and Zhang, L (2020) China's Shenzhen says all arrivals must be tested for coronavirus. Reuters, 23 March. Available from: https://www.reuters.com/article/us-health-Coronavirus-china-shenzhen/chinas-shenzhen-says-all-arrivals-must-be-tested-for-Coronavirus-idUSKBN21B0AY [Last accessed 28 March 2020]

Wyatt, T (2020) Coronavirus: More than 100,000 defy lockdown and gather for funeral in Bangladesh. The Independent, 20 April. Available from: https://www.independent.co.uk/news/world/asia/coronavirus-lockdown-bangladesh-funeral-social-distancing-gathering-a9474596.html [Last accessed 21 April 2020]

Zhu, A (2020) Supporting our global health workers, TikTok. Available from: https://newsroom.tiktok.com/en-us/supporting-our-global-health-workers/ [Last accessed 2 May 2020]

APPENDIX

A. Scenario thinking
B. Forces of disruption
C. Pandemic risk in megacities
D. Innovation

A. Scenario thinking

Scenario thinking is an established method in future studies and industry based on charting out "possible futures" in order to create the possibility of positive change instead of inertia when faced with a challenge because of impending change(s). It emerged because traditional expert based foresight proved quite difficult and because one-dimensional predictions failed again and again. Ogilvy and Schwartz (2004) provide a quick guide to crafting scenarios. The scenarios themselves are narratives and often have an internal deductive matrix at heart with a limited number of dimensions being exposed for effect. Common dimensions expose economics, politics, technology, and social perception. The key is to decide about the critical uncertainties that will impact the decisions the target audience will need to make.

Plotlines can be based on evolutionary change, co-evolution, cyclical change, generations, or other types of transitions. There is usually a wild card scenario, or wild card events (discontinuities) within each scenario.

Scenarios are usually prepared by a group, in order to get the diversity of thinking, but often also to get additional buy-in. Scenarios are then typically run as tabletop exercises where the scenarios are played out with some degree of live action. Such tabletop exercises can last less than a day or up to a week or could also extend over several weeks and months if different groups are involved.

Regardless of the content of the scenarios, to get the

desired effect of a mentality change, a big aim is to communicate awareness around the scenario exercise reflections and findings to a larger group.

B. Forces of disruption

The COVID-19 pandemic has already exposed fault lines that cut across all axis of our society. For a few years now, I have been leaning on my *forces of disruption model* to understand such changes. *Forces of disruption* is a strategic framework in the ilk of others developed initially for strategic management of business challenges but slightly broader in its scope.

Unlike other such frameworks that purely focus on what's best for business, my forces of disruption framework is particularly suited for the considerably more complex task of analyzing the effects of a pandemic. The reason is that it is simple enough to discuss on a broad basis yet encompasses the key elements that have either been immediately disrupted or which potentially could unlock solutions, notably science and technology, policy and regulation, business models and startups, and social dynamics and consumers.

In the following, I'll attempt an extremely brief overview of the four-forces framework. A full framework analysis will be provided in my next book, coming out in early 2021.

First, the *science and technology* fields hold many of the answers that society is looking for in the current pandemic. Scientific progress around vaccines holds the ultimate answer to any sweeping pandemic. Technology that enables work from home has been found to be essential during social distancing. But how to understand the way these domains need to interact with the rest of society? How deep insight does the average policy maker, corporate executive, or citizen need to have in order to efficiently make use of the knowledge emerging from science and technology?

Second, *policy and regulation* are becoming increasingly

crucial in getting a handle on the pandemic. Initially, we call on governments to set the parameters for the public health response. We expect economic rescue measures when significant market disruptions force businesses or entire market segments (e.g., the travel industry) to close down. We expect there to be regulatory safeguards on our health authorities, even as we hope that vaccines can be sped up to meet the need in time.

Ultimately, we also need some sort of global management of the crisis at a political level. A pandemic is most definitely a time when pulling together to agree common rules has its benefits although there are drawbacks. Conversely, as a new normalcy inevitably is called for, what will the new rules of engagement be? This is a negotiated process, where all sectors of society contribute, but ultimately, where policy plays a strong role.

Third, *business models and startups* are crucial aspects of the pandemic response as well as impact. The pandemic has made some business models (e.g., travel and tourism related) near impossible for some time to come. Others (e.g., teleconferencing software, medical equipment manufacturing) are thriving.

Over the past decade, we have looked to startups to solve many of our innovation challenges. The pandemic has exposed the hidden truth about innovation, which is that it cannot simply happen upon demand. This is not to say that innovation will not emerge, simply that it, almost by definition, is not there at the exact moment when you need it (otherwise it would not be considered innovative).

Few startups were ready and able to make an enormous difference when the pandemic hit. Perhaps this was surprising to some? It should not be. Startups are vehicles of innovation they are not magic wands that can be waved and instantly will produce results. Besides, the scale and impact of a pandemic means that startups can only work in consort with larger organizations, typically corporate behemoths, that act as enablers and scale-up partners.

Fourth, *social dynamics and consumers* have surfaced as the ultimate arbiters of any pandemic response, both in terms of public health and the economy and market-related challenges. Businesses could provide any products they want, but consumers need to feel the urge to buy them. Governments could try to suggest social distancing but, ultimately, practicing such rules requires social dynamics that are conducive to following such norms, and encouraging peers to do the same. No amount of policing, and likely not even the military, could keep a population that did not agree with a quarantine at bay. It would lead to protest, revolt and, ultimately, revolution.

Let's try to structure an initial visualization of the key factors at play. We will only nominate the key vocabulary used to invoke a much larger set of actors, factors, issues, and objects at play.

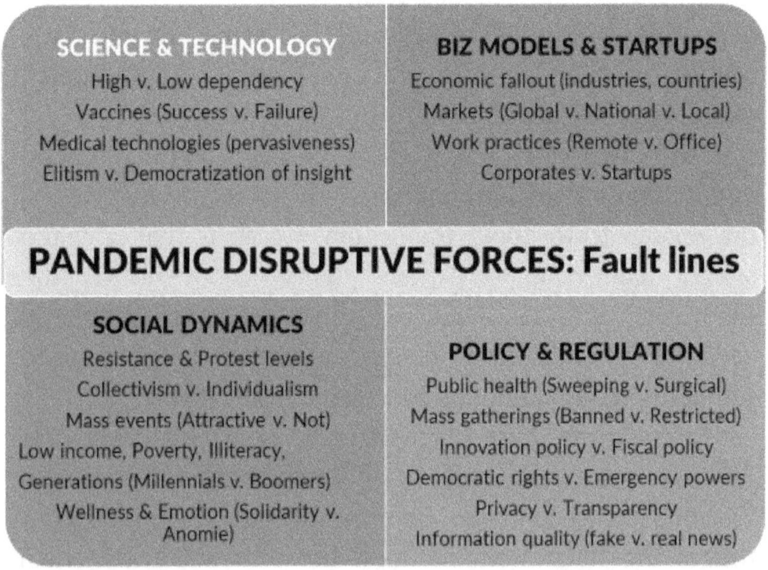
SCIENCE & TECHNOLOGY
High v. Low dependency
Vaccines (Success v. Failure)
Medical technologies (pervasiveness)
Elitism v. Democratization of insight
BIZ MODELS & STARTUPS
Economic fallout (industries, countries)
Markets (Global v. National v. Local)
Work practices (Remote v. Office)
Corporates v. Startups
PANDEMIC DISRUPTIVE FORCES: Fault lines
SOCIAL DYNAMICS
Resistance & Protest levels
Collectivism v. Individualism
Mass events (Attractive v. Not)
Low income, Poverty, Illiteracy,
Generations (Millennials v. Boomers)
Wellness & Emotion (Solidarity v. Anomie)
POLICY & REGULATION
Public health (Sweeping v. Surgical)
Mass gatherings (Banned v. Restricted)
Innovation policy v. Fiscal policy
Democratic rights v. Emergency powers
Privacy v. Transparency
Information quality (fake v. real news)

App Figure 1. Four forces of disruption during a pandemic

Science & Technology

Vaccines, Drugs, Experimental treatments, Telehealth, Medical technology, Ventilators, N95 masks, surgical masks, medical gowns, testing kits, AI, epidemiology, public health, rXiv

Policy & Regulation

Rescue packages, Loans, Quantitative Easting (QE), Quarantines, Stay-at-home orders, Military, Stock markets

Business Models & Startups

Travel industry, Innovation, Small business, Startups, Manufacturing industry, Grocery industry, Airline industry

Social Dynamics & Consumers

Culture, Consumption patterns, Disposable income, Resistance, Protest, Individualism, Collectivism, Illiteracy, Political affiliation, Generational perspective

Did you find that any crucial factors are missing from this picture? If so, that is not surprising. The picture of this pandemic is rapidly emerging. You can contribute to the discussion by participating online (http://www.pandemic-aftermath.com).

The role of open-access repository of electronic preprints (known as *e-prints*) becomes extremely important during a pandemic, when the urgency of sharing information is paramount. Studies that otherwise may not have been issued so fast (and certainly not so widely read) have been pouring out of academia and industry labs and into places like MedRxiv, a pre-print server founded by Yale University, the medical journal *BMJ* and Cold Spring Harbor Laboratory in New York.

Once the salient factors that may go into a discussion of the forces of disruption surrounding the pandemic have been brainstormed and selected, it is time to build the conceptual, and ideally empirical model that will serve to carry out the full analysis. There are two ways of doing so, both of which we explore in Chapters 3 and 4. In the conceptual version, it would suffice to develop simple scoring vectors for each factor, the simplest being 0 and 1, adding a neutral score would make it slightly more predictive, and adding scores between -2 and +2 might be still feasible for quick analysis.

The real issue here is that individuals might need to score these largely based on hunches. The difference between hunches (educated guesses) and real data is not always strikingly different, although sometimes it is, and in this case, it could mean affecting life and death issues.

If we deploy an empirical version of the four forces framework, we would need to only use dimensions for which we have reliable data. The problem with this is that it reduces the amounts of dimensions we would be allowed to include, which may (or may not) drastically reduce the predictive strength of the model, although sometimes missing figures can be approximated or simulated.

However, imagine a scenario where you don't have reliable figures for the number of nurses and you choose to exclude that variable (which is highly predictive on pandemic response success), even though you have a proxy, which would be the number of doctors. The two are not the same, but they correlate.

Pandemic causal effects and loops?

A simple strategic framework is better at surfacing the factors we need to take into account, than it is at delineating causal effects, chains and loops. All dashboards suffer from this predicament, too, by the way. It is far easier to list a myriad of correlating (or not correlating) datasets than it is to figure out which of them predicts the other one.

The truth about social phenomena is that they are typically

not just causal in a very simplistic way. Usually, regardless what spurred the initial push, once the process gets going, a few factors are mutually reinforcing. As we explore in Chapter 3, Yale social scientist Nicholas Christakis is the authority on that aspect. You may know him for his book *Connected: The Surprising Power of Our Social Networks and How They Shape Our Lives* (2011).

The four forces of pandemic disruption

I deploy the four-forces framework throughout the book. Suffice to say that any kind of framework, by design, is a simplification. It models reality by creating ideal typical dimensions that cultivate only the main differences and fault lines. The justification for this approach is that without creating a strawman picture of the world, it becomes near impossible to reason logically around it. Without such a picture, ideally one that resembles the way human actors also see the problem (but in a more structured way), we will simply talk past each other.

At this point, epidemiologists might object and claim they already have all the answers. After all, isn't disease modeling their profession? To this, I will say that nothing about this current crisis is confined to disease modeling. All previous models I've seen have drastically underestimated the factors that go beyond public health and into especially the financial and social dynamics vectors. This is not to say that those models cannot be updated with a revised, more sophisticated picture of the systemic effects given that this crisis truly is global in nature (which makes it somewhat akin to the doomsday scenarios that previous to this only was reserved for Hollywood movies and science fiction books).

Another objection might come from the camp of AI dashboard startups (or larger analytical companies) that claim we already have all this data. Yes, there are literally dozens (now hundreds) of dashboards that bring in various variables and present a picture to the world about the emerging coronavirus implications.

However, each of them suffers from the same problem: they were never intended to scale up to the later stages of an outbreak. Typically, they were designed as early-response systems. They are good at picking up early spikes, not at monitoring a situation where there is a tremendous amount of noise. The quantitative models we have for reducing that noise are far less developed, although I'm sure that they will emerge. That emergence will be part of global society's resilience next time around or even for curbing the second, third, and fourth waves of the current outbreak, and the thousands of micro and meso waves that may or may not turn out to be signals of superspreader events, as the disease washes through the world.

Next, I consider the issue of superspreaders. However, we do not just consider this from an individual perspective, but rather from the perspective of systems that enable superspreading to take place, namely the extreme urbanization that gives birth to megacities.

C. Pandemic outcome in megacities

Over 4 billion people live in cities today. Urbanization characterized the widespread industrial revolution which took place from the mid-19th century until the early-20th century in Britain, continental Europe, North America, and Japan. However, the vast majority of people moved to cities after 1950s post-war economic surge, according to the World Economic Forum. In 2000, there were 371 cities of a million or more people in the world; by 2018, that number was 548.

A megacity is defined by the United Nations as a city that has a population of 10 million or more people. The number of such cities vary by whom you ask, but it is somewhere between 30 and 47 and growing (depending how you count metropolitan sprawl and how recently there was a census). China is in a unique position because of having more than 15 megacities (if you count metro areas), which in pandemic terms would theoretically become one massive pressure cooker, was it not for the fact that their control measures also are draconic.

The emerging importance of cities in China

Before the coronavirus outbreak, few people in the world paid much attention to Wuhan, a megacity in Hubei, a landlocked province in Central China. The province itself is also known for the Three Gorges, a popular destination for Yangtze River cruises and home to the massive Three Gorges Dam. Well, we do pay more attention now. A whopping 9,000 cases of coronavirus in the US could stem from Wuhan alone, according to one study that appeared on the medical preprint publication MedRxiv on March 8, using simulations of transmissibility as well as the number of air travelers between Wuhan and the US over the past few months.

The initial epicenter of the pandemic outbreak has grown rapidly into a megacity over the past decade with a population of just above 11 million, the ninth most populous Chinese city. Chinese authorities famously built two dedicated hospitals in Wuhan in just over 1 week and all told, built 16 such facilities across the city under siege from coronavirus, housing between 500 and 1,000 patients each, receiving a total of 13,000 coronavirus patients. After 2 months of near total isolation, quarantines were lifted in the last week of March 2020, even as more than 2,500 people are still in hospital. Schools have been closed since mid-January and only about 10% of the workforce—healthcare workers, police, and other essential government staff—have been at work.

But a *Lancet* study (Prem, 2020) warns that lifting quarantines too soon could lead to a second serious spike for Wuhan in August. Also, worryingly, 5–10% of patients pronounced "recovered" have tested positive again, prompting the question whether they were false positives due to a faulty test (either the first or the second time or both) or actually have contracted the disease again, which would spell trouble. In fact, one expert claims the nucleic acid tests used in China may only be accurate 30–50% of the time. This also raises new questions about asymptomatic carriers.

A deep distrust has taken root across China toward people from Hubei, according to *The Globe and Mail*, with people being refused entry to hotels and their homes, even being banned from entering Beijing, as large numbers of provincial residence attempt to move around again. As of March 27, the province counts nearly 68,000 confirmed cases with 3,174 deaths from COVID-19 since late last year.

The fact that Wuhan was on a rapidly accelerating urban population growth trajectory is a fact we should pay close attention to. If that factor has any predictive ability in terms of foreshadowing pandemic risk or other challenges, and history tells us it has, we should perhaps monitor other such rapidly urbanizing megacities around the world.

Arguably, in the early stages of an outbreak, the population size doesn't matter. As we have seen, one infected person could infect a few people whether that person lives in a metropolitan area of 100,000 or one of 10 million. Where we need to pay attention is to the stage of potential exponential growth that happens after that. The potential for becoming incubators of disease is much larger in a megacity, but a few factors likely explain how large the risk is. The risk is also likely to vary quite a bit between cities, depending on their situation. We will look at which factors are likely to influence the severity. But let's first consider China itself.

How many cities in China could the average person remember? I'd say most people could readily mention Beijing and Shanghai, if they were in industry, they would add Shenzhen. However, six out of the world' 10 largest container ports are in China, so the country has an outsized importance when it comes to the inner workings of the global manufacturing supply chain. In fact, among the top 15 ports, apart from Dubai (10th), Rotterdam (11th) and Antwerp (13th), they are all in Asia.

Let's quickly summarize a few brief cultural facts about the emerging megacities in China and their coronavirus response, where available.

Southern China's manufacturing sector

Shenzhen, in southeastern China, is a modern metropolis linking Hong Kong to China's mainland. It is known for technology, financial services, logistics, particularly as a global manufacturing center for mobile technology, DNA sequencing, metamaterials, and 3D displays. In fact, it is arguably the world's hardware capital. In Shenzhen, two large hospitals were built only for patients with the coronavirus infection. As of March 23, 2020, all arrivals at Shenzhen's port of entry must be tested for coronavirus, according to Reuters, which one has to assume is an enormous effort on their part. Research published in the journal *Critical Care* recommends to all other Chinese cities that the response has to be citywide, not per hospital, since each hospital is likely to get overwhelmed.

Guangzhou is well known for those who do business with China and for its tricky pronunciation. Guangdong province, where Guangzhou is located, by February 2020 had the second highest number of cases in mainland China after Hebei, the province where Wuhan is located. Despite that, the province lowers coronavirus threat level already on February 24, 2020, in an attempt to restart the Chinese economy, as the number of cases slow, despite infection still spreading. Manufacturers are required to carry out a checklist to ensure facilities are clean and staff are healthy. Plants can then restart.

However, obtaining enough workers is another hurdle,

given the travel restrictions in other provinces and adjacent countries with migrant workers, although one thing seems to be working in the region's favor. The trade war with the US already has reduced the number of factory workers enough that they are less crowded than before that first crisis hit, which may also enable them to practice some degree of social distancing.

Other Chinese megacities

Chongqing, in southern China, is less well known, although being one of the most polluted, it has gotten some press lately.

Hangzhou, another megacity, is best known as the headquarters of Internet industry enterprises such as Alibaba.

Chengdu, a massive Asian tourist destination, is known by animal lovers for its panda breeding conservation center where visitors can view endangered giant pandas in a natural habitat.

Tianjin has the leading port in north China and acts as a commercial gateway to Beijing, which lies at 150 km (93 mi.) inland.

Xi'an is one of the oldest cities in China, one of the Four Great Ancient Capitals, China's second tourist destination after Beijing. It is most famous for its Terracotta Warriors, an international symbol of China's history.

Jinan is a city in eastern China famous for its natural springs.

Nanjing is another of the Four Great Ancient Capitals of China, in fact it was the capital of in total six Chinese imperial dynasties and is hence the home of many human made cultural monuments.

Shenyang in northeast China is famous for its Shaolin monastery temple and agile Buddhist monks so revered by all martial arts aficionados (including my 11-year-old son) and is, fittingly, also the home of the Chinese defense industry in modern times.

Harbin, the northernmost megacity in China, is an important industrial city. With its famously harsh winters, famous ice and snow sculptures and exotic architecture, it has a Russian influence. While it is only somewhat near Russia (at some 2360 km distance), Harbin rose to fame for its proximity to the Trans-Siberian Railway connected through the Trans-Manchurian Railway. Given Harbin's open arms to pro-Tsarist traders and bureaucrats, in 1917, as White Russians escaped the newly formed Soviet Union, Harbin's population exceeded 100,000. Over 40,000 of them were ethnic Russians. Some would say modern Harbin was "built by Russians," although today, the city is practically devoid of Russians. The reason is the Japanese invasion during the Second Sino-Japanese War (1937–1945). In fact, even before that, following the USSR's sale of the Chinese Eastern Railway to Japan in 1935, most Russians left Harbin.

Shantou is known for its tea customs, snacks, seafood, and opera, and was one of the treaty ports established for Western trade and contact. Suzhou, a city just northwest of Shanghai, is known for its canals, bridges and 60 classical gardens, collectively a UNESCO World Heritage Site.

Wenzhou, a Chinese and global manufacturing and commerce hotbed, is famous across China for its savvy businesspeople, who have moved across the world in vast numbers in search of new moneymaking opportunities. There are an estimated 1.6 million people from Wenzhou running businesses in other parts of China, and another 600,000 overseas. One of the largest magnets for the city's diaspora has been Wuhan.

Qingdao, a port city bordering the Yellow Sea, is known for its beer, spelled Tsingtao, the namesake brewery founded here by Germans in 1903 and China's most-selling export beer. The city was under German rule from 1898 to 1914.

Dongguan—a test of China's coronavirus 2.0 resilience

Dongguan, an industrial city in China's Pearl River Delta, although also the home of Cantonese opera, is often called "the world's factory," although the home of 'Made in China' is now largely reinventing itself as a robotics base. However, according to The Guardian, some 75% of its 8.34 million population are migrant workers who return home during the festive period, leaving the city nearly deserted. *The issue of migrant workers is bound to be a tremendously important global issue to sort out in the time to come.* Will migrant worker travel patterns change? Will host cities be able to protect them, given their infamously poor living quarters?

Additionally, Dongguan also has earned the nickname "the Eastern Amsterdam," given that, according to the *Telegraph*, some 10% of the city's more than 8 million population is said to work in the world's oldest profession. The figure is impossible to verify given that prostitution is illegal in China. However, given what we know about the role of the world's oldest profession in transmitting another infectious disease, HIV/AIDS, this city is one to watch.

The picture is mixed, as Dongguan also was recognized by the United Nations Environment Programme as an "international garden city," is widely considered China's "national basketball city" and shares the largest golf facility in the world with neighboring Shenzhen. In fact, the distance between Shenzhen and Dongguan is a mere 62 kilometers. Furthermore, Dongguan is only 50 kilometers from Guangdong's capital city, Guangzhou, it also has a direct high-speed railway to Hong Kong and Macau. There is lots of potential to spread disease between these major population centers which together host near 40 million people.

Quanzhou, on China's southeast coast, historically a primary destination for Arab, Persian, Indian, and southeast Asian ships carrying merchants, is famous for international trade in porcelain and silk. Most notably in recent memory, their five-story coronavirus quarantine hotel, formerly the Xinjia Hotel, collapsed on March 8, 2020, leaving 10 dead and 23 missing.

China's experience with coronavirus will chart the world's experience

The point? Right now, the cultural and economic significance of each of these cities is just about what the informed outsider knows about these cities. The reason is that few foreign journalists are walking about in China at the moment, and likely will for a long time to come. The question is if we will ever have an early warning system for what is brewing in any of these cities, if anything happens again.

However, from the scant evidence we do have, each city responded to the outbreak in its own way, importantly, though, they each seemed to have a citywide response, not hospital by hospital. At this point, we know very little about the relative importance and success rate of central versus local measures of containment.

China is rapidly urbanizing, which is something the whole world should (and will) pay attention to in the time to come, not only for its economic importance but also for its potentially disruptive role in the evolution of a whole host of other phenomena, including infectious diseases. China, in fact, has a plethora of cities that could remain at high risk for pandemics decades to come. We should, perhaps consider ourselves lucky that China still (a) has a strongly controlled state that is well equipped to implement mandatory quarantines, something that is strikingly lacking in many other countries that house megacities; and (b) has a well-developed medical system. Throughout 2020, the importance of these two factors alone became more and more apparent. Should China open up to democracy even further, these megacities would be increasingly out of government stronghold and the risk of infectious diseases getting out of control would be more similar to the West (perhaps higher).

London's history with outbreaks

According to *National Review*, London became the first city to break 2 million people in the early 1800s, and it suffered terrible outbreaks of cholera in the following decades. This led to major sanitation initiatives in the city to improve water quality (Taylor et al., 2015) as well as a slight decentralization effort by the UK government, which is likely why the UK now has at least five major cities. Are we now seeing another urban threat with coronavirus which will lead to similar sweeping changes? Perhaps it's too soon to tell, but let's look at the risk factors.

Pandemic risk in megacities and beyond

Before we attempt to score countries, we will consider cities, focusing on capitals or hubs as proxies for the evolution across the country and in other cities. We start by adding the world's top-10 megacities (i.e., Guangzhou-Foshan, China; Tokyo-Yokohama, Japan; Shanghai, China; Jakarta, Indonesia; Delhi, India; Manila, Philippines; Mumbai, India; Seoul-Incheon, South Korea; Mexico City, Mexico; New York, USA) to the mix. However, there are a full 47 cities with more than 10 million inhabitants in the world. Let's for now add the largest 30 and see where that gets us.

Pandemic outcome for top cities around the world

North America: USA (New York, Los Angeles, Chicago)

South America: Brazil (Rio Di Janeiro, São Paulo), Mexico (Mexico City), Venezuela (Caracas), Buenos Aires (Argentina), Peru (Lima)

Africa: Nigeria (Lagos), Ethiopia (Addis), Egypt (Kairo), Democratic Republic of the Congo (Kinshasa), South Africa (Cape Town), Tanzania (Dar es Salaam), Cairo (Egypt), Angola (Luanda)

Asia: China (Beijing, Shanghai, Guangzhou, Chongqing, Hangzhou, Wuhan, Chengdu, Tianjin, Xi'an, Jinan, Shenzhen, Nanjing, Shenyang, Harbin, Shantou, Suzhou, Wenzhou, Qingdao, Dongguan, Quanzhou), India (Delhi, Mumbai, Kolkata, Chennai, Bangalore), Japan (Tokyo, Osaka), Indonesia (Jakarta), Philippines (Manila), South Korea (Seoul), Pakistan (Islamabad, Karachi), Iran (Tehran), Iraq (Bagdad), Dhaka (Bangladesh)

Europe: France (Paris), Germany (Berlin, Rhine-Ruhr), UK (London), Italy (Milan, Rome), Spain (Madrid), Norway (Oslo), Moscow (Russia), Istanbul (Turkey)

Next, we will rank locations based on the likely severity of the pandemic. This could be a systematic adding of factors from our four-forces framework, but for now, we will simply focus on a schematic estimation. We will also introduce a neutral position, neither (-) nor (+) in pandemic estimation terms. Obviously, short of solid data, the rankings here are so far slightly arbitrary, yet still indicative.

For simplicity each factor will have a value of 1, so that a major economic hub is -1, for instance, given that it adds to the stakes in terms of the degree of mobility its citizens have—increasing their chances of contagion (measured by how much of a transportation hub they are). The exception is the top ten megacities, which we will give -2 on our scale, given their enormous, almost insurmountable challenge should they have a significant outbreak. Pandemic response also has a potential for a +/-2.

We will also grade the national or city governments' response to the pandemic (mostly on speed in terms of implementing public health efforts to counter the pandemic). Failed states will get -2 on transparency and innovation and (likely) on pandemic response/readiness. If the city is only a national transportation hub, I'll give them a neutral score regardless of the city's size, given the outsized importance of imported infections in the COVID-19 transmission patterns so far.

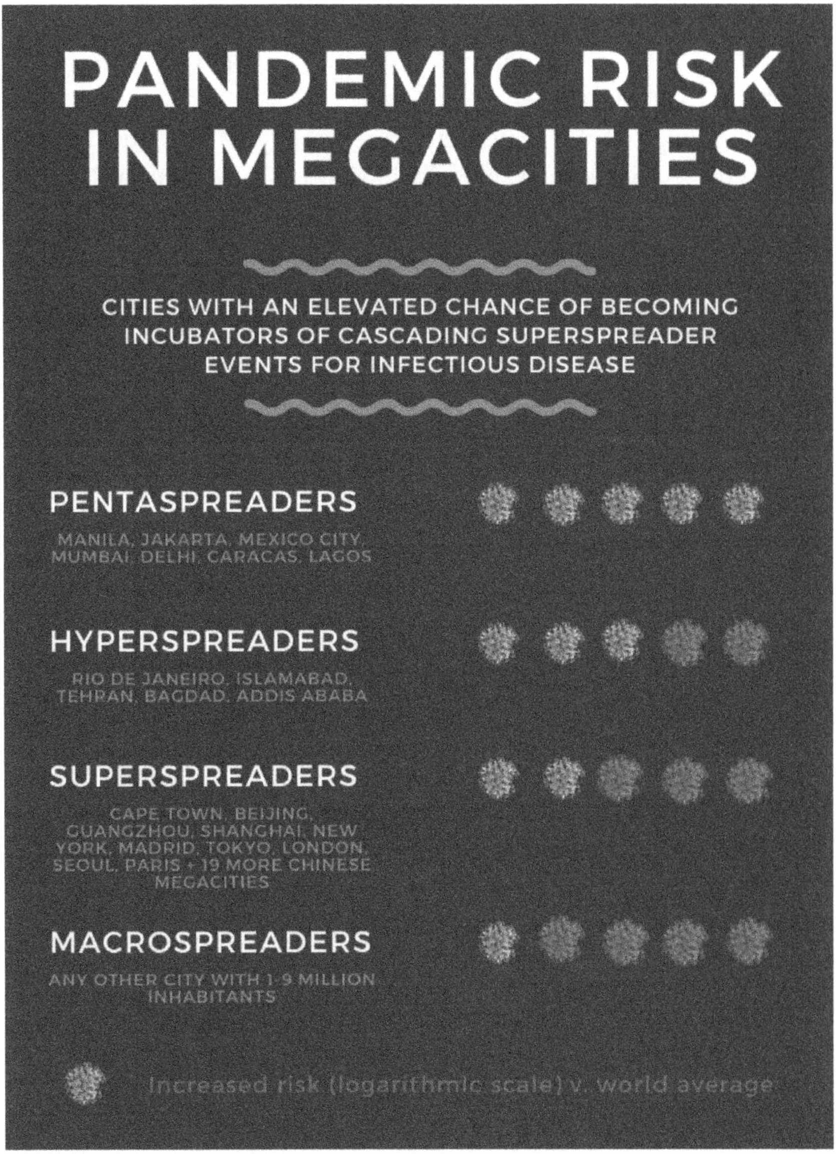
PANDEMIC RISK IN MEGACITIES
CITIES WITH AN ELEVATED CHANCE OF BECOMING INCUBATORS OF CASCADING SUPERSPREADER EVENTS FOR INFECTIOUS DISEASE
PENTASPREADERS
MANILA, JAKARTA, MEXICO CITY, MUMBAI, DELHI, CARACAS, LAGOS
HYPERSPREADERS
RIO DE JANEIRO, ISLAMABAD, TEHRAN, BAGDAD, ADDIS ABABA
SUPERSPREADERS
CAPE TOWN, BEIJING, GUANGZHOU, SHANGHAI, NEW YORK, MADRID, TOKYO, LONDON, SEOUL, PARIS + 19 MORE CHINESE MEGACITIES
MACROSPREADERS
ANY OTHER CITY WITH 1-9 MILLION INHABITANTS
Increased risk (logarithmic scale) v. world average

Pandemic risk in megacities–back-of-the-envelope scores

1. Manila: (-2) Megacity, major population hub, (-1) Health system, (-1) Transportation hub. (-1) Innovation, (-1) Transparency, (-2) Pandemic readiness/response, (-1) Air quality. Total score: -9
2. Jakarta: (-2) Megacity, major population hub, (-1) Health system, (-1) Transportation hub, (-1) Innovation, (-1) Transparency, (-1) Pandemic readiness/response, (-1) Air quality. Total score: -8
3. Mexico City: (-2) Megacity, major population hub, (-1) Health system, (-1) Transportation hub, (-1) Innovation, (-1) Transparency, (-1) Pandemic readiness/response, (-1) Air quality. Total score: -8
4. Mumbai: (-2) Megacity, major population hub, (-1) Health system, (-1) Transportation hub, (-1) Innovation, (-1) Transparency, (-1) Pandemic readiness/response, (-1) Air quality. Total score: -8
5. Delhi: (-2) Megacity, major population hub, (-1) Health system, (-2) Transportation hub, (-1) Innovation, (-1) Transparency, (-1) Pandemic readiness/response, (-1) Air quality. Total score: -9
6. Caracas: (-1) Megacity, major population hub, (-1) Health system, (neutral) Transportation hub, (-1) Innovation, (-1) Transparency, (-2) Pandemic readiness/response, (-1) Air quality. Total score: -7
7. Kolkata: (-2) Megacity, major population hub, (-1) Health system, (-1) Transportation hub, (-1) Innovation, (-1) Transparency, (-1) Pandemic readiness/response, (-1) Air quality. Total score: -8
8. Chennai: (-2) Megacity, major population hub, (-1) Health system, (-1) Transportation hub, (-1) Innovation, (-1) Transparency, (-1) Pandemic readiness/response, (-1) Air quality. Total score: -8
9. Lagos: (-1) Megacity, major population hub, (-1)

Health system, (-1) Transportation hub, (-1) Innovation, (-1) Transparency, (-1) Pandemic readiness/response, (-1) Air quality. Total score: -7

10. São Paulo: (-1) Megacity, major population hub, (-1) Health system, (-1) Transportation hub, (-1) Innovation, (-1) Transparency, (-1) Pandemic response, (-1) Air quality. Total score: -7

11. Lima: (-1) Megacity (barely), major population hub, (-1) Health system, (-1) Transportation hub, (-1) Innovation, (-1) Transparency, (-1) Pandemic readiness/response, (-1) Air quality. Total score: -7

12. Kinshasa: (-1) Megacity, major population hub, (-1) Health system, (-1) Transportation hub, (-1) Innovation, (-1) Transparency, (-1) Pandemic readiness/response, (-1) Air quality. Total score: -7

13. Luanda: (-1) Megacity, major population hub, (-1) Health system, (-1) Transportation hub, (-1) Innovation, (-1) Transparency, (-1) Pandemic readiness/response, (-1) Air quality. Total score: -7

14. Rio de Janeiro: (-1) Major population hub, (-1) Health system, (neutral) Transportation hub, (-1) Innovation, (-1) Transparency, (-1) Pandemic response, (-1) Air quality. Total score: -6

15. Islamabad: (-1) Major population hub, (-1) Health system, (neutral) Transportation hub, (-1) Innovation, (-1) Transparency, (-1) Pandemic response, (-1) Air quality. Total score: -6

16. Tehran: (-1) Major population hub, (-1) Health system, (neutral) Transportation hub, (-1) Innovation, (-1) Transparency, (-1) Pandemic readiness/response, (-1) Air quality. Total score: -6

17. Bagdad: (-1) Major population hub, (-1) Health system, (neutral) Transportation hub, (-1) Innovation, (-1) Transparency, (-1) Pandemic readiness/response, (-1) Air quality. Total score: -6

18. Addis: (-1) Major population hub, (-1) Health system, (-1) Transportation hub, (-1) Innovation, (-1) Transparency, (neutral) Pandemic readiness/response, (-1) Air quality. Total score: -6

19. Wuhan: (-2) Megacity, major population hub, (+1) Health system, (-1) Transportation hub, (-1) Innovation, (-1) Transparency, (neutral) Pandemic readiness/response (bad start, great recovery), (-1) Air quality. Total score: -5

20. Bangalore: (-2) Megacity, major population hub, (-1) Health system, (-1) Transportation hub, (+1) Innovation, (-1) Transparency, (-1) Pandemic readiness/response, (-1) Air quality. Total score: -6

21. Cape Town: (-1) Major population hub, (-1) Health system, (-1) Transportation hub, (neutral) Innovation, (neutral) Transparency, (neutral) Pandemic readiness/response, (-1) Air quality. Total score: -4

22. Beijing: (-1) Megacity, major population hub, (neutral) Health system, (-1) Innovation, (-1) Transparency, (1) Pandemic readiness/response, (-1) Air quality. Total score: -3

23. Guangzhou: (-2) Megacity, major population hub, (neutral) Health system, (-1) Innovation, (-1) Transparency, (1) Pandemic readiness/response, (-1) Air quality. Total score: -4

24. Shanghai: (-2) Megacity, major population hub, (neutral) Health system, (-1) Innovation, (-1) Transparency, (1) Pandemic readiness/response, (-1) Air quality. Total score: -4

25. New York: (-2) Megacity, major economic hub, (-1) Transportation hub, (neutral) Health system, (+1) Transparency, (-1) Pandemic readiness/response, (-1) Air quality. Total score: -4

26. Madrid: (-1) Major population hub, (neutral) Health system, (-1) Innovation, (+1) Transparency, (-1) Pandemic readiness/response, (-1) Air quality. Total score: -3

27. Hangzhou: (-2) Megacity, major population hub, (+1)

Health system, (-1) Transportation hub, (neutral) Innovation, (-1) Transparency, (+1) Pandemic readiness/response, (-2) Air quality. Total score: -4

28. Tokyo: (-2) Megacity, major population hub, (+1) Health system, (-1) Transportation hub, (neutral) Innovation, (neutral) Transparency, (+1) Pandemic readiness/response, (-1) Air quality. Total score: -2

29. Shenzhen: (-2) Megacity, major population hub, (+1) Health system, (-1) Transportation hub, (neutral) Innovation, (-1) Transparency, (+1) Pandemic readiness/response, (-2) Air quality. Total score: -4

30. Chongqing: (-2) Megacity, major population hub, (+1) Health system, (-1) Transportation hub, (neutral) Innovation, (-1) Transparency, (+1) Pandemic readiness/response, (-2) Air quality. Total score: -4

31. Dongguan: (-1) Megacity, major population hub, (+1) Health system, (-2) Transportation hub, (neutral) Innovation, (-1) Transparency, (+1) Pandemic readiness/response, (-2) Air quality. Total score: -4

32. Chengdu: (-1) Megacity, major population hub, (+1) Health system, (-1) Transportation hub, (neutral) Innovation, (-1) Transparency, (+1) Pandemic readiness/response, (-2) Air quality. Total score: -3

33. Tianjin: (-1) Megacity, major population hub, (+1) Health system, (-1) Transportation hub, (neutral) Innovation, (-1) Transparency, (+1) Pandemic readiness/response, (-2) Air quality. Total score: -3

34. Xi'an: (-1) Megacity, major population hub, (+1) Health system, (-1) Transportation hub, (neutral) Innovation, (-1) Transparency, (+1) Pandemic readiness/response, (-2) Air quality. Total score: -3

35. Jinan: (-1) Megacity, major population hub, (+1) Health system, (-1) Transportation hub, (neutral) Innovation, (-1) Transparency, (+1) Pandemic readiness/response, (-2) Air quality. Total score: -3

36. Nanjing: (-1) Megacity, major population hub, (+1) Health system, (-1) Transportation hub, (neutral) Innovation, (-1) Transparency, (+1) Pandemic readiness/response, (-2) Air quality. Total score: -3

37. Shenyang: (-1) Megacity, major population hub, (+1) Health system, (-1) Transportation hub, (neutral) Innovation, (-1) Transparency, (+1) Pandemic readiness/response, (-2) Air quality. Total score: -3

38. Harbin: (-1) Megacity, major population hub, (+1) Health system, (-1) Transportation hub, (neutral) Innovation, (-1) Transparency, (+1) Pandemic readiness/response, (-2) Air quality. Total score: -3

39. Shantou: (-1) Megacity, major population hub, (+1) Health system, (-1) Transportation hub, (neutral) Innovation, (-1) Transparency, (+1) Pandemic readiness/response, (-2) Air quality. Total score: -3

40. Suzhou: (-1) Megacity, major population hub, (+1) Health system, (-1) Transportation hub, (neutral) Innovation, (-1) Transparency, (+1) Pandemic readiness/response, (-2) Air quality. Total score: -3

41. Wenzhou: (-1) Megacity, major population hub, (+1) Health system, (-1) Transportation hub, (neutral) Innovation, (-1) Transparency, (+1) Pandemic readiness/response, (-2) Air quality. Total score: -3

42. Qingdao: (-1) Megacity, major population hub, (+1) Health system, (-1) Transportation hub, (neutral) Innovation, (-1) Transparency, (+1) Pandemic readiness/response, (-2) Air quality. Total score: -3

43. Quanzhou: (-1) Megacity, major population hub, (+1) Health system, (-1) Transportation hub, (neutral) Innovation, (-1) Transparency, (+1) Pandemic readiness/response, (-2) Air quality. Total score: -3

44. London: (-1) Major economic hub, (-1) Transportation hub, (+1) Health system, (+1) Innovation, (+1) Transparency, (-1) Pandemic readiness/response (herd mentality policy

backfired and lost 1 month of time), (-2) Air quality. Total score: -2

45. Seoul: (-2) Megacity, major population hub, (+1) Health system, (-1) Transportation hub, (+1) Innovation, (+1) Transparency, (-2) Pandemic readiness/response, (-2) Air quality. Total score: -4

46. Paris: (-1) Major population hub, (+1) Health system, (-1) Transportation hub, (neutral) Innovation, (+1) Transparency, (neutral) Pandemic readiness/response, (-1) Air quality. Total score: -1

What I find interesting in this analysis, is that, all things considered, Wuhan comes out in the middle, neither the world's most risky place for pandemics, nor among the better megacities. The biggest and densest megacities in Asia fare the worst in this model given their compounded risk. A surprising number of Chinese megacities also don't do as poorly given the draconic governance options. The real question seems to be what happens in the "meaty middle" where risk is very high and the total numbers of people affected represents a good part of world population.

There are a number of special circumstances to note, which may be part of a more detailed analysis. New York and London have outsized economic importance for the world's economy because of their financial districts. Cape Town and Addis are gateways to Africa and their fate will largely decide that continent's fate with COVID-19. A major outbreak in Rio De Janeiro could sink not only Brazil but a huge part of South America. A massive outbreak in India's megacities Mumbai and/or Delhi would be devastating and put the entire 1.4 billion population at risk over some time (1–2 years).

These scores would need to be continuously updated to reflect the situation on the ground as things change with the Pandemic response, for instance, but the basic risk profile stands.

The final score could be multiplied with infections or death toll averages for the sample above (controlled for population) to find how much it would deviate from each other.

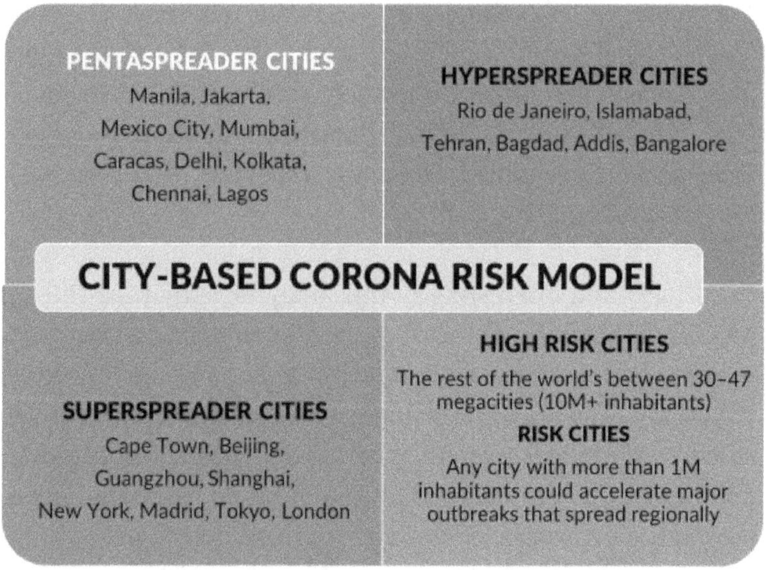
PENTASPREADER CITIES
Manila, Jakarta, Mexico City, Mumbai, Caracas, Delhi, Kolkata, Chennai, Lagos
HYPERSPREADER CITIES
Rio de Janeiro, Islamabad, Tehran, Bagdad, Addis, Bangalore
CITY-BASED CORONA RISK MODEL
SUPERSPREADER CITIES
Cape Town, Beijing, Guangzhou, Shanghai, New York, Madrid, Tokyo, London
HIGH RISK CITIES
The rest of the world's between 30-47 megacities (10M+ inhabitants)
RISK CITIES
Any city with more than 1M inhabitants could accelerate major outbreaks that spread regionally

App Figure 2. City-based corona risk model

Pentaspreader cities

Manila, Jakarta, Mexico City, Mumbai, Caracas, Delhi, Kolkata, Chennai, Lagos

Hyperspreader cities

Rio de Janeiro, Islamabad, Tehran, Bagdad, Addis, Bangalore

Superspreader cities

Cape Town, Beijing, Guangzhou, Shanghai, New York, Madrid, Tokyo, London

So far, the implication of the analysis is that if we want to understand 80% of what's happening with COVID-19 across the world, we need only look at what's happening in London, New York, Beijing, and Delhi.

The further implication could be that, if we stem the tide

in those cities, we would be able to control the outbreak going forward. The reason being that those cities control the bulk of global economic power, cultural significance, and social dynamics (as well as the top compound risk for a major outbreak) and would be able to mobilize to "save the rest" should that become necessary.

Leaving the accuracy of this analysis apart, I see absolutely no evidence that this kind of macro-level thinking has been happening at any level of government or intergovernmental organization over the past few months. I sincerely doubt that the WHO, the world's pandemic watchdog has observation delegations in each of these superspreader cities, not even in hyperspreader cities or even in pentaspreader cities that have exponential potential for spread of disease for years to come.

More than delegations, we should have a joined up worldwide mitigation strategy to avoid these cities' outbreaks from spilling over into major population centers even beyond their metropolitan borders.

This is, in fact, the kind of effort the United States government would have spearheaded a few decades ago when they still saw themselves as the world's police. Who's our police now that we need it, for the first time, arguably since the 1918 influenza pandemic?

Nothing out of the UN has signaled this kind of global strategic risk overview. Or, at least, no media has reported anything of the sort. To my knowledge, no think tanks, no independent intellectuals have been putting together a similar analysis (if so, I'd like to get in touch with them). Yet, without this kind of strategic risk picture, we are going blindly into the near future.

Moving on, let's look at the professional groups and other social groups that are the most likely superspreaders.

Professionals and social groups: most likely superspreaders

Health workers
Commuters
Executives
Sports fans

Finally, we will look at highly specific locales where we might have reason to believe that contagion could spread rapidly, even though these might be quite isolated from the rest of society, namely total institutions such as jails and refugee camps, as well as societal institutions such as hospitals and elderly homes. The negative impact, and the network effect, of a superspreader would be most deeply felt there.

Hotspots for contagion

Jails
Refugee camps
Hospitals
Schools
Elderly homes
Sports stadiums
Megachurches
Railway stations
Airports
Airplanes
Subways
Exhibition centers
Gyms

I have not yet seen any analysis of relative risk in each of these locales, but that would seem to be pertinent public health information going forward. I believe the scientific literature operates various scales of mass events and this scale could perhaps be adapted to estimate risk levels. The total number of people gathered at once or passing through the same physical space and the overall density with which it happens on a regular basis are clearly factors but not the only factors. Does risk get compounded if one individual regularly visits more than, say three to five of these locales?

Precise "surgical" action instead of mass quarantines

Let's just say, for the sake of argument, that this analysis was all we had. The logical consequence would be that we would try to reduce spread among health workers, commuters, executives, and sports fans in the megacities of New York, London, and Delhi. For the sake of argument, let's assume we had this knowledge on February 1, and had been able to bring any activity we deemed necessary in those three cities to a halt. How many lives would have been saved? Also, if our analysis is correct, we would not have had to shut down these cities, only do surgical actions, such as force commuters to work from home, test all health workers before they went into work, force executives to stop traveling, and put a ban on big sports events. *Maybe next time?*

Let's now look at the evolving infection rates and death toll in these three cities. As of May 2, New York city has 18,491 deaths, India has 1,323 deaths most in the state of Maharashtra which includes the megacity of Mumbai and 4,122 infected cases and 64 dead for Delh (MOHFW, 2020), UK has 28,205 deaths, with London as the epicenter (JHU, 2020).

Revised analysis—quantifying megacity risks

Next, let's do a more solid job, using the data from only the identified factors in our four-forces model for which we have solid comparative data, to see whether a different picture emerges or whether the two pictures (the simple conceptual model v. the empirical model) are relatively similar. To simplify matters in our narrative, we will only validate the ranking within the top 10 in our initial analysis (I'll try to have the larger picture in a future review).

Government response: I'll look at the date of the pandemic countermeasure compared to (a) the number of infected, (b) the death toll, and (c) the total population.

Four forces of pandemic superspreading events

Science & Technology
#Scientists per capita, #Clinical trials, Availability of Medical technology

Policy & Regulation
Global Health Security Index ranking (country), Pandemic response, City rankings (population, urban density, innovativeness)

Business Models & Startups
Size of economy (GDP), #startups (according to Crunchbase)

Social Dynamics & Consumers
Consumption market size

Empirical sub-indicators of Pandemic acceleration risk
Urban Density: Demographia World Urban Areas: 2019 (http://demographia.com/db-worldua.pdf)
World Air Quality Index: https://waqi.info/

As data is still emerging, I have not finalized the analysis, but would be happy to do so in a future project in the coming years, should there be demand for it.

Non-fiction books on the pandemic threat

A dozen or so popular books have been on the pandemic threat:

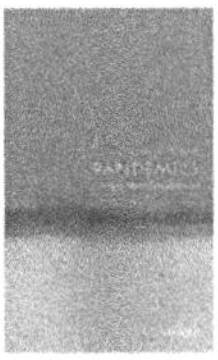

Pandemics: A very short introduction (Oxford University Press, 2016) by Christian W. McMillen (Paperback). The book is an account of pandemics throughout human history from a history professor.

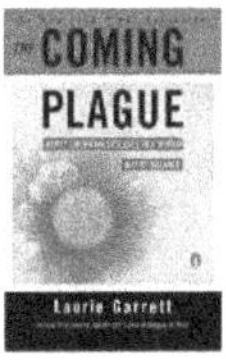

The Coming Plague: Newly Emerging Diseases in a World Out of Balance (Anchor, 1995) by Laurie Garrett (Hardcover). The book, from a Pulitzer-winning journalist and commentator on pandemic readiness, traces the patterns lying beneath the new diseases in the headlines.

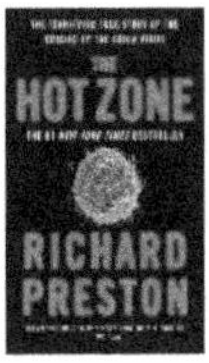

The Hot Zone: The Terrifying True Story of the Origins of the Ebola Virus (Harvard Business Review Press, 2020) by Richard Preston (Paperback). The book is the story of the deadly virus (Ebola) that emerged from Africa's rain forests.

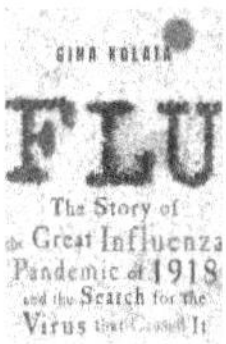

Flu: The Story of the Great Influenza Pandemic of 1918 and the Search for the Virus That Caused It (Atria Books, 2001), by *Gina Kolata* (Paperback). The book is about the causes of the Spanish Flu and the possibility it could happen again.

The Great Influenza: The Story of the Deadliest Pandemic in History (Penguin, 2005), by John M. Barry (Paperback). Arguably the definitive account of the 1918 Flu Epidemic.

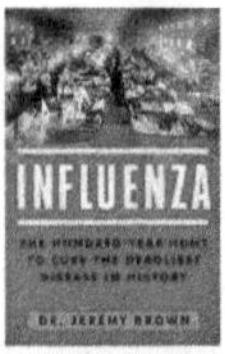

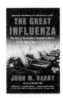

Influenza: The Hundred Year Hunt to Cure the Deadliest Disease in History (Atria Books, 2018) by Dr. Jeremy Brown (Hardcover).The book written by an ER doctor, explores the complex history of the flu virus, from the origins of the Great Flu that killed millions, to vexing questions such as: Are we prepared for the next epidemic, should you get a flu shot, and how close are we to finding a cure?

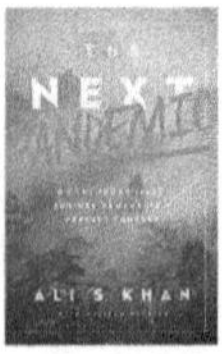

The Next Pandemic: On the Front Lines Against Humankind's Gravest Dangers (PublicAffairs, 2016) by Dr. Ali Khan & William Patrick (Paperback). The book is a firsthand account of disasters like anthrax, bird flu, and others—and how we could do more to prevent their return and also an urgent lesson on how we can keep ourselves safe from the inevitable next pandemic.

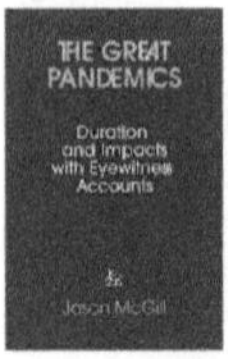

The Great Pandemics: Duration and Impacts with Eyewitness Accounts (Auroch Press, 2020), by *Jason McGill* (Paperback). The book outlines a plan to prevent worldwide infectious outbreaks, including better public spending, communication, innovation, etc.

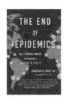

The End of Epidemics: The Looming Threat to Humanity and How to Stop It (St. Martin's Press, 2018), by Dr. Jonathan D. Quick and Bronwyn Fryer (Hardcover). The pamphlet attempts to both provide a deep historical perspective by analyzing ancient text for clues on the geopolitical, economic, social, and psychological effects of a pandemic and relate it to contemporary geopolitical configurations and technology.

D. Innovation

Astonishingly absent in the crisis so far, beyond the Imperial College studies on COVID-19, is the perspective of science-based modeling, or novel technological approaches that are so prevalent in other parts of society, or indeed that rose to prominence around other outbreaks such as Ebola. This seems to indicate that AI, at least in the form that we can immediately harvest, is less mature than its proponents would have it. Similarly, statistics-based epidemiology is also noticeably weak, with predictions that either are bombastically wrong or tentative to the extreme compared to what one might expect. Perhaps good data is not yet there? Or, is this voice being suppressed?

What are the major innovations that are rolling in to help in the coronavirus crisis? A few categories of innovations have emerged: (1) treatments (including drugs), (2) vaccine developments (including from smaller biotech companies and startups), (3) medical device innovations (improvised ventilators or new consortia who produce such equipment on months' notice as well as mobile patient transportation units used for emergency medivacs under both civil society and army control), (4) COVID-19 testing tools and protocols, (5) online disease discovery and tracking tools, and (6) video-conferencing tools (digital startups such as Zoom have become unicorns overnight). Let's briefly consider a few examples.

Treatments

The most promising drug currently being tested is *Remdesivir*, US pharma company Gilead Sciences' treatment for Ebola virus disease and Marburg virus infections. In January, Gilead reported the drug had shown to be active against SARS and MERS in animal models. Remdesivir has already been administered based on compassionate use both in the US and elsewhere. Seven trials of Remdesivir are ongoing, including two investigator-led Chinese studies, two phase-3 trials being run by Gilead in the US, Europe, and Asia, and a National Institute of Allergy and Infectious Disease (NIAID) test in around 800 patients with a broad spectrum of symptoms. Gilead's severe COVID-19 study includes 2,400 participants from 152 different clinical trial sites all over the world. Its moderate COVID-19 study includes 1,600 patients in 169 different centers, also all over the world. Whilst Remdesivir is no panacea, it might have some effect. On May 1, the US approved emergency use of the drug on severely ill COVID-19 and hospitalized patients.

Ongoing COVID-19 vaccine efforts

Vaccine efforts are an obvious example. The WHO R&D blueprint (2020) has signatories from around the world. Over 500 clinical trials of potential COVID-19 treatments and interventions have been launched worldwide, according to TranspariMed (2020). Among those, some 40 clinical trials for a vaccine are ongoing, but what's at stake here isn't just the science, but the financing, the partnerships, and the worldwide rollout.

The Coalition for Epidemic Preparedness Innovations (CEPI), a nonprofit global partnership between public, private, philanthropic, and civil society organizations dedicated to the development of vaccines against emerging infectious diseases, has nearly $30 million so far invested in several candidates, including the first to be injected into trial participants. The eight COVID-19 vaccine development projects CEPI is invested in include Curevac, Inovio Pharmaceuticals, Moderna, Novavax, The University of Hong Kong, The University of Oxford, The University of Queensland, and a consortium led by Institut Pasteur (Cepi.net). Gavi, the Vaccine Alliance, is working on vaccine preparedness of health systems in lower-income countries and to ensure continued immunization efforts against other diseases (e.g., measles, polio, yellow fever, and diphtheria) continues so there are not more crises to fight at the same time and finally, exploring mechanisms and incentives to "ensure vaccines are available to the most vulnerable, no matter where they live" (gavi.org). Worldwide vaccine rollout cannot be assumed otherwise.

The organization plans to advance the top six of these candidates into larger efficacy trials with thousands of participants. CEPI has announced $2B is what's needed to get the job done. As of April 16, 2020, the total sum pledged toward the US$2 billion target stands at US$765 million.

Biomedical Advanced Research and Development Authority (BARDA), part of the US's HHS Office of the Assistant Secretary for Preparedness and Response, is contributing hundreds of millions of dollars to two top vaccine candidates: one made by Johnson & Johnson's Janssen division and another developed by Moderna in collaboration with the US government that was injected into the first trial participants last month at the Kaiser Permanente Washington Health Research Institute in Seattle.

China, on its end, has as of March approved two vaccines for human trials, by a Beijing-based unit of Sinovac Biotech and by the Wuhan Institute of Biological Products, an affiliate of state-owned China National Pharmaceutical Group. Traditional vaccine has trials first in small animals, then move to primates, then to the humans, but at least one of the Chinese vaccines has moved straight to human trials. Many experts in the west say that's a bold move that can backfire.

Antivaxxers who already fear the real prospect of mandatory vaccines in many countries, are watching this process closely. One might imagine what a global backlash against vaccines in general would do to the public health situation, should any of the COVID-19 vaccines go array in terms of human safety.

In Israel, the MIGAL research institute's researchers have developed an effective vaccine against avian coronavirus Infectious Bronchitis Virus (IBV), to be adapted soon and create a human vaccine against COVID-19 (migal.org.il/en). There have been misleading reports shared thousands of times on Sri Lankan Facebook about the readiness of this vaccine, according to the fact checker AFP (2020).

In the US, existing mandatory vaccines include the measles, polio, and hepatitis A and B, vaccines that kids need to get in order to attend school. As of January 2018, France, for instance, now mandates 11 vaccines (for instance adding whooping cough, hepatitis B, measles, mumps, and rubella), up from three (diphtheria, tetanus, and poliomyelitis). The WHO recommends that countries have 95% vaccine coverage.

The sci-tech approaches taken by each of these vaccine manufacturers vary from DNA to RNA vaccines to enlisting spike proteins or even other viral compounds (e.g., adenovirus) in the fight and include the use of nanoparticles straight out of nanoscience textbooks about to be written as well as trying to derive a coronavirus vaccine from other somewhat similar vaccine paths (e.g., IBV).

Data from the Trials Tracker run by Oxford University (covid19.trialstracker.net) combines the WHO's International Clinical Trials Registry Platform (ICTRP) with the US-based ClinicalTrials.gov, which is great because the WHO service is no longer publicly available due to web traffic overload.

Medical device innovations

As of April 2020, ventilators have been on everyone's mind for months. This previously not much featured piece of medical equipment is last resort hospital care 101. To deploy it, one has to insert a long plastic tube through the trachea and vocal cords that allows a machine to deliver puffs of highly oxygenated air to the lungs. The machine itself then controls the release of oxygen and, essentially breathes for the patient. The process works quite well for severe pneumonia patients.

Ventilators, which cost between $25,000 and $50,000, and are only used in respiratory emergencies are, understandably, are not plentiful under normal circumstances. For example, before the COVID-19 crisis, the UK government had only 8,175 ventilators.

The Penlon's Prima ES02 model was approved on 16 April, stemming from 'Project Oyster' by the VentilatorChallengeUK consortium launched on March 30, which includes High Value Manufacturing Catapult, Ford, a number of UK-based Formula 1 (F1) teams and Siemens. The UK National Health Service (NHS) ordered 15,000 units immediately. Another model, Project Penguin, is being manufactured by Smiths Medical. Independently, Dyson's CoVent ventilator prototype, still awaiting approval as of mid-April, has a 10,000-units standing order from the government, pending regulatory approval.

The VentilatorChallengeUK consortium is also working with University College London (UCL) to develop a continuous positive airway pressure (CPAP) device for the NHS. In parallel, University of Warwick and Queen's University Belfast are running a clinical trial that seeks to enroll 4,000 patients to find ventilator alternatives for coronavirus patients. The study is based on the theory that noninvasive interventions (including CPAP or BPAP masks driven by oxygen or high-flow oxygen through the nose) at an earlier stage may reduce the need for invasive ventilation with a mechanical ventilator.

According to NPR (2020), ventilator mortality rates are unclear but vary between 50–80% in various studies and anecdotal evidence from practitioners. Intensive Care National Audit and Research Center (ICNARC, 2020) in the UK report that among the 98 patients who received advanced respiratory support—defined as invasive ventilation, BPAP, or CPAP via endotracheal tube, or tracheostomy, or extracorporeal respiratory support—66% died.

The ventilator itself can do damage to the lung tissue based on how much pressure is required to help oxygen get processed by the lungs. It also opens the door for a range of respiratory diseases. If there was a way to safely deploy noninvasive mechanical breathing instead of and earlier than ventilators, that could be highly impactful, especially in the developing world but also in improving outcomes all around. However, this would break with standard respiratory treatment protocol.

Transporting patients with infectious diseases is challenging. In a massive epidemic, if helicopters, aircrafts, and ambulances have to be disinfected after each transport, the whole system may collapse or will at least be very inefficient. Epiguard is an innovation from a Norwegian startup who have created a flexible patient transport unit to be used for transport of patients with infectious diseases including coronavirus, Ebola, measles, tuberculosis, or multiresistant bacteria. The hard-top polycarbonate, reusable specialized isolation unit (SIU) is a self-contained patient transportation chamber which can be secured safely with any vehicle or stretcher that could be used in ambulances and on helicopters and airplanes (epiguard.com).

The isolator can be configured to either protect the surroundings from the patient (via underpressure), or to protect the patient from the surroundings (via overpressure). EpiShuttle has glove ports to provide medical personnel access to the patient's entire body, which allows for food, medicine, and equipment to be safely put into the isolator compartment. The isolator enables intensive care treatment of the patient, with possibility for procedures such as intubation, inserting of central venous lines, and urinary catheters, through use of its interchangeable operator ports.

The National CBRNE Centre for Medicine in Norway has deployed the EpiShuttle to all five university hospitals in the country. The EpiShuttle is currently in use with the World Health Organization (WHO) in the Democratic Republic of Congo (DRC) as part of its response to the country's Ebola crisis. EpiGuard was founded at the Oslo University Hospital, Norway, in 2015 by a group of doctors, together with cofounders Inven2, Eker Group, and Hansen Protection (epiguard.com) and is supported by the European Innovation Council (EIC), an ambitious EU agency that aims to do for startups and spinoffs what the grantmaking European Research Council does for basic research. An EpiShuttle costs around $40,000.

A similar approach, although significantly costlier and more impractical, is taken by the US military. The Transport Isolation System is an infectious disease containment unit that can be secured inside aircraft to minimize the risk of contagion to the aircrew while at the same time allowing for medical care. The Transport Isolation System was first implemented after the Ebola outbreak and will now be used for COVID-19 medivac procedures by the US Air Force, although as of April 3, 2020, it hasn't yet been tried.

The US Defense Department is currently developing another system called the Portable Bio-Containment Module which is similar to a shipping container and larger than the Transport Isolation System.

The differences in approach between Epiguard and the Americans are striking. Epiguard is essentially a bed with a dome around it for lack of a better way to describe it, or perhaps more like a bobsled, for those who have seen those. Epiguard is designed to be used in a small hospital helicopter. The TIS is a near container-size compartment, which admittedly can hold two patients (or four ambulatory patients) but that would require an airlift. The large

McDonnell Douglas/Boeing C-17 Globemaster III military transport aircraft can only transport two TIS units at one time, so this is incredibly resource intensive. The Portable Bio-Containment Module will be even bulkier.

Air filtration is another emerging market in the post-COVID-19 world. A company founded in 2013 by biomedical engineer and former Imperial College postdoc Hugo Macedo, called Smart Separations (smartseparations.com), has an experimental ceramic filter device (e.g., a microsieve) purifying indoor air by heavily reducing carbon particulates, dust, pollen, odors, and chemicals in air more efficiently and affordably than current methods. Many industries still rely on outdated cloth filters. However, this new platform could also filtrate blood, stem cells, water, air, milk, wine, and more to keep impurities out of the substances we rely on every day. Their niche is the underexplored microfiltration market, where manufacturing cost-efficient filters with a pore size of between 1 and 50 micrometers is distinguished from molecular filtration (gas, water, proteins) and macro filtration (sifting flour on top of a cake).

Already before the crisis, air filtration was an established €15 billion global market, according to the EU project's description (Cordis, 2020). The company envisions improving indoor air quality through integration with domestic appliances (in the short term) and removal at source through industrial emissions reduction (long term). What about the office air purification retrofitting market? Or the airplane air purification market? The bolt-on capability of their technology to current systems is exciting. Newly emerging niches seem quite promising for this company.

COVID-19 testing tools and innovations

Testing, testing, testing, has been the WHO's mantra throughout the crisis. Around the world, there have been shortcomings and shortages around tests, test equipment, personnel, and testing sites. A variety of tests exist, but broadly, there are two types, a diagnostic test useful for patients who currently may have the disease, called a PCR test (reverse transcription polymerase chain reaction, i.e., RT-PCR) and a serological test that can detect past viral infections and would be instrumental to tackle the issue of asymptomatic transmission by figuring out who actually have had the disease but may not be aware of it. Until recently, only Singapore conducted serological tests for COVID-19, and based on a test that's not been validated for clinical use, according to Nature (2020). On April 15, Abbot Laboratories, the American medical devices and healthcare company, launched a serological test in the US, expecting to ship close to 1 million tests to US customers this week, 4 million during April, and ramping up to 20 million antibody tests in June.

On March 27, 2020, Abbott received emergency use authorization (EUA) from the US Food and Drug Administration (FDA) for the fastest available molecular point-of-care test for the detection of novel coronavirus (SARS-CoV-2; formerly called 2019-nCoV), delivering positive results in 5 minutes and negative results in 13 minutes (but even the company admits that false negatives are possible with lower viral loads). During the first 2 weeks, 566,000 units were shipped, and the company aims to deliver 50,000 tests per day to start with and 5 million tests in April, which would be a game changer to remedy the US testing deficit.

There are only 200 of the other testing tool, the existing m2000, Abbot's large, high-volume laboratory instrument already used for other testing, in hospital, academic center and reference labs throughout the US. However, it enables 150,000 laboratory tests to be made quickly, with tests already sent to hospital and academic medical center labs in 18 states including Illinois, California, New York, Massachusetts, and Washington.

According to The COVID Tracking Project

(covidtracking.com/data), which collects data directly from all US states and territories, there were 3,401,064 total test results (Positive + Negative) as of April 16.

Even the mighty US CDC botched the rollout of their first diagnostics test, which arguably could be said to have cost thousands of lives.

British company diagnostics.ai, employs artificial intelligence to analyze the molecular structure of the test sample (a newer method called Real Time PCR or Q-PCR) but is able to pool the results, making the process more efficient.

Some 1,600 test kits of the SHERLOCK test, codeveloped by CRISPR pioneer Feng Zhang at the Broad Institute of MIT and Harvard in Cambridge, Massachusetts (and attributable to the biotech startup, Sherlock Biosciences, Inc., Zhang has cofounded), are now circulating labs around the world to see if it is ready for prime time, given that Zhang's lab has no access to patient samples.

Online disease discovery and tracking tools

Infectious disease modelling has become a critical piece in the public health tool kit. This is especially true during epidemics and emergencies.

Boston-based Healthmap attempts to build a comprehensive view of the current global state of infectious diseases. Founded in 2006 by a team of researchers, epidemiologists and software developers at Boston Children's Hospital, Healthmap is an established system utilizing online informal sources for disease outbreak monitoring and real-time surveillance of emerging public health threats. It brings together disparate data sources, including online news aggregators, eyewitness reports, expert-curated discussions, and validated official reports. Does it work? The interactive visualization (healthmap.org/COVID-19/) tracing the spread of the disease from January 15 to present is cool and the visual is pleasant, but doesn't add much to what one can read from other overviews such as Google News (news.google.com/covid19/map). The issue with all of these dashboards is the quality of the data, not the quality of the visualization.

In truth, it has been confusing over the past few months. There are "too many" signals and articles to gain a comprehensive view, but also too many inputs missing from the picture (right now it only tracks news stories as well as infection cases, but not recovered cases or deaths), even compared to what you would find in a regular search engine session. This is not Healthmap's flaw alone, of course, but it points to some of the weaknesses with the methods deployed.

In theory, the automated process, monitors, organizes, integrates, filters, visualizes, and disseminates online information facilitating early detection of global public health threats. In practice, it is still a demo tool which might work better for more established flu outbreaks that are seasonal but where it might be difficult to figure out when it will begin and end in a particular part of the country.

Healthmap uses various online news aggregators as well as public health websites as sources, including ProMEDMail, WHO, GeoSentinel, OIE, FAO, EuroSurveillance, Google News, Moreover, WDIN, Baidu News, and SOSO Info, operating in nine languages.

Healthmap has earlier been used to trace the emergence of West Nile virus in New York City using satellite data, predicting patterns of Lyme disease based on climate change, and to analyzing patterns of influenza epidemics. It may evolve to be useful for coronavirus but is not currently adding much to the picture.

Massachusetts's Governor Baker just went back to using volunteers (people) as contact tracers given that no online tool even comes close to doing the job of tracking exactly who has been exposed to COVID-19, let them know, and ask them where they have been the past 2 weeks. Other countries do have some digital tools to bring to bear, notably using cell phone tracking, but this hasn't happened at least in Massachusetts.

Johns Hopkins' map, or the COVID-19 Dashboard by the Center for Systems Science and Engineering (CSSE) at Johns Hopkins University (JHU), has been criticized for its enormous red dots that cloud each map, but that's sort of unfair given the unprecedented spread which truly does leave a big mark. Most of these dashboards use roughly the same sources, although not exactly the same. Johns Hopkins claims to use the following data sources: WHO, CDC, ECDC, NHC, DXY, 1point3acres, Worldometers.info, BNO, the COVID Tracking Project (testing and hospitalizations), state and national government health departments, and local media reports.

The more important issue with such dashboards is what they leave out. Let me take an example. As I zoomed in on Norfolk, Massachusetts, where I live, I noticed that Suffolk, the county to the east, which includes Boston, had more cases. But before making too much out of that, it would have been useful to know what I found out by using a search engine, which is that Suffolk has a population of 803,907 (2019) and Norfolk a population of 706,775 (2019). Also, what about how many tests were carried out, recovered cases, I could go on. What this dashboard can do is tell me, based on the data it has, where are infections increasing, how does the outbreak differ across countries,

Nextstrain (nextstrain.org/ncov/global) is an open-source project to harness the scientific and public health potential of pathogen genome data. Nextstrain presents a single, continuously updated overview of both endemic viral disease (seasonal influenza, dengue) as well as emergent viral outbreaks (Avian influenza, Zika, Ebola), all based upon the same underlying bioinformatics architecture. As for COVID-19, it breaks down the genome of the virus, alongside an animated map showing the routes by which it traveled from country to country.

The tool is perfect if you want to geek out on "pathogen phylogenies," or to say it in a simple way, who infected who in an epidemic, and with which mutation of the pathogen. The significance of this tool is to show genetic data to identify whether, when, and how countries are getting hit with multiple introductions of the virus, or even more useful, to show how *local* outbreaks are connected.

There are numerous questions about how Nextstrain gets its data, and the quality of that data. That information is not as transparent as with Healthmap and the Johns Hopkins tool. Their data seems to be largely sourced through an outfit originally known as a Global Initiative on Sharing All Influenza Data (now simply known as GISAID), a public-private partnership formed in 2008 between the German government and the nonprofit organization Friends of GISAID that provides public access to the most complete collection of genetic sequence data of influenza viruses and related clinical and epidemiological data through its database. The problem with COVID-19 data is that we have relatively few samples and those samples may not be thoroughly analyzed nor is it certain that they tell the whole story. Other data needed to piece together an outbreak would include patient risk factors, travel history, and case reports, according to Duncan MacCannell, the chief science officer for the Center for Disease Control's Office of Advanced Molecular Detection, as quoted by Wired (2020).

London School of Hygiene and Tropical Medicine also has their tracker, the only unique aspect being the ability to overlay other diseases (SARS, H1N1, Ebola) on to the map.

Finally, a review article in Nature (2019) points out that extensive online communities and forums such as Twitter, Virological, FluTrackers, ProMED, Nextstrain, HealthMap, and Microreact allow rapid dissemination of unpublished results and analyses.

WeBank, China's first and leading online bank, where Tencent, the world's largest video game company, is the largest shareholder have quickly gained traction with their activity tracker making use of what the investment community calls alternative data.

Researchers on WeBank's AI Moonshot Team took a deep-learning system developed to detect solar panel installations from satellite imagery and repurposed it to track China's economic recovery from the novel coronavirus outbreak. The team used its neural network to analyze infrared images from various satellites, including the Sentinel-2 satellite. What emerged? Hot spots indicative of actual steel manufacturing inside a plant. Painting a picture of business recovery from counting cars in large corporate parking lots. Beyond satellite data, WeBank also took daily anonymized GPS data from several million mobile phone users in 2019 and 2020 and used AI to determine which of those users were commuters. The company also mined social media platforms for mentions of companies that provide online working, gaming, education, streaming video, social networking, e-commerce, and express delivery services.

What the exact results were is less interesting from my point of view, given how it will evolve, but it is important to consider how much the alternative data supply will increase if such data analysis tools go mainstream and gain acceptance as investment grade data. This process would likely accelerate with the deepening crisis, plus the need for intermittent scale-ups /and scale-downs, which I consider in the scenarios.

The innovative AI use from Asia follows what the Chinese venture capitalist Kai-Fu Lee argued in his book *AI Superpowers* (2018) where he predicted that Chinese AI capabilities would be at the forefront of important societal processes way before the US or Europe and that China will be the next tech-innovation superpower. Compare that with the manual contact tracing and testing failures happening on those two continents.

Nine days before the World Health Organization warned about the novel coronavirus, according to the *US News and World Report* (2020), BlueDot, a Toronto-based startup providing "outbreak risk software," spotted the threat posed by coronavirus. BlueDot (bluedot.global), a startup founded back in 2008 that has so far raised $9.5 million, used data from hundreds of thousands of sources, such as statements from official public health organizations, media, health reports, and demographics as well as airline information.

Its tagline promises it "protects people around the world from infectious diseases with human and artificial intelligence," specifically helping "governments protect their citizens, hospitals protect their staff and patients, and businesses protect their employees and customers."

The startup relied on Dr. Kamran Khan's, one of the cofounders, expertise in treating SARS patients as an epidemiologist and physician.

According to the *Toronto Star* (2016), BlueDot claims it was able to predict the outbreak of the Zika virus in Florida, 6 months before it occurred. Their model used Brazilian flight itineraries, temperature maps, population densities, ranges for known and possible Zika-transmitting mosquitoes, as well as other data to make the predictions.

BlueDot lists ASEAN, the Singaporean Ministry of Health as well as the Canadian and Philippine government as clients. Betakit (2019), the Canadian startup news site claims they have also been used by several hospitals across North America, 12 public health agencies around the world, and within Air Canada. BlueDot was previously the commercial arm (spinout) of an academic research program called BioDiaspora. In fact, the company was formerly known as BioDiaspora, Inc. and spun off from St. Michael's Hospital in partnership with MaRS Innovation.

When we expect innovation to happen overnight, it is

interesting to ponder that both Healthmap (2006) and BlueDot (2008) were founded decades ago and lived a relatively anonymous existence until the current coronavirus crisis hit. Those who expect miracles from innovation better ponder what this means for supporting innovation in the future. Let me spell it out just in case: innovation takes time and you never really know when you might need it—until you suddenly do.

For an overview of many such dashboards, the University of Michigan library's Community Health research guide has a great list. Tracxn (2020), the Indian startup tracking platform lists Metabiota, Unite Us, BroadReach, Biospatial, and 30 others as BlueDot's competitors, so the field of disease tracking is growing.

Metabiota, founded in 2008, is a San Francisco-based startup founded by Nathan Wolfe (@virushunter), the virologist, and the Lokey Business Wire Consulting Professor in Human Biology at Stanford University, as well as the author of *The Viral Storm: The Dawn of a New Pandemic Age* (2011). Metabiota, which has the Silicon Valley-style funding amounts ($34.8M so far), also has its own disease tracker (metabiota.com/epidemic-tracker) with "over 120 Pathogen Profiles," "operations in nearly 20 countries," and with the "largest infectious disease catalog in the industry, including a 1 million-year stochastic event catalog informed by over 20 million simulations" and is "the only model of its kind to capture both high-probability and low-probability events," covering "century of human outbreak events."

The PR is much more hyperbolic with Metabiota than with Healthmap and BlueDot. The reason it's gotten less "play" during the current disease is that its business model seems to only allow a peak into their model while the true value is only gained by taking a business subscription. Interestingly, though, one could argue that, medium term, their model is likely to be what governments turn to when the appetite for "death counts" has ceased to get mainstream media headlines. Listed brand name clients currently include USAID, World Bank, and Wellcome Trust.

But how good is Metabiota's forecasting? If we take the Metabiota Risk Report No. 3: February 25, 2020, they predict "with 95 percent confidence" that there would be between 81,500 and 295,000 cases by March 3, the median being 127,000 cumulative cases. On 3 March, the WHO reported there were 90,893 reported cases of COVID-19 globally, and 3,110 deaths, so perhaps not that far off. It must be said, this was a risk report Metabiota strategically have chosen to release, and the prediction was only for 1 week ahead, but in a crisis, there may be actors willing to pay for that service if it can be proven relatively accurate over time.

Having a critical view of these dashboards, I will still say that spending a few moments scanning a variety of online dashboards is far, far more informative than turning on the TV and listening to a bunch of talking heads sensationalize based on the needs of the hourly news cycle.

Videoconferencing tools

Videoconferencing rapidly became the new norm as the coronavirus epidemic became a reality. It happened fast, but not without challenges.

According to Encyclopedia Britannica, the first concepts of video conferencing were developed in the 1870s, as part of an extension of audio devices. It didn't catch on that early, though. Throughout the 1960s and '70s, the Norwegian company Tandberg was the pioneer. However, the original company went bankrupt in 1978 after a sharp financial downturn. At the time, its main competitor was Polycom and other competitors were HP, Sony, Radvision, VTEL, and Aethra.

In the early 2000, however, Skype is the real story because of the popular adoption of its proprietary Internet telephony

(VoIP) network. The Swedish startup launched in 2003 so that people far away will get in contact without needing to "waste money" using telephone lines. Having enjoyed substantial momentum among the early Internet users, Skype was sold to eBay in September 2005 for approximately $2.5B and in May 2011 Microsoft purchased Skype from eBay for $8.5B USD.

In November of 2009, long-time partner Cisco acquired Tandberg for $3.4B and by 2011, only the Cisco brand remained, eventually becoming the product Cisco Telepresence Manager.

The major news story so far around the future of work is the emergence of the Zoom videoconferencing solutions. Zoom was founded in 2011 by Eric Yuan, a former Cisco WebEx engineer and executive, who reportedly spent over 2 years struggling with visa issues—he was rejected eight times in total, finally receiving a US visa on his ninth try, according to Make-It (2020). He came to the US in 1997 and landed a job at the startup WebEx, which was bought by Cisco in 2007 for around $3 billion.

Even though Zoom had its initial public offering already in 2019, at a price of $36 per share and raising $752 million, it was coronavirus that would make the real difference. In the spring of 2020, the company started providing its videoconferencing tools to K-12 schools for free as schools closed down due to coronavirus, putting it squarely positioned in the rapidly emerging online teaching and instruction market in the US and beyond. As of April 15, 2020, it is trading around at $152.53 per share with a market valuation of roughly $42 billion, meaning the stock trades at 300 times trailing free cash flow as of this writing.

It went from a few hundred thousand users to millions of users in a few weeks. It is the subject of national security concern due to a lack of cybersecurity protections including encryption. The last few weeks have exposed privacy issues as "Zoom bombing," where hackers inexplicably jump into a

Zoom call, have increased in frequency. Some governments (including India, Taiwan), agencies (NASA), companies (Google, SpaceX) and school systems (NY Department of Education) banned it when the news broke, others have embraced it. Many of the security flaws in Zoom are, understandably, being addressed on the fly.

Beyond videoconferencing, there are many other startups and initiatives being developed. One example, Wemunity, is based on the idea of creating a community of people who already are immune using a social media approach. Wemunity is an open-source project initiated by Deloitte Digital "where we explore how immunized citizens can be utilized strategically in response to viral epidemics," particularly in local communities (wemunity.org). Its Facebook group has 299 members as of April 17, 2020, so major global traction it has not yet achieved. Another obstacle with this approach is that it is based on self-reporting, and before the medical facts around coronavirus immunity have been properly established. Having said that, the idea of immunity certificates is being proposed in Germany, the US, and other countries, and the concept of local volunteerism is a powerful one, which will become needed in this and other pandemics.

Lastly, Israel, a hotbed for medical innovation has at least 30 innovations relevant to coronavirus, ranging from diagnostics, tests, treatments, care management, or vaccine candidates via tests to medical devices, according to Israel 21c (2020), the online news magazine.

The relative absence of innovation

We are, by now, slowly starting to see a set of beneficiaries to the evolving situation. The business of portable disinfection UV light scanners (and their dangerous knock-offs) predictably thrives and is likely to see significant incremental product extensions into all sizes and price points. On the down are things like movie theaters and obviously anything travel-related, although the smart players should be busy reinventing themselves. E-commerce thrives in all its forms, at least until supply chain disruption catches up with that channel as well. E-work solutions, especially novel teleconferencing solutions like Zoom thrive, as well. E-learning thrives as does any online education tool. However, the challenge of maintaining the attention of learners over time persists.

Regulatory approvals speed up (for now), especially for anything that can be perceived as marginally helpful to the pandemic management effort. Childcare startups thrive and are likely to explode and morph into many forms, offline and online, if the work-at-home orders stay in place around the world.

Biotech startups thrive (beyond immunology); the whole sector is likely to see a lift just like it does immediately, following every pandemic. Telehealth applications may have an opportunity now, especially with e-consultation and perhaps e-surgery. Whether this finally is a boon for e-health as such remains to be seen.

Finally, 3D printing might be a beneficiary of this pandemic, as there likely will be a push to move manufacturing closer to home.

Innovation in corporations?

As was widely reported, luxury goods company LMVH, home of high-end perfumes such as Dior and Louis Vuitton, Belvedere vodka, Moët champagne, and Hennessy spirits, converted their factory practically overnight to produce hand sanitizer for French hospitals and public health facilities. Chairman and CEO and majority owner Bernard Arnault, the third-richest person in the world, with a net worth of $97.7 billion, according to Bloomberg, could afford to do this and got massive PR from it, as my inclusion of this example illustrates.

An article in the Wall Street Journal (2020) claims "corporate innovation flourishes" in the coronavirus fight, pointing to innovations from "shoes to masks." But while it is true that churning out useful, improvised medical, personal protective equipment and hand sanitizer from firms that did no such thing in the past is *incrementally* innovative (which is, admittedly, sometimes better than radical innovations) and may help stem short term shortages, I'm not sure it qualifies as a big leap forward.

Other news stories point to companies donating food or supplies to shelters or students as innovation even though that clearly is a mix of PR and charity and has little to do with invention. Why can't we have a clear definition of innovation and not water out the concept with unrelated activity?

On the contrary, I would say that corporations have been astonishingly slow to innovate, but I wouldn't call that a surprise. Also, industry and government alike have put their faith in the just-in-time principle applied to what we now know is incredibly fragile global supply chains, meaning even essential manufacturing and food production has relied on weekly supplies for key ingredients, materials, or components instead of paying the money to have even a basic storage facility. The same goes for private (and public) hospitals.

Moreover, I think we should not put so much faith in short-term innovation based on flawed interpretations of Greek thinker Plato's idea that necessity is the mother of invention.

The challenge is that true change requires patience. "As people work from home, eschew air travel, forego commutes and conduct meetings on Zoom and Skype, carbon emissions have dropped precipitously, proving that conducting business and curing climate change aren't mutually exclusive," writes Erica Ariel Fox in *Forbes* (2020). Yet, could we say this is "proven"? Some would argue it is simply a *short-term necessity* that has come at great cost. The true effect hasn't come yet: What will happen once social distancing is relaxed? If there is no governance framework, no "work at home" policy change or aggressive emission targets by industrialized and emerging economies alike, this will only become nature's "breather" before it chokes.

As Fast Company (2020) points out, large companies need to learn to innovate frugally in the time to come and must "unlearn" how they practiced innovation in the past 100 years, giving the example of MIT's $100 ventilator compared to "the $30,000 commercial ventilator." Well, that ventilator doesn't exactly do what the commercial one does, but that's another story. "U.S. firms can no longer rely on top-down strategies, costly R&D projects, and rigid highly structured innovation processes. They urgently need to adopt a new, bottom-up approach to frugal and flexible innovation," writes Navi Radjou.

In truth, there will need to be a bit of both. Pharmaceutical innovation may need to become more frugal, but it is also true that if we are going to expect miracles like vaccines developed in months, not years, then basic science funding and commercial R&D labs need to be bigger, not smaller than before *and* they need to be more efficient, collaborative, and distributed.

Scenarios means different things to different people. McKinsey's Global Health + Crisis Response Team initially issued three potential scenarios (on February 28) where a Quick recovery is the least likely, has a Global slowdown is their base case, and a Global pandemic and recession is their conservative case. Their evolving analysis is quite tentative and hard to follow, which is a bit surprising, but should perhaps tell us that the picture is still murky if you apply a consultant lens.

Similarly, Deloitte (in collaboration with Salesforce) has come up with 3-5-year scenarios for our pandemic future. In (1) The Passing Storm (effective response, economic rebound in late 2020) seems overly optimistic, (2) Good Company (a surge of public-private sector partnerships) is needed and is quite realistic, (3) Sunrise in the East (with East Asian nations handling the disease and recovery best) is interesting for its emphasis on the importance of centralized government coordination in times of crisis, and (4) Lone Wolves (waves of disease, isolationism, surveillance) is intriguingly probable and scary at the same time (Deloitte, 2020).

ACKNOWLEDGMENTS

I want to thank my excellent book editor, Nick Courtright, skilled developmental editor Kyle McCord, inspiring interior book designer Cameron Finch, and diligent proofreader Courtney King Bain at Atmosphere Press, without whom this book could not have been written, edited and produced in less than three months.

I thank my family for having put up with my endless observations and attempts to discuss the vagaries of the coronavirus epidemic over the past months.

At the end of the day, I had no choice but to write this book. My thoughts kept coming back to what was happening, and I somehow felt that my experience in a multitude of ways compelled me to sit down and reflect immediately. The more I understood about coronavirus, the more I realized that the rewriting of the rules that society are built upon has, again, begun. Just like previous times, it will be shocking, disruptive, and painful, but also liberating, thought inducing, and transformative. I also realized that due to the accelerated pace, this process is going to happen over the next decade, not over the next hundred years. This awoke the social scientist in me, not just the technology futurist.

Thank you so much to those who have taught me about scenario building, science and technology, public health, international institutions, policy making, and disruption along the way.

A special thanks to Ken Ducatel (now Director at DG DIGIT, European Commission) who hosted me at Institute for Prospective Technological Studies (IPTS) in Seville, Spain, back in 2003, honing my skills in foresight. Many thanks to Tore Tennøe, Director at the Norwegian Board of Technology, who paid for the trip and gave me a summer to specialize in technology foresight.

Thanks to MIT, who have given me the experience, networks, and tools to analyze and influence innovation at the highest levels and have enabled me to begin to understand where science and technology is taking us—or could take us if we so wish.

Thanks to Ketil Thorvik whom I met back in Trondheim, Norway in 1998 and wrote the first regional foresight study, Trøndelag 2030 with. Back in 1998, 2030 seemed like a comfortably remote time frame to draft scenarios—well over 30 years out. Today, it is only a decade away, and we still have no idea what we will be faced with. Then, like today, we need to turn to our imagination. If we cannot imagine our future, even as our visioning may uncover things that are not all what we hoped for when we were young and optimistic, what kind of human beings are we?

I remain optimistic that with resolve, we can bring COVID-19 and whatever else may be added to our burdens, to merely represent a chapter in a book about our century, not to a lingering, dystopian future we need to constantly be afraid of awaking. I hope this for my children, and I hope this for myself and, lastly, I hope this for the human race.

Lastly, I want to thank the front-line workers in the battle against COVID-19, specifically our medical professionals as well as our service workers, who tirelessly enable us to buy groceries and get our packages and shipments delivered. I'm sure that in the months and perhaps years ahead there will be many more to thank. I also want to acknowledge that, as I outline in my book, any crisis is always hardest on the weakest amongst us, those that already have enough challenges to bear. Whether you are immunocompromised, elderly, or have any number of preexisting conditions or live in places that predispose you for coronavirus vulnerability because of poor air quality, poor health security, or poor leadership, I dedicate this book to you.

ABOUT ATMOSPHERE PRESS

Atmosphere Press is an independent, full-service publisher for excellent books in all genres and for all audiences. Learn more about what we do at atmospherepress.com.

We encourage you to check out some of Atmosphere's latest nonfiction releases, which are available at Amazon.com and via order from your local bookstore:

Great Spirit of Yosemite: The Story of Chief Tenaya, nonfiction by Paul Edmondson
My Cemetery Friends: A Garden of Encounters at Mount Saint Mary in Queens, New York, nonfiction and poetry by Vincent J. Tomeo
Change in 4D, nonfiction by Wendy Wickham
Disruption Games: How to Thrive on Serial Failure, nonfiction by Trond Undheim
Eyeless Mind, nonfiction by Stephanie Duesing
A Blameless Walk, nonfiction by Charles Hopkins
The Horror of 1888, nonfiction by Betty Plombon
White Snake Diary, nonfiction by Jane P. Perry
What?! You Don't Want Children?: Understanding Rejection in the Childfree Lifestyle, nonfiction by Marcia Drut-Davis
Peaceful Meridian: Sailing into War, Protesting at Home, nonfiction by David Rogers Jr.
Evelio's Garden, nonfiction by Sandra Shaw Homer
Difficulty Swallowing, essays by Kym Cunningham
A User Guide to the Unconscious Mind, nonfiction by Tatiana Lukyanova
Breathing New Life: Finding Happiness after Tragedy, nonfiction by Bunny Leach

ABOUT THE AUTHOR

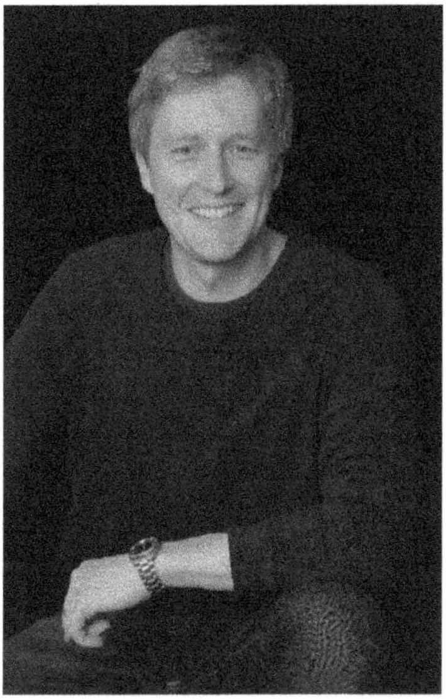

Trond Arne Undheim is a futurist, speaker, entrepreneur, and former director of MIT Startup Exchange, based outside of Boston. Trained as a social scientist with a career in technology and innovation, he is the CEO and cofounder of Yegii, a search engine for industry professionals, providing collective intelligence. He holds a PhD on the future of work and artificial intelligence and cognition. Undheim is the author of *Leadership From Below* (2008) and *Disruption Games* (2020). His next book will be on the future of technology.

Previous scenario building experience include conducting the first regional foresight study in Norway, called Trøndelag 2030 (1998). He has also conducted foresight work at the Norwegian Board of Technology (2002–2004), during which he had a research sojourn at The Institute for Prospective Technological Studies (IPTS), one of the seven Research Institutes of the European Commission (EC). He has also led as well as participated in several foresight projects while working at the European Commission. He has cofounded think tanks, several startups, and he has experience from consulting work in public health including projects on infectious diseases like Ebola and HIV/AIDS. He was a Senior Lecturer in Global Economics and Management at the MIT Sloan School of Management.

CPSIA information can be obtained
at www.ICGtesting.com
Printed in the USA
LVHW091341050720
659734LV00001BA/14

9 781648 261909